CANCER DIAGNOSED:
What Now?

CANCER DIAGNOSED: What Now?

Cancer treatment:
a survey of the literature and guidelines to
effective treatment

What every patient and
every doctor should know

Dr Willem Serfontein

Copyright © 2011 by Dr Willem Serfontein.
Second Edition

Library of Congress Control Number:		2011900481
ISBN:	Softcover	978-1-4568-5073-9
	Hardcover	978-1-4568-5074-6
	Ebook	978-1-4568-5075-3

All rights reserved. No part of this book may be reproduced or transmitted in any form or by any means, electronic or mechanical, including photocopying, recording, or by any information storage and retrieval system, without permission in writing from the copyright owner.

FORTIFOOD HEALTH SERVICES (PTY) LTD
P.O. Box 2458, Zwavelpoort, Pretoria, 0036, South Africa
Tel.: +27 12 8110432 Fax: +27 12 8110433
E-Mail: Fortifood@Telkomsa.net
Website: www.fortifood.co.za

This book was created in the United States of America.

To order additional copies of this book, contact:
Xlibris Corporation
0-800-644-6988
www.xlibrispublishing.co.uk
Orders@xlibrispublishing.co.uk

Contents

Introduction 19
Some conventional medical cancer myths 21
Some alternative medicine cancer myths 25
Integrity, honesty and politics in medicine 28
Examples of biased comments on the use of natural substances 36
Comments by the "experts" 38
The response by conventional medicine 41
The external vs. the internal approach 46
The problem of acidity 48
Some important steps in the treatment of cancer 51
The ten warning signs of cancer 53
When medical treatment fails 58
Cancer, causes, definition, properties 66
Some of the secondary causes of cancer 71
Some of the properties of cancer cells 82
Pain control in the cancer patient: the dangers of narcotics 90
The stages of cancer 93
Understanding the four phases of treating cancer 99
Remission 102
Building the immune system: Preventing the return of the cancer 105
Different types of cancer 110
Conventional medical treatment of cancer 113
Alternative cancer treatments 128
Is my treatment working? 143

How to balance foods to maintain alkalinity 146
Understanding the phases of treating cancer 152
The dangers of swelling and inflammation 156
How to read patient reports and testimonials 158
Cure rates: the great deception factor 159
Choosing a treatment strategy: some general remarks 162
The spiritual aspect 169
The cancer diet 170
Overview of treatment protocols of some types of cancer 189
The cardinal rules of alternative cancer treatment 228
Some general remarks on cancer and carcinogenesis 235
Evaluation of some cancer protocols 239
Treating the healthy cells in the cancer patient 362
Some general remarks on cancer 365
Thirteen vital steps for the cancer patient 374
The cancer patient's rights 382
Abbreviations 385
References 387

SUMMARY: The book is not a prescription for the treatment of cancer but seeks to provide important information from the literature which is essential for the patient and his/her doctor in order to select the best treatment options for his/her problem. It dispels both conventional medical myths and alternative cancer myths about cancer and provides an overview of the process of carcinogenesis which can be readily understood by the non-professional reader.

It discusses the alarming increase in cancer deaths and suggests that this is partly due to dishonest practices in medicine and the profit-driven pharmaceutical drug market.

It also draws attention to the biased approach to the use of natural substances in the treatment of disease and specifically to the treatment and prevention of cancer . . .

It focuses on the vast corruption in the public media due to the pressure of advertising dollars and how this has ultimately influenced medical thinking.

It also underlines the fact that the solution to the cancer problem has been known since the fundamental discoveries of Dr Otto Warburg in the first half of the previous century but this has not been applied in practice as a result of pressure by certain sections of the pharmaceutical industry in order to preserve their drug-based approaches to disease treatment.

Dr Warburg's work, conducted over a period of nearly 50 years, conclusively shows that low intracellular oxygen levels are the primary cause of cancer, all the other accepted "causes" of cancer such as smoking, foreign chemicals etc being of a secondary nature. Thus there is only one fundamental cause of cancer—oxygen deficiency inside the cells—and until this problem is addressed, no real advance towards a final solution of the cancer problem can be expected.

The book provides important statistics on the cancer incidence and deals with the shortcomings of the accepted medical treatments of cancer (chemotherapy, radiation therapy and surgery). It specifically provides authoritative information from reliable published sources on the long term efficacy of chemotherapy in the treatment of cancer which has a real success rate of less than 5 % of patients treated, as shown by several major referenced studies.

An important cumulative message conveyed by all the research information now available, is that cancer cannot be cured by the removal (physical or otherwise) of the cancerous growth, but that the conditions in the patient must be changed in such a way that growth of the cancer cells is suppressed. In this regard the role of certain polyunsaturated fatty acids, which according to Prof Peskin and others, act as "magnets" which pull oxygen molecules over cellular membranes to the inside of cells, is of prime importance. In addition, the role of the immune system in curtailing the growth of cancer cells—especially during the early phases of the disease—is discussed.

Various alternative cancer treatments are presented in some detail and guidelines are provided for the selection of certain treatments and combinations of treatments in specific situations as documented in the literature.

The importance of diet in the treatment of cancer is stressed and various cancer diets from the literature are provided. The role of certain foods in maintaining alkalinity is also discussed.

Finally, an overview of treatment protocols of some types of cancer is presented as well as an evaluation of some cancer protocols as presented in the literature.

DISCLAIMER

This book is not a prescription for the treatment of cancer. It seeks to provide important information from the literature which is essential for the patient and his/her doctor in order to select the best treatment options for his/her problem. The ultimate treatment strategies must be decided on by the patient in consultation with his/her doctor, with the clear understanding that each cancer patient is different and that treatment should be individualized.

Due to patient variability, it is impossible to guarantee success in any particular case. I am not a clinician. My task as a medical scientist is to present the latest evidence to clinicians and patients for their evaluation.

It is essential for the patient to understand what his chances of recovery are using conventional or natural methods. These are presented in an unbiased form, but the views expressed may not be popular with all adherents of either discipline.

The views expressed are those of the different authors in the references cited, with my own analysis of the facts added. I strongly advise against self-treatment without medical guidance. At the same time, it is necessary that the patient understands the issues involved and then participates in the decision-making process.

Further reading

The enormous amount of published information on cancer treatment creates a serious problem for the patient who, in a short time, must make life and death decisions. The amount of information is simply staggering. In addition to the conventional treatment methods (surgery, radiation therapy, chemotherapy, and hormone treatment), there are some 300 different published alternative cancer treatments, not all of which have a sound scientific basis. This document lists the essential steps that the patient and his/her doctor should take into account in selecting a treatment protocol. Since the publication of *Beating Cancer*, I have had numerous enquiries about recommended treatment protocols. This document is aimed at providing that information.

In addition to the many literature references cited, the following sources should also be consulted:

- *Beating Cancer*, 2002. W.J. Serfontein, Cape Town: Tafelberg Publishers.
- *The Cancer Tutor*, http://www.cancertutor.com/.
- Bollinger, T. 2007. *Cancer: Step outside the Box*. USA: Infinity Partners.
- Henderson, Bill. 2007. *Cancer-Free*. USA: Booklocker.
- Young, R.O. & Young, S.R. 2001. *Sick and Tired*. USA: Woodlands Publishing.
- Diamond, W.J., Cowden, W.L. & Goldberg, B. 1997. *An Alternative Medicine Definitive Guide to Cancer*. Tiburon, California: Future Medicine Publishing.
- Moss, R. 2002. *The Cancer Industry*. Equinox Press.
- Moss, R. 2000. *Questioning Chemotherapy*. Equinox Press.
- Hauser, R.A. & Hauser, M.A. 2002. *Treating cancer with Insulin Potentiation Therapy*. Oak Park, Illinois, USA: Beulah Land Press
- Haley, D. 2002. *Politics and Cancer*. Potomac Valley Press, 3rd edn.

In researching the material for this book, I have drawn freely on a large number of published articles and books, especially *The Cancer Tutor* (see above); the book by Cameron and Pauling, *Vitamin C and Cancer;* the book by R Moss, *The Cancer Industry*; the books by Robert O. Young, *The pH Miracle* and *Sick and Tired?*; the book by Robert R. Barefoot, *The Calcium Factor*; the book by Bill Henderson, *Cancer Free*, and many other sources.

I would strongly urge the serious cancer student to buy these books—they are a goldmine of valuable information. I am grateful to the authors of these different sources for much of the basic information on which the book is based. Naturally, I have added my own comments and in many instances I have changed dosage levels of the materials used. In general, I have also adapted the information and sources of material to South African conditions.

Foreword

I would like to congratulate Dr Serfontein on this excellent work, which will certainly make a substantial contribution to the field of Alternative Medicine. In today's society CANCER is an extremely relevant and often politicized topic. I think the most difficult question for any patient who has just been diagnosed with cancer is "What do I do now?" There are so many opinions, and so much information available on the internet, all of which must be considered by patients faced with this dilemma.

This book has truly succeeded not only in describing the different options available to patients as they attempt to distinguish fact from fiction, but also in exposing the veiled agendas and profit-oriented goals of major pharmaceutical companies ('Big Pharma').

One of the major difficulties I have encountered, practicing Insulin Potentiation Therapy (IPT) for nearly four years in South Africa, is that of Medical Insurance Companies (Medical Aids) being preoccupied with their own financial gains, without any real empathy for their clients (the patients), who contribute so much to these funds. In South Africa, cancer therapy is monopolized by the Oncology establishment under the umbrella of the South African Oncology Consortium (SAOC). The SAOC is the only establishment allowed to advise Medical Aids which treatments should be paid for and which not. If you are a medical doctor, but not a member of this elite club, the cancer patients you treat cannot be refunded by their Medical Aid for alternative forms of therapy. The question rightfully arises: what has happened to the patients' right to choose their own therapy?

If, as a patient, I pay my medical insurance premium and don't have cancer, I am paying the same premium as anyone else, which entitles me to the same "oncology cover" as all other members. However, the moment I am diagnosed with cancer, I can only claim Medical Aid cover for treatments that have been approved by the SAOC. *Why, if I do not desire to be exposed to the devastating side effects of conventional therapy, do I not have the right to choose alternative treatment? Why can my oncology allowance for the year not be paid out to me as a lump sum?* If I then choose to spend this on a holiday rather than endure conventional chemotherapy, I should surely have the right to do so. I have paid for my medical insurance just the same as anyone else. Until this fundamental flaw in our medical insurance system is changed, people will suffer at the hands of conventional medicine as they already do, just because of a refusal to recognize alternative therapies as the legitimate right of every patient.

Another organisation that is supposed to assist patients is the Cancer Society of South Africa (CANSA). However, they are just an extension of the SAOC. Provided treatments meet SAOC guidelines, they will be summarily promoted by CANSA. Furthermore, patients are advised to avoid other alternatives. *IPT* has been especially targeted by CANSA since its establishment in South Africa in 2006. All the supposed cautions against IPT are based on 'hearsay' without any attempt to support these allegations with scientific evidence. No scientific research has been published anywhere in the world that substantiates these so-called 'warnings'.

Cancer has its roots in a global imbalance within the body, affecting the *immune system* which is compromised by numerous factors rendering it unable to identify and destroy the defective cancer cells. The focus of any active cancer treatment should be to selectively target the cancer cells and preserve, or even improve the ability of the immune system of the patient to eradicate the disease. However, most conventional cancer therapies cause severe injury to the immune system, which in the long term may cause just as much damage as the underlying disease.

The important question I tell my patients to ask themselves over and over again is: "What is the potential impact of the proposed therapy on my body and immune system?" The less the damage, the safer the treatment is likely to be, with fewer of the serious side-effects which significantly impair quality of life.

Cancer is the only disease that is treated with medication which can cause cancer in its own right. Treatment of a healthy patient with cancer drugs may result in the development of cancer later in life as a direct result of the treatment. Therefore, the less you expose yourself to these harmful drugs, the better.

You must also ask yourself how much precious time and quality of life may be lost because of the chosen treatment. And when people tell you "the side-effects are not so bad", do not only ask patients who endured those treatments, but also their families who cared for them and experienced at first hand the suffering of their loved ones.

My advice to anyone reading this book is: never be bullied into a treatment by the typical rhetoric "if we don't treat you now, it will be too late". Do your homework first, by reading this book. *FIGHT FOR YOUR RIGHT TO CHOOSE*. It is your constitutional right and is being denied you by the South African Medical Insurance industry and the SAOC. You paid your premiums and they owe you compensation, as well as the right to choose the treatment that you would prefer.

Always remember, the effectiveness of medical anti-cancer treatment should not be measured by the degree of organ damage that can be induced, but rather by the extent to which organ function can be preserved.

You didn't choose your disease, but you can surely select your therapy!

GOOD LUCK.

Dr. E. Pretorius MB ChB (Pret), MBA (Texas),
Dipl Candidate (ACAM) IPT (Mexico)
Tel: 012 6546074
Fax: 012 6547587
MP 0366803 PR No: 1557882

Preface: Second Edition

This book first appeared in 2002 as *Beating Cancer* (Tafelberg Publishers). Since that time, new developments have appeared, especially in the field of alternative medicine, which necessitate an update of the original book. In addition, *Beating Cancer* has stimulated both patients and doctors to rethink their own views about cancer. This in turn has generated a flood of e-mail and telephone enquiries which I find strenuous to handle in view of the time needed to do justice to these questions, some of which are of fundamental importance.

The objective of this book is not in the first place to provide new information on the treatment and management of the cancer patient. It is intended as a guide to the non-professional person who has just been diagnosed with cancer and is at a loss how best to handle the situation in the midst of a bewildering mass of conflicting advice received from conventional doctors on the one hand, and proponents of alternative medicine on the other. In this book I express views critical of the current cancer establishment. I trust that in the long term I shall be able to convince the reader that my criticism stems not from bias against the conventional medical establishment, but rather from a heart-felt desire to be openminded and honest in the interest of patients.

I have at times leveled severe criticism at the "Cancer Establishment" for their lack of openmindedness and honesty on their part in dealing with the very promising field of alternative medicine, and I have attempted to expose the fact that the actions and pronouncements of that Establishment are often guided by a hidden agenda involving a widespread network of financial interests. That does not mean that the ordinary doctor or even oncologist is corrupt, although their actions and advice often seem to be colored by just such interests. They do what they do as they are part of a questionable system which compels them to follow what has become known as "standard medical practice". It is important to realize that the system has developed over a period of nearly one hundred years, having been initiated by J.D. Rockefeller in 1911 to ensure his own financial interests in the growing pharmaceutical market. Thus medical practice was put firmly on its present course of drug-based medicine, which has grown into the system as we know it today, making it very hard and even hazardous for any member of the profession to "step outside the box", as Dr. Bollinger says in his book. I firmly believe that the way forward is to combine the best of orthodox medicine with alternative medicine (including the increase of oxygen levels in cells) for the benefit of the patient. The emerging cancer treatment protocol of Insulin Potentiation Therapy (IPT) and use of certain essential fatty acids (EFA) in the treatment of cancer are excellent examples of this.

Introduction

There are few things that instill more fear in the hearts of human beings than the verdict "you have cancer". For most patients, this is the equivalent of a death sentence, because of the extremely high mortality rate associated with most cancers—despite conflicting reassurances by medical doctors and costly treatment using orthodox methods. This fear is aggravated by the fact that patients generally have no understanding of the disease and also do not understand that successful treatment consists of much more than orthodox medical treatment. The situation is further complicated by the existence of two schools of thought: on the one hand the conventional approach by medical doctors and oncologists based mainly on surgery, radiotherapy, chemotherapy (and hormone treatment in the case of hormone sensitive cancers) which the medical establishment assures us offer the best chances of recovery despite considerable evidence to the contrary. In fact, there is evidence that these methods do not have a real cure rate of much better than 5 % of patients, except in a few rare cancers, which will be discussed later. Attempts to portray the prospects of conventional treatments in an exaggeratedly positive form (necessitated by the dictates of the conventional Establishment) are becoming more and more transparent. These further create uncertainty in the minds of enquiring investigators, as many of them have friends who have died of cancer, in spite of intensive treatment by means of conventional methods and assurances by oncologists that the treatment offered was the best available. And yet these methods are not entirely without merit, and can sometimes be combined with appropriate alternative treatments to the advantage of the patient, as I will show later.

On the other hand, a rapidly growing number of natural treatments (perhaps more than 300 at the present time) which have collectively become known as "alternative medicine". Proponents of these methods are on the whole violently opposed by the conventional medical establishment and accused of "quackery" without critical evaluation of the evidence or clinical testing. The harsh dismissal of alternative methods often goes to extremes, such as drug authorities banning these methods and the products on which they are based from the public arena; in some cases even physically destroying the products and imprisoning the owners. While some of these methods (perhaps 10) appear to have real value in the management of many types of cancer, some of the others are truly based on hearsay medicine and are rightly regarded by many as quackery. Nevertheless, the small numbers of these treatments that do merit attention are such that dramatic results have been achieved by using them correctly. In this book I will try to explore this in greater detail, and to suggest improvements. I will be discussing a few of the most important alternative treatment methods in a general way, since these can be used for a wide variety of cancers.

I do, however, include brief discussions on the most important types of cancer in order to highlight that which is peculiar to that particular cancer and which treatment methods should be preferred, according to published information. I also devote some attention to which treatment methods may or may not be combined (based on published information) since this is a very important matter. As I am not a clinician, I will not discuss treatment in detail, but rather leave that to the discretion of the patient and his/her doctor.

I will also try to suggest how the most promising of the alternative methods can best be combined with standard orthodox treatment, where this is indicated according to literature sources. I expect to receive severe criticism from extremists in both schools of thought. This is, however, necessary in order to clear the air and prepare our minds for future, more constructive thinking.

Unfortunately, it will also be necessary to delve among the cobwebs of politics and even outright hidden corruption in medical circles, especially in the higher echelons of the profession, and examine how this relates to the interaction that without doubt exists between the top structures of the pharmaceutical giants ("Big Pharma") and the leaders in the medical profession, who determine in practice what "standard medical treatment" supposedly comprises. Invariably, such treatment is based on drugs, especially of the patentable variety which sell for exorbitant prices, much to the benefit of "Big Pharma". Thus it is the system that is corrupt and not individual doctors, who simply have to toe the line or suffer the consequences.

Some conventional medical cancer myths

1. **All alternative cancer treatments are old wives' tales and devoid of any serious scientific backing.**
   This is clearly a myth that can be easily exploded by anyone who is prepared to do some serious reading. This should include a survey of the Internet and the many good books referred to in the Introduction above.

2. **Cancer is an acute illness that appears suddenly.**
   The popular concept of cancer is that it is a mysterious disease that appears out of the blue and kills the patient. Hence also the popular notion is, even among some doctors, that if you can remove or otherwise kill the growing cancer mass, the cancer will disappear.
   Many patients have had their cancers for years and the only recent development was its discovery. Cancers develop because the inner terrain (biochemical milieu) in their bodies allowed the cancer to develop over time; these conditions are lifestyle related and have been with the patient for a long time. There are only a few cancers that grow so quickly that treatment decisions have to be taken in a hurry. The vast majority of cancers are of a chronic nature which allows the patient adequate time to seek several opinions and to read as much as possible on the subject.

3. **Cancer can be killed by a "magic bullet".**
   This myth is encouraged by Big Pharma and the popular press, who frequently report that a new drug that kills cancer cells has been discovered, and that now the prospects of solving the problem are brighter than ever before. These "magic bullets" gradually pan out and we never hear of them again. There are many such examples.
   A solid tumor mass is made up of a heterogeneous mass of different cancer cells and even some normal cells. The cells on the outside of such a

cancerous mass are frequently different from those on the inside, and these again may be different from cells in metastases (remote new growths) that may have developed from the primary tumor. These cells all have different antigens on their cell surfaces and are in different stages of cellular respiration and fermentation.

That is why the patient may get tumor regression of one cancerous lesion with high dose conventional chemotherapy while another lesion (eg perhaps a metastatic lesion) continues to grow. This is in contrast to IPT where three or more different drugs are used simultaneously, thus reducing the chances of some lesions continuing to grow while others recede. The conclusion is that cancer can only be controlled by using the diverse killing power of IPT combined with increased cellular oxygenation, whilst at the same time correcting the abnormal body biochemistry which allowed the cancer to develop in the first place.

4. Solid cancers can be removed by surgery.

Usually the doctor assures the patient after surgery that he "got everything" and that there is no more cancer. This only means that he cannot find any more cancer by means of the methods of cancer detection usually used by doctors in such situations. This means that there was no further visual evidence of cancer based on the CT scan and mammogram or whatever other detection methods were used. These patients very seldom have comprehensive cancer tests done such as the AMAS and Navarro tests as well as other evidence of abnormal bio-chemistry. Surgery should therefore not be relied upon as an absolute method of disposing of the cancer. It cannot remove cancer cells that are not in the tumor mass and, of course, it does nothing to correct the faulty biochemical milieu which allowed the cancer to develop in the first place.

5. The oncologist knows best how to treat cancer.

This is hammered into medical students in medical school by medical institutions and universities the world over. Oncologists do know a lot about cancer, but their primary recommendation is usually high-dose conventional chemotherapy. Nobody ever says a word about the fact that authoritative studies in Europe and Australia have shown less than 5 % of real benefit. It is difficult to believe that highly trained oncologists the world over continue to prescribe conventional high-dose chemo in the face of well-documented evidence that it brings little real benefit to the patient. I predict that these oncologists will one day—in the very near future—regret what they are now professing.

It is nonetheless wise to have a good oncologist on board and to let him make all the initial investigations. But unless your oncologist has real knowledge of all the other treatment options, you should not follow his advice but rather consult widely with other specialists. IPT, the essential fatty acid protocol and the CsCl/DMSO protocols should be seriously considered along with the other options mentioned in this book.

6. Nutritional products interfere with the effectiveness of chemotherapy.
Virtually every cancer patient is told by his/her oncologist that antioxidants will make the chemotherapy treatment that he/she is offering ineffective. The truth is that conventional chemotherapy does not need antioxidants to make it ineffective—it is by itself and inherently ineffective at curing cancer, as shown by the authoritative studies discussed later in this book. Sadly, oncologists who make such unsubstantiated claims about natural products know nothing about these products and quite often do not take the trouble to find out. Frequently patients do, however, decide to use such nutritional supplements on the basis of advice obtained from other specialists, and when they then confront their oncologist with a much reduced cancer, the oncologist would typically ask them what they did and try to find out more details about the natural treatments used. But very seldom will they approach the natural therapists responsible for details about the treatment.

Many studies have been published on the effects of natural products on the successes or otherwise of conventional chemotherapy. Here is a summary of some of the results of the effects of natural products when used in conjunction with conventional chemotherapy:

- It potentiates the killing effects of conventional chemotherapy (eg IPT)
- It enhances the survival of patients
- It makes patients feel better
- It improves the inner terrain of patients, making it less favorable for growth of cancer cells.

More information is available in this regard. (30) Oncologists often claim that natural products have unfavorable effects on the effectiveness of chemotherapy. As Dr. Hauser remarks (*Ibid.*, p 214), these oncologists should now say to which one of the above effects they mostly object.

The overall conclusion (with the exception of a few minor published negative side-effects, (30) must be that natural products increase the effectiveness and decrease side-effects of chemotherapy with a few minor exceptions.

7. **Diet has no effect on cancer—eat what you want.**

This is one of the outstanding blunders of the medical profession which, I predict, they will greatly regret in years to come. Common sense indicates that diet is all-important, because it creates the internal terrain in the body, which is one of the principal determinants of whether cancer cells will develop and grow. There may be room for discussion on exactly what constitutes an optimum diet, but there can be no doubt that a quality-wrong, unhealthy diet is an important cause of cancer.

8. **My friend had the same type of cancer as I have and was cured after treatment using a particular protocol. It should therefore also work for me.**

This is a serious mistake. Your body has its own inner biochemical terrain which is the determining factor in the development of cancer. There is no strict scientific procedure by means of which you can predict whether your body will respond to a particular treatment. The nearest you can get to that ideal is a method based on behavioral kinesiology which determines your response to 12 different treatments.

The surest way at this point in time is simply to test the various protocols (starting with IPT and CsCl/DMSO) and to find out what is working for you.

9. **Mammography will detect early cancer.**

While often relied on for that purpose, this is not true (*Int J Health Services* 2001, 31: 605).

10. **Cancer is caused by genetic abnormalities.**

This myth has been around for a long time. The originator of this hypothesis later retracted and reversed his position. The fact that cancer's prime cause is not genetic was later confirmed by the world's largest cancer research centre in Houston, Texas (*Townsend Letter*, Aug-Sept 2007, p 81).

11. **High fiber diets protect against colon cancer.**

This is not necessarily true, at least not according to some investigators (*Lancet* 2000, 356: 1286).

Some alternative medicine cancer myths

1. **If, after treatment or for some or other reason, the outward signs of cancer are no longer there, you are cured and you need not be further concerned.**

    This is a very dangerous myth, because many cancers go into remission only to return, frequently after a long time. Therefore, after initial successful treatment, you should continue with treatment for at least 1-2 years, and consider using one of the other alternative methods discussed in this book.

2. **All chemotherapy is bad.**

    When fundamental issues like the current one raging between conventional medicine and alternative medicine occur, one of the great dangers is that extreme statements are made which may harden into radical approaches. Conventional chemotherapy has earned itself a thoroughly bad image as a result of recent studies which have convincingly shown that real benefits for patients are less than 5 %. That does not mean that all chemotherapy is ineffectual.

    Firstly, there are a few cancers for which conventional high-dose chemo has been shown to work, as discussed elsewhere in this book. Secondly, and perhaps more importantly, modified chemotherapy in the form of IPT is one of the most powerful tools against cancer that we have at present. Therefore the word "chemotherapy" (meaning to cure by means of chemical agents) should not scare you off as such. It all depends on how it is used.

    The bottom line is therefore that chemotherapy has its place depending on how it is used.

3. **Cancer is an immunodeficiency disease.**

    Most cancer patients get cancer at a stage of their lives when, initially at least, they still appear healthy and show no evidence of immunodeficiency, such as frequent colds and infections. When first diagnosed, they therefore have no signs of immuno-insufficiency. The problem, according to Dr. Hauser, seems to be that although there is no immuno-insufficiency as a whole in well-nourished patients, the cancer patient's immune system does not recognize the cancer cells as foreign to the body. This could theoretically be corrected by means of a vaccine, but such a vaccine is not yet available and is unlikely to appear in the near future, in view of the very diverse nature of the more than 100 different types of cancer and the fact that it does not address the principal cause of the disease.

In general, though, it is not wise to rely only on the immune system to fight a life-threatening cancer. In such a situation, the effects of the immune system need to be augmented and supported by a powerful cancer-killing protocol such as increased cellular oxygenation, IPT and/or CSCl/DMSO. This does not mean that the immune system is of minor importance. It is not, but it mostly plays a surveillance role in preventing the cancer from developing in the first place and inhibiting regrowth of cancer cells. Many of the alternative therapies discussed in this book depend on the stimulation of the immune system.

4. All allopathic medicine is bad.

Here again good, balanced judgment is called for. There are times when surgery, radiation and/or high-dose chemotherapy may be called for, even if only as a temporary, emergency measure. There are also many allopathic drugs that are useful in treating the cancer patient, eg to control pain. Therefore, not all allopathic medicine is ineffective, but it should be used judiciously.

5. All cancer patients should go vegetarian and use a lot of plant and fruit juices.

This is not necessarily true for all cancer patients. Cancer patients as a group have high insulin levels which accompany the cancer process. Insulin has a stimulating effect on cancer and makes cancer cells more receptive to treatment with drugs, eg chemotherapy drugs (IPT). On the other hand, between IPT treatments and to prevent cancers from forming, insulin levels should be kept low. Juices, especially fruit juices with their high sugar content, will cause insulin levels to rise. In this context, vegetable juices are much better, because of their lower sugar content and also because they help to detox the patient. For some reason, fruit juices seem to be particularly contra-indicated in metastatic cancer. Experts like Dr. Hauser state that, in all his experience and that of his colleagues, no one has ever seen a patient with metastatic cancer go into remission on a juice diet or with herbal remedies alone. Yet many alternative cancer therapies are based on a vegetarian type of diet with plant and fruit juices. The Gerson diet is a good example (see later). This may not be appropriate for all cancer patients. If high insulin levels are part of a patient's biochemistry, a much lower carbohydrate intake may be indicated. On the other hand, for the person with low insulin levels when diagnosed with cancer, a Gerson type of vegetarian diet with a high intake of juices may be more appropriate. The best way to find out is with the aid of a glucose-insulin tolerance test and metabolic typing, which is *inter alia* based on a personal questionnaire to be filled in by the patient. Clearly, there is no such thing as *one diet fits all*. Typically, according to Dr. Hauser (*Ibid.* p 216), a vegetarian type of juicing diet with a high patient blood pH level (alkaline), and a low urinary pH (acidic), would be appropriate. For cancer patients with the opposite metabolic indicators, a high protein, low carbohydrate diet would be indicated. The bottom line then is that cancer patients should eat according to their metabolic type.

6. **Fish oil supplements alone protect against cancer.**
There is evidence against such a view (*Townsend Letter*, Aug-Sept 2007). The w-3 fatty acids in fish oil need to be balanced by the correct quantities of unadulterated w-6 fatty acids (eg first virgin cold pressed sunflower oil; see later).

There are many other myths in circulation regarding cancer, but these are the important ones. Until we get rid of all myths and other unjustified beliefs and practices relating to cancer treatment (often inspired by outside financial interests), we have little hope of ever winning the war against cancer.

Integrity, honesty and politics in medicine

Ideally, this is not something we should be discussing here, as honorable people with no hidden agendas cannot imagine that these factors could play a role in the medical treatment of sick people. Unfortunately, we do not live in such an ideal world, and unless the cancer patient is aware of the extent to which these factors do play a role in medical treatment, he/she cannot make the life-and-death decisions about treatment options. It is also vitally important for the patient to understand that, when things are not what they appear to be, the fault does not lie in the first instance with his/her medical doctor or oncologist. These are mostly honorable and dedicated people who are honestly trying to do their best for the patient, within the constraints imposed on them by the health authorities who decide what "standard medical treatment" should be. These decisions are made by a few of the top figures in the highest echelons of the profession and are rigorously enforced all the way down to the individual practitioners by means of a system that has evolved over more than 100 years. This makes it very difficult, if not impossible, to identify the real culprits.

The method by which such enforcement takes place is by no means direct—only a few of the top members of the profession who are really ignorant or corrupt enforce such decisions for their own benefit. Enforcement down the line on the practicing physicians takes place by means of a system of "peer pressure", the main impetus of this being pressure by certain financial interests over a very long time.

I have recently seen a very apt representation of how this takes place. In a presentation, entitled "How a paradigm is formed", scientists hypothetically placed five monkeys and a "leader monkey" in a cage. In the middle of the cage was a ladder, with bananas on the top of the ladder. Every time a monkey went up the ladder after the bananas, the "leader monkey" soaked him and the rest of the monkeys with cold water. After a while, every time a monkey tried to go up the ladder, the others beat up the one on the ladder without the active participation of the "leader monkey". After some time, no monkey dared to go up the ladder regardless of the temptation (increased number of bananas). The scientists then decided to bring in another "outside" monkey. The first thing the new monkey did was to try to go up the ladder.

Immediately, all the other monkeys beat him up. After several severe beatings, the new monkey learnt not to climb the ladder, though he never knew why. He was now simply doing as the others were doing. Then a second "out-side" monkey was brought in and the same thing occurred; the first outside monkey now enthusiastically participating in the beating of any monkey who tried to go up the ladder. Then more "outside" monkeys were brought in (numbers 3, 4, 5, etc.) until the new monkeys outnumbered the original monkeys, all now toeing the same line. Ultimately, what was left was a group of new monkeys that, even though they had never received a cold shower, continued to beat up any monkey who attempted to climb the ladder.

If it were possible to ask one of these monkeys why they beat up all those who attempted to climb the ladder, the answer would be: "I don't know—that's how things are done around here."

And that is how things are done in the conventional medical establishment.

Interestingly, the unholy collusion between Big Pharma and Big Medicine goes back nearly 100 years, to the extent that the present generation of doctors and oncologists don't even realize that they are part of a system designed to reap maximum financial benefits for both these partners from the problems created by disease. As summarized by Ty Bollinger in his book, John D. Rockefeller (the business tycoon), aiming to dominate the upcoming pharmaceutical markets purchased a controlling interest in the pharmaceutical giant IG Farben in Germany. After the war the financial tangles grew to include Bayer (of aspirin fame), all of this with firm American interests involved. In order to achieve his objectives, Rockefeller needed to "re-educate" the medical profession towards prescribing more drugs, so he hired Abraham Flexner, a layman, to travel the country and assess activities at the various medical schools. In actual fact, very little assessing and much more steering took place, with the results of this study being a foregone conclusion.

Eventually, Flexner submitted a report to the Carnegie Foundation. As expected, the gist of this report was that it was far too easy to start a medical school and that most medical schools were not teaching "sound medicine", meaning they were not pushing enough drugs. Flexner also suggested some form of control over medical schools, allowing only those that conformed to the privileges of being an accredited medical school. This was accepted by Congress. The American Medical Association (AMA) became the watchdog and was empowered to determine which medical schools were properly following the standards of conventional medicine. In this manner, a person with no scientific or medical training (Flexner) was able to restructure the entire medical training system in the USA (and ultimately in most of the Western World) in favor of drug-oriented conventional medicine, the harmful effects of which have lasted for nearly 100 years and will probably continue for a long time to come.

Thus the concept of "standard medical treatment" was born and taken over by many other Western nations.

The predetermined objective of the Flexner Report was to label doctors who did not toe the line and who did not prescribe drugs as "charlatans" and "quacks". Medical schools that offered courses in "quackery" (natural medicines and homeopathy) were told to either drop these or lose their accreditation. In this manner, the total number of accredited medical schools was halved between 1910 and 1944 ([1](#)). The result was, as originally planned by Rockefeller, that all accredited medical schools became heavily oriented towards drugs and drug research.

Ultimately, Rockefeller's plan was a shining success. Whatever conflicts of interest existed between Big Pharma (according to Young and Bollinger) and medicine ("Big Medicine" according to the same authors), were gradually reduced to the benefit of Big Pharma, due to relentless pressure on the practice of medicine ([1](#)), ([13](#)). In this process, the American Cancer Institute (ACI), the National Cancer Institute (NCI) and American Medical Association all became eroded, in time, to nothing more than Government agencies with close but mostly hidden ties to Big Pharma. Part of this programme provides for the suppression of natural products for the treatment of disease and, specifically in the case of cancer, of the environmental links to cancer and especially to preventing the public from learning about this relationship.

Because Big Medicine has chosen drugs and the development of new drugs to solve unsolved medical riddles like cancer, they can at best address symptoms (eg cancer as experienced by the patient) and never the true causes, since the true causes are related to natural products and not to drugs. Cancer—and for that matter all the other major diseases that plague mankind—are not simply signs of a deficiency of certain drugs!

In this manner they will never solve the cancer problem. Since 1971 when President Nixon proclaimed his war on cancer, $2 billion (note *billion*) has been spent on drug-related cancer research, much of that huge amount of money devoted to the development of drugs and ending up in the coffers of Big Pharma.

Dr. John Bailer, who spent 20 years on the staff of the National Cancer Institute and who was editor of its journal, declared at the annual meeting of the American Association for the Advancement of Science:

> *"My overall assessment is that the national cancer program must be judged a qualified failure"*

And that is putting it mildly. In the meantime, they are also waging a relentless war against all other alternative approaches to cancer treatment, including the use of natural products. Part of that war consists of preventing the public from knowing these facts and discrediting and casting suspicion on natural products in the treatment and prevention of disease. You need only look around you to see how it is done. Just read the press and see how often unfavorable but twisted reports about the dangers of vitamins (Vitamin C seems to be a favorite) appear. You will never see anything good about these natural products unless you read the Internet, where the Anti-Natural Product Cartel has less influence.

You might ask how it is possible that even respected scientists are guilty of joining this charade. The answer is that the system has evolved over such a long time (nearly 100 years) that nobody really realized what was happening and, like the monkey example above, everyone simply accepted that "This is how things are done here".

As pointed out by Dr. Bollinger in his book (1), the Cartel of Big Pharma and the associated big chemical companies could not have created a more favorable climate for themselves. They first of all make big profits from carcinogenic chemicals used to boost agricultural production and used as medicines. They make even more profit from selling expensive, patented but ineffective drugs used by the pharmaceutical industry in treating the multitude of diseases, including cancer, resulting from exposure to the drugs, and finally they sell even more drugs to control the side-effects of these drugs.

In the meantime, they have enslaved the "free press" by spending billions of dollars on advertising, by threatening to withdraw these dollars from any magazine that does not toe the line, or newspaper that dares to publish unfavorable comment on their drugs or, indeed, favorable reports on natural products which compete with their drugs in the marketplace. When last did you see a favorable report in the popular press on the use of a natural product in the treatment of disease?

The corruption is not limited to discrediting natural products and suppressing information. It goes so far as deliberate dishonesty in drug testing with the objective of speeding up the process of registration in order to earn even greater drug profits. There are many examples, adequately listed and discussed in the books mentioned previously (1). I will mention only one striking and authenticated example:

Dr. H. Ley is a former FDA commissioner, who testified in this regard before a Senate Committee in Washington. One case described by him involved a trialist (a professor) who had tested almost 100 drugs for 28 different drug companies. The fees for such clinical testing are considerable, often in the region of $1000 per patient, each trial usually involving several hundred patients. This is obviously a lucrative business and the trialist will do his utmost to satisfy the particular drug company. In this case, patients who died left the hospital or dropped out of the study (40) and were silently replaced by others without notification in the records. Forty-one patients reported as participating in the study, were in fact dead or not in the hospital during the studies. More details are available in the US Senate reports (Competitive Problems in the Pharmaceutical Industry). Such dishonesty in drug testing is not all that rare. An internal affairs Food and Drug Administration (FDA) report revealed that 1 in 5 doctors commissioned to carry out field research on new drugs *invented* the data they sent to the drug companies and pocketed the fees. This is not surprising, since doctors specializing in the conduct of such trials may earn up to a million dollars a year.

There are many other ways in which Big Pharma infiltrates the medical profession and influences medical thinking. A few years ago Dr. M. Angell, a former editor of the prestigious *New England Journal of Medicine*, wrote an article entitled "The Truth about Drug Companies". In this article she states:

> "... *over the past two decades the pharmaceutical industry has moved from its original high purpose of discovering and producing useful new drugs. Now primarily a marketing machine to sell drugs of dubious benefit, this industry uses its wealth and power to co-opt every institution that stands in its way including the US Congress, the FDA, academic and medical centers and the medical profession.*"

I could continue in the same vein and cite much more detailed evidence of the widespread corruption in the medical profession as described in the books listed above. This has been done in an excellent manner by the authors in their respective books, and there is therefore no need to repeat it here. Some of the subjects discussed in these books include:

- The cancer industry survives and thrives by perpetually searching for the "cure" but never finding it. Recall President Nixon's promises of 1971.
- The cancer industry is built on the foundation of treating the symptoms of cancer, while doing nothing to treat the actual cause, which is not drug-related.
- The *Journal of the American Medical Association* (JAMA) reported in February 2002 that 87 % of doctors involved in the establishment of national guidelines on disease have financial ties to Big Pharma.
- Doctors, *inter alia* by prescribing the toxic drugs prescribed by the system, are the third leading cause of death in the USA.
- In America, a doctor risks jail time and the possibility of having his license revoked if he recommends or uses alternative cancer treatments, no matter how strong and convincing the evidence in favor of such treatments may be.
- Prescription drugs kill more than 100 000 Americans each and every year.
- There is much pressure, in virtually all Western countries, to have vitamins and minerals classified as drugs which can only be procured when prescribed by a doctor. This has the advantage of placing these products under the control of the Establishment while at the same time earning huge sums of money.

The staggering success of Rockefeller's original scheme of steering the medical profession towards drugs (especially the drugs used to treat cancer) has yielded enormous profits for Big Pharma. The following table gives some idea of the amount of money spent annually on the treatment of cancer in the USA alone (1)

Breast cancer	$ 6.6 billion
Colorectal cancer	$ 6.5 billion
Lung cancer	$ 5.0 billion

Prostate cancer	$ 4.7 billion
Bladder cancer	$ 2.2 billion
Uterine cancer	$ 1.6 billion
Melanoma	$ 1.1 billion
Leukemia	$ 1.1 billion
Kidney cancer	$ 1.0 billion
Ovarian, stomach, pancreas and cervical cancer, each approximately	$ 1.0 billion
TOTAL COST	$33.8 billion

The following example gives an indication of where this huge amount of money goes. We can get an answer to this question by considering the costs associated with the treatment of just one type of cancer: *non-small-cell lung cancer*, which kills more people than any other cancer. These patients and/or their insurance companies pay $175 000 per year per patient for treatment, over half of which goes towards the costs of the chemotherapy drugs used in the treatment (*Aust Health Rev* 1982, 5: 213). Drug treatment for breast cancer (the second biggest killer of women) ranges from $5 000—$25 000. For terminal cases of breast cancer, medical aid schemes pay on average $50 000—$62 000 per case (*Med Care* 1995, 33: 828).

Approximately half of these funds go towards drug costs, but in spite of the astronomical costs, very little is achieved in terms of alleviating suffering and reducing mortality. The huge profits of the drug companies keep the system going. The doctors who perform cancer treatments and the scientists who develop the drugs and conduct research are not the ones who benefit or control the medical approaches to cancer. It is the larger power structure of the cancer establishment that effectively controls the shape and direction of cancer prevention, diagnosis and treatment. According to Dr. R. Moss (3), the field of cancer care in the Western World is organized around a medical monopoly that ensures the continuous flow of money to Big Pharma, research institutes and (in the USA) to government agencies such as the FDA, the National Cancer Institute and the American Cancer Society. In his book previously referred to (*The Cancer Industry*) (3), Dr. Moss calls this the "Cancer Industry" with its extensions to the corporate media, public relations groups, the media and even some doctors and scientists who specialize in killing cancer by means of drugs. The tentacles of this huge organisation in fact extend to world-famous cancer centers such as the

Memorial Sloan-Kettering Hospital in New York, and even to the popular press, and also embrace other major health problems such as heart disease and diabetes. Thus, by analogy to Dr. Moss's proposals, we are now justified in talking of the Diabetes Industry, the Heart Industry, etc.

One may well ask: what holds such a huge structure together and functional? The answer is quite obvious: money, and the fact that the system is self-propagating by means of peer pressure analogous to the monkey example previously given.

Thus the campaign started in 1911 by Rockefeller, to ensure the interests of the chemical industry in the form of a drug-orientated approach to all health matters, is seen to have succeeded beyond his wildest expectations after 100 years. The fact that this is not in the real interest of public health does not appear to count at all. We may therefore expect to be burdened by this approach to health matters for many more years to come.

There are numerous other examples of independent thinkers and innovative geniuses who were scorned and even threatened with death for promoting ideas that ran against the "system" and against what at the time was considered to be the absolute truth. The following are some examples:

- Jacques Cartier discovered in the early 19th century that scurvy was caused by a deficiency of Vitamin C and that it could be cured by extracts of tree bark and needles from pine trees. He reported this to doctors on his return to Europe, but was laughed at. Nearly 200 years later, medical "experts" discovered the relationship between Vitamin C and scurvy.
- Galileo was scorned and threatened with death for his belief that the sun (and not Rome) was the centre of the planetary system. This went directly against the "system", which at that time was the Roman Catholic Church.
- Ignaz Semmeweiss, a Hungarian gynaecologist, was expelled from medical society and driven out of Vienna for suggesting and proving that puerperal fever could be drastically reduced if doctors only took the trouble to wash their hands.
- The discoverers of aviation, Wilbur and Orville Wright, were dismissed as "hoaxers" by *Scientific American*, the US Army and many other American scientists.
- William Harvey was ridiculed for his suggestion that blood was pumped from the heart to the tissues by means of the vascular system. There are many other examples.

Examples of biased comments on the use of natural substances

I have recently had firsthand experience of how the system works in practice.

In the first instance, my advice was sought in connection with an article by the Cochrane Institute (4) regarding the alleged toxicity of vitamins. The Cochrane study collected evidence of 68 clinical trials (232 000 patients). From these the authors identified 47 trials (180 939 patients) that they arbitrarily considered to have a low risk of yielding erroneous results ("the low bias trials"). When the data from these 47 trials were pooled, it was found that taking anti-oxidants increased the risk of death by 5 %. Vitamin E alone increased the risk by 4 %, while synthetic beta-carotene increased the risk by 7 % and Vitamin A by 16 % (4). Vitamin C and selenium had no effect on mortality, according to this study, which is directly the opposite of what other studies have shown (5).

A major flaw of the Cochrane study was the decision to calculate the results after arbitrarily excluding the "high bias risk" trials and then to present the results as representative of the entire field population of 68 studies. The authors fail to mention that had these studies been included, there would have been no significant effect of antioxidants on mortality. The argument for excluding these trials would have been more acceptable if the end point of the study had been based on subjective symptoms such as fatigue, depression, pain, etc. where subjective factors and personal bias could play a role. In this case, subtle imperfections in randomization methodology and researchers' awareness of treatment assignments could influence the outcome. These are so-called soft end points. But it is totally unimaginable that in the case of a hard end point such as death, as in this study, these factors could have played a role. The exclusion of 21 trials from the study was therefore unjustifiable and represents the introduction of a serious bias.

Another serious error was the way beta-carotene was combined with Vitamins E and A in some trials. It is now well known and accepted that beta-carotene increases the risk of lung cancer *in smokers,* possibly because of a toxic interaction between compounds in tobacco smoke and beta-carotene. In non-smokers, however, it has no effect on mortality. Pooling the results of all the beta-carotene trials (whether or not the participants were smokers) is therefore not permissible, because this implies that beta-carotene supplements are bad for everyone, not only smokers. Moreover, by including beta-carotene along with the other antioxidants in smokers, other antioxidants may be erroneously implicated for what was entirely due to beta-carotene.

Also, the conclusion that Vitamin A increases the risk of death is wrong and in direct contradiction of a major study in which the dramatic life-saving effects of the vitamin were convincingly demonstrated. In one study (n = 18314 of pooled participants), cigarette smokers were given a placebo or a combination of Vitamin A and beta-carotene. In another Vitamin A study included in the survey, 109 elderly nursing home residents were given a single massive dose of 200 000IU of Vitamin A or a placebo. The patients were then observed for infection. During the follow-up period, the death rate was higher in the Vitamin A group than in the placebo group (11.3 % vs. 7.1 %). However, a closer scrutiny of the trial setup revealed that the participants in the Vitamin A group were on average nearly 5 years (4.8yrs) older than those in the placebo group. At the high average age of the participants, 4.8 years may make a meaningful difference, and the observed higher death rate may in fact have been entirely due to the age difference. In addition, one might question the wisdom of giving such a massive dose of Vitamin A to elderly, debilitated people rather than indicting all doses of Vitamin A for all people.

One cannot avoid the suspicion that the organizers of the survey were in subtle and perhaps not so subtle ways trying to prove that nutritional supplements are harmful. This is strongly supported by the absence of comments by the authors concerning selenium. They devote very little attention to the results of their own survey and to the numerous other studies that have conclusively demonstrated the remarkable beneficial effects of selenium (also an antioxidant). In the Cochrane survey, selenium supplementation produced a statistically significant 9 % reduction in mortality when the results of all 67 trials were pooled. When the "high bias risk" trials were excluded, the beneficial effect of selenium was even more pronounced (10 %). This was mentioned neither by the authors of the survey, nor by the "experts" who commented in the sensation-seeking popular press on the significance of the survey for the ordinary health conscious consumer of vitamins.

Comments by the "experts"

What caused the wave of criticism against vitamin supplementation in the popular press was the finding of the Cochrane Study that supplements containing Vitamins A, E and beta-carotene (antioxidants) increased mortality risk. One headline in a popular magazine suggested that all vitamins are toxic, and that if you take your daily vitamin supplement (which you have been doing for many years) you may be shortening your life.

Even the life-saving Vitamin C has not escaped attention. A pharmacologist (Dr. Straughan), reacting to the Cochrane findings, stated that we do not need more than 200mg of Vitamin C daily, and that there is no evidence that large doses of vitamins are advantageous. This statement must be evaluated in the light of the wide range of published evidence which indicates otherwise (7). In evaluating the Cochrane findings, it is first and foremost necessary to ask how much was administered for how long and especially in what combination. Fat soluble vitamins such as those mentioned tend to accumulate in the body and may therefore cause toxicity if excessive doses are taken, and especially in the wrong combination. For example, what does "Vitamin E" mean in the Cochrane context? The Vitamin E complex in nature consists of a mixture of at least 8 different vitamins (vitamin isomers), each with different functions and some with complementary roles. When just one of these is given in excessive doses, the delicate balance between the vitamins may be upset, with harmful health consequences. Most commercial Vitamin E preparations consist of only one of these vitamins (eg d-a-tocopherol). Alpha tocopherol has a number of positive effects on the cardiovascular function. Taking large amounts of alpha tocopherol in isolation, however, may deplete the closely-related gamma tocopherol which may be even more important for the heart. It is extremely unlikely that under the conditions of the Cochrane meta-study due attention was given to this matter by the widely differing studies which comprise the meta-study, since virtually all the commercial Vitamin E preparations contain only the alpha isomer. The same can be said about the widely-differing population groups that have contributed to the meta-study, which includes 47 different studies conducted on widely differing populations and different races and countries. To take the questionable statistical results of a survey of such widely differing groups and to apply these to individuals in a particular setting is simply wrong, and to extend the results to include all other "vitamins" and to imply that our trusted vitamin supplements have suddenly become toxic, is highly irresponsible, especially in view of the avalanche of published scientific studies and the views of world authorities on the subject which indicate otherwise (7).

It is true that beta-carotene supplements have been shown to increase the lung cancer incidence in smokers by 16 %. But here again, as in the case of Vitamin E, we are dealing with one of 600 different arytenoids that occur in nature. The lesson must surely be that beta-carotene should not be given alone in large doses, especially in smokers. It does not mean that beta-carotene is "toxic" and that it should therefore be avoided.

In the Cochrane Survey, selenium supplementation produced a statistically significant 9 % reduction in mortality when the results of all 67 trials were pooled. When the "high bias risk" trials were excluded, the beneficial effect of selenium was even more pronounced (10 %). This was not mentioned by the authors of the survey and also not by the "experts" that commented in the popular press on the significance of the survey for the ordinary health-conscious person. The overall and lasting impression gained from the conclusions of the Cochrane Study is that somewhere along the line one or more of the key persons were anxious to scare away the public from using these very beneficial natural substances. This same sentiment was echoed very strongly by the popular press. One popular magazine even asked, by way of a headline: "Death by vitamins?"(*YOU* Magazine, 2007). When these misleading statements first appeared in the popular press, I attempted in vain to put the record straight by presenting the abovementioned facts by way of comment. My contributions were summarily refused by a number of newspapers and magazines, with the explanation that the topic is now already "old". Yet these same publications hurry to publicize every bit of information that reflects badly on natural products (vitamins, minerals, etc), whether or not such information has any real scientific basis and whether it is "old" or not.

Another good example of official prejudice against the use of natural substances to treat patients is to be found in the studies on Vitamin C in cancer patients.

Dr. Ewan Cameron, a renowned surgeon and oncologist at the Vale of Leven Hospital in Scotland, and Prof. L Pauling, twice Nobel Laureate and internationally acclaimed scientist, studied the effects of high-dose Vitamin C therapy in cancer patients. These two experts reported on the survival times of 1000 terminally ill cancer patients given high doses (10 000mg) of Vitamin C and those of a control group of 1 000 patients with similar types of cancer and initial status treated by the same physicians in the same hospital and who had been managed identically except for the supplemental Vitamin C (7). All participants were considered untreatable, meaning that further conventional treatment was no longer deemed beneficial. The controls were matched to the treatment group with respect to age, primary tumor type, and clinical status of untreatability. An outside doctor who had no knowledge of the survival times of the Vitamin C patients was employed to examine the case histories of each of the 1 000 controls and to record for each the survival time (time in days between the date of abandonement of all conventinoal forms of treatment and date of death). The results were beyond the best expectations, according to the trialists. After approximately 400 days in the trial, the last of the control patients died, but at that stage 16% of the Vitamin C patients were still alive. At that stage, the average time of survival after the date of untreatability was 4.2 times greater in the Vitamin C patients than in the controls. At 600 days, five of the ascorbate patients were still alive and at that time the survival rate ratio was 5.6 in favor of the ascorbate patients. The 100 ascorbate patients lived on average 300 days longer than the matched controls. The trialists also recorded that ascorbate patients lived happier lives during the terminal period (7). Five ascorbate patients who lived beyond 600 days and were still taking their daily Vitamin C were considered cured. A five percent cure rate may not appear impressive, but if applied to the population of cancer patients in the USA, it means that 20 000 of these patients can be saved every year.

In this study, many different types of cancer were included. The effect of Vitamin C appeared to be particularly strong in the case of bladder, colon and breast cancer. More similar trials were conducted at the Vale of Leven, and the overall conclusion by the trialist was that the survival time of terminally ill cancer patients who were beyond conventional medical treatment and who were treated with 10g per day of Vitamin C, was more than 300 days longer than that of matched controls.

Similar studies have been conducted independently elsewhere in the world, with similar or better results. A notable example is the study in Japan where more impressive results were obtained. (8)

The response by conventional medicine

A double blind study by Dr. Moertel and his associates at the Mayo Clinic had the published objective of repeating the Vale of Leven study (9). The trialists concluded their paper with the remark that they "cannot recommend the use of high-dose Vitamin C in patients with advanced cancer who have previously received radiation or chemotherapy".

There were, however, significant differences between the Moertel *et al.* study and the Cameron-Pauling studies:

- *Previous treatment by immune-destroying radiotherapy and/or chemotherapy.* In the Cameron-Pauling study, only 4 % of the Vitamin C patients had previously been treated with chemotherapy, whereas in the case of the Moertel study 87 % of the patients had previously been treated by means of radio—and/or chemotherapy.
- *Abrupt termination of Vitamin C therapy.* Previous work by Pauling on the pharmokinetics of Vitamin C showed that Vitamin C is converted into a significant number of unidentified metabolites and that these play a role in the vitamin's therapeutic action. For this reason, unfavorable effects are seen in patients who had been treated with Vitamin C when such therapy is abruptly terminated.
- *Treatment time.* The Vale of Leven study showed that cancer patients on Vitamin C therapy started to derive benefit only after approximately 2 months or more. Yet most of the Moertel patients were treated for shorter periods than that.

All these factors could have played a role in Moertel's study to cause bias in the trial. It was previously determined that Vitamin C therapy would be continued in the Moertel trial as long as there was no evidence of increased cancer growth or loss of weight. If this occurred in any patient, the Vitamin

C would be immediately stopped. In many patients these effects could only be expected to be reversed to some extent after 2 months of treatment. In the Moertel trial, this must have occurred in many patients, who were therefore withdrawn from the study and recorded as failures of Vitamin C treatment.

The authors of the Creagan-Moertel paper do not mention these complicating factors, although the title of their paper ("Failure of high-dose Vitamin C therapy to benefit patients with advanced cancer, a controlled trial") directs attention towards the ineffectiveness of Vitamin C. This was in fact, for the abovementioned reasons, not a trial of Vitamin C therapy. It is difficult to escape the conclusion that the trialists were very much expecting their study to yield negative results. Whatever the real causes were, the trial was conducted in such a manner that the results were predictably negative.

These are just two examples of how the evidence is skewed—either deliberately or as a result of a lack of knowledge—to turn public and medical interest away from natural products in the prevention and treatment of disease.

There are many more such examples, including the laetrile story (10). It should be noted that the same forces that operate in shaping medical thinking, of which the abovementioned are some examples, also operate in the arena of the press, presumably to condition the public mind as well. This has very much to do with the enormous amounts of advertising money that the press earns from advertising medical information and products

One of the problems in properly evaluating alternative treatment methods is that practically the only patients that are treated by alternative methods are the ones given up on by the conventional doctors. These are the ones that have been sent home by their doctors to die, which usually happens after the patient has had one or two courses of chemotherapy. It is well known that chemotherapy does serious harm to the immune system, thereby virtually ensuring that the patient will not recover in spite of temporary remissions. In spite of this, many of these patients (up to 50 %) have been saved in the past by natural treatment methods (11). This is because well-designed natural treatments usually include several products, including one or more to stimulate the immune system.

Why is it necessary for the cancer patient to know all this? The reason is that, after failed medical treatment, the patient who now contemplates alternative treatment needs to have all the critical information that is necessary to select one of the most powerful alternative treatments and to know how to combine this with other supportive treatments, eg to strengthen the immune system. There are only a few treatment options that can achieve a cure rate of up to 50 % in these patients.

The abovementioned information may be summarized as follows:

- Almost 100 % of newly diagnosed cancer patients undergo orthodox treatments first, on the advice of their doctor and/or oncologist.
- The vast majorities of these patients die or are sent home and later die as a result of their cancer (including metastases) and their orthodox cancer treatment, which frequently includes at least one course of chemotherapy.
- Only a very small percentage of those sent home to die ever undertake alternative treatments at this late stage, due to lack of information and a true factual perspective of their situation.
- The vast majority simply goes home and dies.
- Only a very small percentage of those who undertake some alternative treatment choose a treatment strong enough to give them a 50 % chance of survival.
- If they choose the best possible alternative treatment for their situation in the first place, a true cure rate of at least 90 % is easy to achieve according to the *Cancer Tutor* (11). This cure rate is also possible with conventional methods such as chemotherapy, provided these are used in combination with natural substances such as insulin and DMSO (IPT or IPT and DMSO Potentiation Therapy or DPT—see later).

Insulin allows small amounts of drugs (eg chemotherapy drugs) to target cancer cells because of its effects on cell membranes, thus increasing the effectiveness of such drugs enormously. DMSO does the same, but it actually binds to chemotherapy drugs and then carries the drugs into the cells because of the high affinity that DMSO has for cancer cells.

IPT and DPT may actually be combined, which even further increases the effectiveness of the drug.

Because of the effectiveness of these combinations, very low doses of chemotherapy (about 10% of the normal toxic doses given) can be used to achieve much greater effects and no toxicity.

It sounds incredible, but it is true that in this manner the cure rate of chemotherapy can be increased from the normal 3 % to 90 % without toxicity! I will be discussing these aspects more fully in a later section.

> *The only remaining question then is: why is it not used? Why, if all of this is true, has it not been properly evaluated and publicized by the orthodox establishment?*

The answer is simple: money and lack of information.
The situation can be summarized as follows:

- Everybody in the Western World gets the bulk of their information from the media (television, radio, newspapers, magazines, medical journals, etc.). These media also earn massive dollars annually from advertising pharmaceutical products, which gives the advertisers a considerable amount of leverage over the media. It is a simple fact of life (which I have personally experienced more than once) that newspapers, journals, etc. that publish articles that reflect unfavorably on the interests of the particular advertiser will lose that particular client.

    This introduces a heavy bias in the press, slanted in whatever way the advertisers choose, and this happens without direct pressure in the form of threats.

- The pharmaceutical industry spends more than $3 billion per year on advertising in the media in the USA alone. This gives them considerable leverage over what appears in print and what does not.
- The vast corruption in the media due to advertising dollars has been around for a long time. Way back in 1940 a book by Morris Beale appeared which gives a lot of information in this regard (12). Even before the advent of television the media clearly understood that they had to refuse to say things in the media that are true but cut into the profits of advertisers. A prominent journalist summed up the situation as follows:

    We are the tools . . . of rich men behind the scenes. We are the jumping jacks, they pull the strings and we dance. Our talents, our possibilities and our lives are all the property of other men. We are intellectual prostitutes.

This, unfortunately, is true. It was true in 1940 and it is true now.

- As a result of the huge amount of advertising money involved ($3 billion a year in the USA alone), journalists are required to be utterly loyal to the interests of Big Pharma. (1). A single verbal slip

by a journalist in print, on or off the air, could cost him/her their job. Prior approval by the advertisers is required before a particular journalist can say something even mildly critical of Big Pharma.
- The conventional medical treatments of cancer (chemotherapy, surgery, radiation therapy and others) and their proponents have also been taught over the years to be equally subservient to Big Pharma, to the extent that Big Pharma wields significant influence in what is taught in medical schools. Medical doctors are under the control of the American Medical Association in the USA and are not allowed to use natural substances in the treatment of cancer, regardless of scientific evidence to the contrary. A similar situation exists in most other Western countries. Therefore, medical doctors in the Western World are taught nothing but medicines, which are prescription drugs produced by Big Pharma. At most, these medical doctors are allowed to use some natural substances in the treatment of some symptoms.
- Vitamin companies are allowed to advertise their products, but not specifically for the treatment of disease. In this manner the media receives no advertising dollars in competition with drugs. Hence the stringent requirement that those vitamin manufacturers are not allowed making claims, no matter what strong clinical support they may have.

Summarizing all the evidence above, it is quite clear that commercial interests have quietly taken over medical thinking on all the major diseases that plague mankind. The whole scene is manipulated in such a manner that the average person and even many professionals never hear anything about alternative cancer treatments, but all the good things and many more about orthodox medicines and "breakthroughs" that regularly occur without any of the promised benefits ever being seen.

Commercial interests are further solidified by cross-ownership of shares and cross-board directorships between the top echelons of the pharmaceutical industry and major government and business interests (1, 11).

The external vs. the internal approach

The traditional medical approach to the treatment of cancer has been to cut it out, to drug it out (chemotherapy) or to burn it out (radiation)—in other words, diseases are treated by removing the external signs. Such procedures do not address the fundamental causes of the disease and offer, at best, only temporary relief. This is dictated by the conventional view of the human body as consisting of a collection of individual parts, and as each part becomes diseased, it should be replaced, treated or removed. This concept evolved from the mechanical approach to physical systems in the material universe, in which the different constituent parts function independently from one another. It has its origins in the Newtonian physics of the nineteenth century. This is the external approach to disease on which much of the present day medical treatment is based.

However, biological systems do not function in this way. A living entity like the human body functions as a single whole entity in which the constituent parts are intimately related via the neuro-endocrine-immune complex on the basis of "each one for all and all for each one." In a way, a disease in one organ is actually a disease of the whole.

In the case of cancer treatment, there is a place for both the external and internal approaches, since a cancerous growth can no longer be regarded as part of the whole, due to its autonomous nature and the fact that it contributes to the mass of cancer cells that the immune system has to deal with. Once a defined tumor mass has been identified, it has to be physically removed, as it no longer responds to normal regulatory mechanisms. However, in this manner the fundamental cause of the disease has not been removed and new growths may therefore appear. It is at this stage that the real treatment of the patient should begin. In this regard some alternative treatment methods have far more to offer than the conventional methods, which do not address this side of the problem at all.

Dr. Vincent was hired by the French government to determine why cancer occurs more in certain areas of France than others. He found that water quality is an important factor in the occurrence of clusters of cancer cases. Chlorinated and fluorinated drinking water have been shown by others to increase the risk of cancer substantially. My own experience in Africa has shown that the composition of the soil is another important determinant of cancer. The presence of adequate levels of calcium, magnesium, selenium and other minerals in the soil is of prime importance.

All of these together define what has become known as the biological terrain in a patient. In pioneering work, Dr. R. Greenberg of the Whole Health Center in the USA defined several factors that determine a patient's internal terrain. Acidity (acid base balance) and oxidation reduction status were found to be important determinants of the internal terrain.

This determines how we view disease and how diseases develop. Diseases will develop in an organism where the biological terrain is favorable for their development. This applies in the case of most diseases, including infections as well as metabolic diseases such as cancer. This is the direct opposite of what Pasteur suggested initially, namely that infections arise primarily from outside sources.

The problem of acidity

Increased acidity exists in all cancer cells and appears to be an important contributory cause of the disease. By removing the cancerous cells by conventional methods, this aspect of the disease remains intact, thereby creating the conditions necessary for the growth of new cancer cells.

The problem of systemic acidity reaches beyond cancer cells and cancer. Robert O. Young deals with this matter in a very elegant way in his book (13) in which he relates all disease to unbalanced acidity. I urge you to buy this book and study it carefully. It is a virtual gold mine of information and addresses a very real health problem in all Western societies. The following is a summary.

Acid stress of the body's pH balance is sufficient to provoke the body into producing disease symptoms. The vast majority of people suffer from ongoing, self-generated acid stress that underlies most symptoms, but also significantly promotes the development of such major diseases as AIDS and cancer. In this manner, a whole chain reaction is set up, including the growth of pleomorphic micro-organisms, which in turn contribute to the process of carcinogenesis. The body attempts to maintain blood pH values at around 7.4. Variations *above* this do occur, but very much more common and infinitely more harmful are variations *below* this value. Many enzymatic reactions that regulate cellular metabolism are sensitively dependent on pH and, as the acidity increases, many of these are compromised. When this occurs, the body does everything in its power to correct the fault by drawing on its buffering systems and mobilization of alkaline minerals from the bones, such as calcium, magnesium, potassium and sodium. If the overload is too great for the body to balance, excess acid is dumped into the tissues for temporary storage. Next the lymphatic system must neutralize what it can. If the lymphatic system becomes overloaded and/or vessels are not functioning properly due to lack of exercise, acid deposits will build up in the tissues, setting the scene for various diseases. In this regard, the blood must be distinguished from the tissues. When the body is compensating, blood pH may rise somewhat, but the tissues may remain highly acidic. This also leads to disease, and irritation and inflammation may develop. In addition to all these problems, acidity and lack of oxygen create ideal environmental or inner terrain conditions for the development of a variety of pathogenic micro-organisms which may further be responsible for many disease symptoms.

The initial acidification of the body is caused *inter alia* by an improper diet loaded with acid-forming foods.

Digested foods are "burned" (assimilated) in the body leaving "ashes" or food residues. These ashes can be acidic, neutral or alkaline depending on the mineral composition of the food. The alkalinizing elements (ashes) are calcium, magnesium, potassium and other minerals as previously mentioned. Acidifying "ashes" are formed by dietary sulphur, phosphorus, chlorine and iodine. These acidifying elements occur in relative high amounts in foods of animal origin.

A major means of ensuring a proper acid balance in the body is a proper dietary ratio of acid to alkaline foods. After many years of research, we now know that the optimal ratio is 80:20, meaning four parts of alkaline foods to one part of acid food. This is of particular importance in the cancer patient, where there is an overgrowth of pleomorphic organisms which multiply rapidly adding their quota of acids to the pool. When the patient is acidic, the higher the level of alkaline foods in the diet, the faster will be the recovery from disease.

Examples of strongly acidifying foods are fish and fries, hamburger and fries, steak and potatoes, while sprouted grains, fresh vegetables and low sugar fruits are examples of alkalinizing foods. In general, animal, dairy, processed, fermented and refined sugar foods are acid-forming, as are most grains except buckwheat. All vegetable juices are highly alkaline. The most alkaline juices are those of green vegetables and vegetable tops (eg beet greens). Vegetable soups, especially those made with onions, garlic and cucumber, are strongly alkalinising. Low sugar fruits (lime, lemon, avocado, tomato) are alkalinizing. Please consult Robert O. Young's book for more details on acidifying and alkalinizing foods (13).

I have personal experience of how the effects of alkalinisation on disease patterns may be seen in whole populations. Some years ago I was involved in a study on the geographical distribution of AIDS in Sub-Saharan Africa. These Studies and other information revealed that AIDS was widespread in Sub-Saharan countries, with incidences ranging from 20-45 % and on the increase, much higher than in Europe or elsewhere in the world. There is, however, one exception: Senegal. The incidence in that country is exceptionally low, being of the order of 0.5 % and stable at that level. The Senegalese have very much the same lifestyle as other African countries where the AIDS incidence is 20-40 times higher, including the fact that they are a highly sexually active society. Remarkably, that country also has the world's lowest cancer incidence (14). This appears to be the result of a geological freak which ensures that a highly alkaline, selenium enriched environment exists in Senegal.

Senegal is essentially a dried up Cretaceous and early Eocene sea. When this sea dried up, sedimentary rocks were formed from the dissolved minerals in the sea water. As a result, calcium phosphates were precipitated in the form of a rock known as phosphorite. The drinking water in Senegal is entirely dependent on ground water obtained from soil rich in phosphorite and especially the minerals calcium, magnesium and selenium. In the light of what was said above about alkalinity and cancer, it can be stated that Senegal has the ideal environment protect against cancer. The very low cancer incidence in Senegal has been previously documented (15).

Intracellular acidity is also promoted by lactic acid which accumulates in cells with a predominantly fermentation basis of energy production as discussed elsewhere in this book.

Some important steps in the treatment of cancer

In addition to removing the cancerous growth as such (where possible) and its causes (eg increased cellular acidity and decreased levels of undulated w-6 fatty acids), the correct treatment must also include reactivation of the patient's own defense mechanisms, including the immune system, which normally removes cancerous cells as soon as they develop, and which protects the body against further insults. It must also include steps to correct other metabolic errors, such as redox irregularities that may be present. These processes depend on the integrated action of the neuro-endocrine-immune system. The entire system in turn depends critically on the availability of the correct mix of nutrients, including certain vitamins, minerals, amino acids and other biological molecules. In this regard, Vitamin C appears to be of particular significance.

Cancer is a symptom of a disease. By treating the symptom of the disease (such as the killing of cancer cells), we will never be able to cure the disease entirely, with the exception of those cases where the body itself can make the necessary corrections.

In this book, I present certain avenues of approach that have helped many others free themselves of this scourge. These include:

- The creation of a biochemical milieu that will be unfavorable for the growth of cancer cells. This includes *inter alia* the correction of systemic acidic conditions prevailing in the body, but also specifically in the cancer cells. It also includes steps to correct glucose and insulin metabolism. The biochemical milieu in the body must be such that excessive levels of blood glucose and insulin are avoided
- The effective reversal of cachexia

- Improved immune function
- Lowering the dissemination of cancer cells to distant sites in the body (metastases)
- Increasing oxygen levels inside cells, which is critically dependent on the presence of unadulterated w-6 fatty acids in • the cellular membranes as discussed below
- Early detection and treatment
- The correct anti-cancer diet, including the correct mix of w-3 and w-6 fatty acids.

The ten warning signs of cancer

Early detection and treatment are essential for the most effective treatment of cancer, regardless of the protocol followed. The patient himself is in the best position to notice the earliest manifestations of the disease. If you notice any of the following signs, you should immediately contact your doctor for further investigation:

- A lump or thickening in the breast or testicles
- Any lesion (eg on the skin) that does not heal
- A change in a wart or mole may be indicative of melanoma. Skin cancers may appear, as dry, scaly patches; or as pimples which do not go away, or as inflamed or ulcerated areas. Warts and moles which bleed or grow should be checked
- Sores in the mouth that persist
- A sore throat that persists, hoarseness, a persistent lump in the throat or difficulty in swallowing may indicate cancer of the larynx and should be investigated
- A change in bowel or bladder habits as well as continuing urinary difficulties, constipation, diarrhea, bloodedness with gas pains, rectal bleeding or blood in the stool all may indicate cancer and should be investigated
- Constant indigestion or trouble swallowing, nausea, heart burn, bloating and loss of appetite may all be symptoms of the upper gastrointestinal tract cancers (esophagus, stomach) and should not be ignored
- Unusual bleeding or discharge from the vagina are seen in the early stages of uterine cancer or the later stages of cervical cancer
- Difficulty in urinating may indicate prostate cancer in men
- A persistent cough could indicate lung cancer.

Cancer signs, symptoms, causes, statistics

Type	Some Symptoms	Possible causes	5-year survival*
Bladder	Blood in urine (bright red rust colored); pain, burning (urination), frequent urination; urge to urinat but unproductive; urine cloudy	2-3X higher in whites, in men, in smokers, truck drivers, in workers exposed to chemicals	80 %
Breast	Lump or thickening in breast, discharge from nipple, change of skin (redness, swelling, warm feeling, enlarged lymph nodes under arm, high blood oestrogen levels	Age, early menstruation, late menopause, childless or first child after 30, breast cancer in family, wearing bra	83 %
Colorectal	Rectal bleeding, red blood in stools, black stools. Abdominal cramps, alternating constipation and diarrhea, loss of appetite and weight, weakness. Pallid complextion	Polyps, ulcerative colitis. Crohn's disease, family history, residence in industrial area. Lack of fibre in diet	61 %
Kidney	Blood in urine, dull pain in back, lump in kidney area, high blood pressure, redblood cell count abnormal	Twice as high in men, smokers, overweight, coke oven and asbestos workers	58 %
Leukemia	Weakness, paleness, fever, flu-like symptoms. Bruising with prolonged bleeding, lymph nodes. Enlarged liver, spleen areas, pain in bones and joints, frequent infections, weight loss, night sweats	Exposure to ionising radiation and chemicals, genetic predisposition	69 %

Type	Some Symptoms	Possible causes	5-year survival*
Lung	Persistent cough, increased sputum, sometimes blood smeared, persistent ache in chest, lung congestion, lymph nodes in neck enlarged.	Smoking, secondary smoke, toxic exposure (asbestos, chemicals)	13 %
Melanoma	Change in mole or bump on skin, bleeding or other changes (size, shape, color, texture) of existing mole	Lack of w-6 fatty acids. Sun exposure, particularly during childhood, sun burning of freckling easy, 40 times higher in whites	87 %
Lymphoma	Painless swelling in lymph nodes of neck, under arm, groin; unexplained fatigue, weight loss, itchy skin, rashes, small lumps in skin, bone pain, swelling in some part of the abdomen; liver and spleen enlarged	Lowered immunocompetence (AIDS), non-Hodgkins lymphoma after organ transplants, exposure to chemicals	51 %
Oral	Feel lump in mouth with tongue, sore spot (lip, pharynx) during eating in mouth; ulceration of lips, oral cavity tongue, dentures no longer fit well, oral pain, bleeding, foul breath, loose teeth, and changes in speech.	More in men; tobacco, chewing tobacco, toxic exposure	
Ovarian	Mostly few symptoms, abdominal swelling, sometimes vaginal bleeding, digestive discomfort	Age, never pregnant, residence in industrial area, family history of breast, ovarian cancer.	44 %

Type	Some Symptoms	Possible causes	5-year survival*
Pandreas	Upper abdominal pain, unexplained pain, weight loss, pain near center of back, loss of appetite, intolerance of fatty foods, yellowing of skin, abdominal mass, enlargement of liver, spleen.	Age, smoking, high fat diet, higher in black people	3 %
Prostate	Urination difficulty, bladder retains urine, frequent urgency to urinate; burning painful urination, sometimes bloody urine, tenderness over bladder, dull ache in pelvis and back.	Age; higher in black people	86 %
Uterine	Abnormal vaginal bleeding of fresh blood or watery discharge in post-menopausal women; collection of fluid in uterus, painful urination, pain during intercourse, pain in pelvic area.	Cervical cancer: smoking, sex before 18, may sexual partners, higher in black people.	68 %
Endometrial cancer	Early menstruation	Never pregnant, oestrogene exposure, HRT (hormone replacement therapy) without progesterone, Tamoxifen, diabetes, gall-bladder disease, hupertension, obesity.	

NOTE: *The table above is a condensed version of that given by Diamond, Cowden and Goldberg in their book previously referred to (69).

* The five year survival figures are those reported following conventional treatment. This does not reflect cure rates or survival rates. The actual survival rates are very much lower than the figures shown in the table.
* Note that in all cancer, a lack of essential fatty acids (especially w-6) is an important cause.

When medical treatment fails

Cancer mortality statistics over the last century do not reflect kindly on currently accepted medical treatments of cancer. The future also does not look bright unless we change our thinking about cancer. Unless we approach the problem in a much more open-minded fashion, we are heading towards a steadily increasing cancer death rate, which in the near future is expected to exceed that of heart disease, making cancer the number one killer of mankind.

Over a period of only 90 years in the previous century, cancer deaths, as a percentage of total mortality, increased from 3.4 % in 1900 to 25 % in 1990. According to several surveys, including one in the UK, the Western World is heading for a cancer epidemic (16). While currently one in four people will die of cancer, every second person will die of the disease by the year 2017, less than 10 years from now (17).

Children seem to be particularly badly affected. The National Cancer Institute (USA) reports a 28 % increase in the incidence of childhood cancers from 1950 to 1988, only 38 years. Cancer now kills more children between the ages of 3 and 14 than any other illness (Hankey, B., Natl Cancer Institute, and Statistics Branch).

In 1971, with his War on Cancer programme, US President Nixon claimed that within five years a cure for cancer in the form of drugs that would kill cancer cells would be available. Such drugs did become available, but now, after 47 years, more than $40 billion on research and more than $1 trillion on treatments later, the situation is not better than in 1971. Against the more common cancers in the USA (lung, liver, bone, brain, colon, breast and prostate) no progress has been made in conventional medicine's super-expensive war on cancer since it was declared in 1971 by President Nixon.

In fact, the overall death rate from cancer has risen by 8 % since the War on Cancer was started.

Millions of people have died with no relief in sight from traditional therapies.

A report in the *New England Journal of Medicine* in 1986 assessed the progress against cancer in the US over the years 1950 to 1982. Some progress is reported on the treatment of a few very rare forms of cancer, which account for 1-2 % of total cancer mortality, but the report notes that the overall cancer death rate had increased substantially since 1950 and then concludes:

> *". . . some 35 years of intense effort focused largely on improving treatment, must be judged a qualified failure . . . we are losing the war on cancer."*

If a solid tumor is found early and then removed, it will regrow or appear elsewhere about 50 % of the time. Once a cancer has spread to other sites, chemotherapy and radiotherapy will heal it permanently only about 3 % of the time. These facts clearly demonstrate that in spite of billions of dollars spent on conventional cancer treatments, these methods simply do not work, except in a very small percentage of patients. There are even indications that untreated patients may live longer than those treated with chemotherapy.

In this regard, chemotherapy is rapidly coming to be regarded as the scapegoat by those who are prepared to examine the facts objectively. Statistics indicate that chemotherapy will cure only 3 % of the most dangerous and prevalent types of epithelial cancers (mainly blood and lymph cancers).

Why do we not hear about this, and why do oncologists persist in prescribing chemotherapy?

They are simply part of the system, and going against the system has many serious implications for them. For example, they will certainly lose their research money (flowing from President Nixon's war and other government sources); if they treat patients correctly according to their convictions, they may even be jailed and have their medical licenses withdrawn—at least in the USA.

The fact that the three traditional methods of cancer treatment may cause the spread of cancer to distant sites in the body significantly increases the risk associated with such treatments and also substantially contributes to the high overall cancer mortality rate. Dr. Israel notes in his book that several studies have shown that cancer patients who have had radiation therapy are more likely to have their cancer spread to other sites in their bodies. An article appeared (18) which states:

> "... secondary cancers are known complications of chemotherapy and radiation therapy."

Surgery too, is often responsible for the spread of the primary cancer, since an apparently unimportant part of, or carelessness in the procedure can spill millions of cancer cells into the patient's bloodstream to lodge elsewhere. This also applies to all biopsies.

In the meantime, however, some alternative anti-cancer treatments have become available which do appear to hold promise. Unfortunately, the further development of these methods is hampered by unnecessary infighting amongst the cancer therapy establishments, further aggravated by the very significant influence of outside financial interests. It seems that the time has come for all of us to set aside petty differences and to seriously re-examine our thinking, options and attitudes.

Unfortunately, though, this is not obvious to everyone. Even a chairman of the American Cancer Society has commented: "Everyone eventually dies of something." While this is true, we do not have to die unnecessarily and pre-maturely.

On the other hand, misleading reports create a false sense of optimism when there is in fact very little to be optimistic about. Such misleading statements are designed by some researchers in an attempt to justify research grants. Even the National Cancer Institute in America is guilty of such misleading statements. For example, it claims that because the breast cancer survival rate increased from 60 % in 1960 to 75 % in 1993, the survival rate had improved by 15 % over that period.

There are two things wrong with this statement. Firstly, *survival* does not mean *cure*. (*11*) According to this system, a patient who lives five years and one day will be counted as cured. This system is often used by the medical establishment to claim success in clinical trials when such claims are not warranted. Survival in this context means five-year survival, which is by no means the same as cure, especially in this instance where slow-growing breast cancer is concerned. These patients may live 15 years or more after diagnosis before death. Breast cancer is now being diagnosed much earlier, so that if more cases are diagnosed earlier, then more patients will be alive five years later.

The success record of conventional chemotherapy in the treatment of most tumors is equally bleak (*19*).

From 1950 to 1980 and beyond, there has been a steady and relentless increase in the cancer death rate in America in spite of the widespread use of chemotherapy. This does not mean that conventional treatment methods are totally ineffective; it simply means that each year more people die than can be "cured" by these methods, and this gap increases from year to year. It also means that these methods are not addressing the fundamental causes(s) of the disease, but at best have temporary effects which in time are superseded by the onward march of the disease.

The statistics tell us that we are losing the war on cancer, and numerous studies support such a conclusion. For example, the number of newly diagnosed cancer cases, as well as cancer deaths, continue to escalate unabated, and this applies to most types of cancer. Since 1950, the overall incidence of cancer has increased by 50 %, that of prostate cancer by 100 % and that of breast and colon cancer by 60 %. According to Dr. S. Epstein (Chairman of the Cancer Prevention Coalition), the overall incidence of cancer has increased by 24 % and the cancer death rate by 30 % between the years 1973 (when Nixon's anti-cancer programme was effectively initiated) and 1999. Breast cancer (54 %) and prostate cancer (105 %) are notable. Different surveys show slightly different figures, but the trend remains the same and stresses the point that very little progress (if any) has been made over the last 50 years.

At this point, it may be useful to consider the views of several Nobel Prize winners and internationally recognized experts on the merits of present-day medical treatment of cancer.

What world class authorities say

Dr. Otto Warburg (Nobel Prize, 1940 and 1966):

. . . but nobody can say that one does not know what cancer and its primary causes are. On the contrary, there is no disease whose prime cause is better known so that today ignorance is no longer an excuse that one cannot do more about prevention. That prevention of cancer will come there is no doubt, for man wishes to survive. But how long prevention will be avoided depends on how long the prophets of agnosticism will succeed in inhibiting the application of scientific knowledge in the cancer field.

In the meantime, millions of men must die unnecessarily.

The words "prophets of agnosticism" are particularly significant in the present-day situation where we are increasingly witnessing the impact of outside financial interests on scientific thinking.

Dr. Linus Pauling (twice Nobel Prize winner), when asked about the war on cancer, declared:

> *Everyone should know that the war on cancer is largely a fraud and that the National Cancer Institute and the American Cancer Society are derelict in their duties to the people who support them.*

Dr. James Watson, (Nobel Prize for discovering the structure of DNA and the genetic code) served for two years on the National Cancer Advisory Board in the US. When asked about the National Cancer Program and the war on cancer, he declared:

> *It's a bunch of shit.*

Dr. Glen Warner, oncologist:

> *We have a multibillion dollar industry that is killing people, right and left, just for financial gain. Their idea of research is to see whether two doses of this poison are better than three doses of that poison.*

Dr. Robert Atkins, well-known internationally for his books on nutrition and his novel ideas about fats and heart disease, made himself thoroughly unpopular with the medical establishment when he showed, by means of a clinical study backed by the medical establishment, that his fat-based dietary approach was much more effective in correcting the risk factors for heart disease than the official low fat diet recommended by the medical profession. He commented as follows on cancer:

> *. . . there have been many cancer cures and all have been ruthlessly and systematically suppressed with a Gestapo-like thoroughness by the cancer establishment. The cancer establishment is the not too shadowy association of the American Cancer Association, the leading cancer hospitals, the National Cancer Institute and the FDA. The shadowy part is the fact that these respected institutions are very much dominated by members and friends of members of the pharmaceutical*

industry who profit so incredibly much from our profession-wide obsession with chemotherapy.

Many other scientific celebrities have made similar strong-worded declarations on the direction that medical research on cancer is taking.

Amid this gloomy picture, there is some hope for the future. Firstly: prevention. Leading cancer experts from Harvard University have presented convincing evidence in the *New England Journal of Medicine* that 90 % of all cancers are environmentally induced and therefore preventable ([20]). These as well as other studies highlight the role of nutrition in preventing cancer. In spite of these significant findings, which have now been known for many years, present-day medical treatment of cancer completely disregards nutrition as a role player in the treatment and prevention of cancer.

The conventional methods most commonly used for the treatment of cancer are surgery, chemotherapy, radiation and hormone therapy. These forms of treatment are all aimed at killing cancer cells or at interfering with the proliferative aspects of the disease. None of these methods include correction of the patient's nutritional status, and none of these methods are sufficiently selective—they also kill significant numbers of normal cells, causing much pain and distress to the patient in addition to damaging the immune system, sometimes irreversibly. The greatest drawbacks of these methods are that they do not attend to the extremely important aspect of nutrition and the patient's inner terrain, and they also do nothing to strengthen the patient's natural resistance mechanisms.

This is particularly serious in the case of the chemotherapy drugs. The well-known oncologist and cancer researcher Prof Braverman, in a critical review, comments as follows:

. . . many medical oncologists recommend chemotherapy for virtually any tumor, with hopefulness undiscouraged by almost invariable failure ([21]).

Traditional chemotherapy may be of value in the case of some rare forms of cancer such as testicular cancer and certain leukemias, but it helps only 3 % of patients with the major forms of cancer ([19]).

From the available evidence, it would appear that the effectiveness of chemotherapy can be greatly increased and toxicity diminished by means of IPT and possibly also by means of DMSO Potentiation Therapy (DPT). For reasons not entirely understood, these very promising avenues have not yet been explored by the conventional medical establishment. In fact, the use of IPT has been strictly forbidden by the medical authorities in America in the past, with the result that the only doctors who practice this very promising new approach are now based in Mexico. This is such an important new development that I will return to it later in this book.

These are the facts that we have to face and deal with if we wish to make progress in future. The following steps are now of vital importance:

- The medical and scientific communities must stop infighting, which is often based on personality clashes rather than scientific facts.
- The medical community must take serious cognizance of some of the more promising alternative methods, and consider ways and means by which these may be combined with conventional methods. For example, the CsCl/DMSO protocol and IPT and the regulation of intracellular oxygen levels by means of certain fatty acids (Warburg) represent such combinations which appear to have merit and which are now awaiting well-designed large scale clinical trials. Many others may be cited and this aspect will be dealt with in more detail later.
- Drug regulation authorities must abandon their bitter prejudice against all alternative approaches, including diet, and allow these to be investigated in an open-minded manner in clinical trials. Their strict ban on the use of these methods has resulted in the near-complete absence of reliable clinical studies on the use of alternative methods in cancer treatment. The absence of supporting clinical studies is in turn used by the same authorities as evidence that natural methods of cancer treatment are ineffective. In this manner a particularly vicious circle is created, much to the disadvantage of many patients and much to the benefit of the pharmaceutical industry.
- In particular, the authorities must abandon their prosecution and persecution (sometimes even with brutal force) of those doctors who use alternative methods.
- There are various reports available now of where official bodies have undertaken to test some of the alternative methods by means of trials of their own. Unfortunately, these trials were designed and performed in such a manner that the negative outcomes reported could have been predicted even before the trials started. Good examples are the flawed Vitamin C trial by the American Cancer

Association under the guidance of Dr. C. Moertel (9) and the laetrile studies conducted by the same institutions. This will be discussed in greater detail later.
- Above all, financial interests should not be allowed to play a role in drug evaluation trials and therefore in medical treatment.

Cancer, causes, definition, properties

Before reading the rest of this section, I suggest that you consider what Virchow ("the father of pathology") said many years ago:

> "... *germs seek their natural habitat—diseased tissue—rather than being the cause of the disease; mosquitoes seek the stagnant water, but do not cause the pool to become stagnant* ..."

A heated debate on the origin of infectious disease, started in 1860 between two Frenchmen, Louis Pasteur and Antoine Beauchamp, continues to this day. The outcome of this duel, which was initially won by Pasteur, had a major effect on the course of medical practice eversince.

Pasteur promoted the germ theory of disease, which postulated that infectious diseases arise from monomorphic microbes outside the body, and that each microbe has a constant shape and color and is responsible for one particular disease. He also believed that each disease was caused by just one unique microbe which entered the body from outside, thus focusing much attention on killing the microbes as a means of combating the disease. Initially he did not consider such factors as host resistance and the internal milieu of the patient as of any significance. This has created a multibillion dollar pharmaceutical industry to supply the necessary germ-killing drugs.

Beauchamp, on the contrary, hypothesized that diseases arise from pleomorphic (more than one form) microbes inside the body. These pleomorphic organisms can go through various stages of growth and can mutate into various growth forms, including pathogenic forms, depending on the inner terrain of the patient. In this manner he focused attention on the condition of the host (the inner terrain of the patient) rather than on the microbes. The existence of such pleomorphic organisms in cells has been observed and described by several authors, including Claude Bernard, another famous Frenchman, and Enderlein, a famous German professor of microbiology, who used special dark field microscopy which allowed him to see these living pleomorphic organisms in live human blood. Others who have contributed to the pleomorphic theory include the Canadian biologist G. Naessens, who used ultraviolet light microscopy that easily allows identification of a cancer micro-organism in the live blood of cancer patients.

Dr. Royal Rife made a further important contribution by developing a machine which, by means of a small electric current and magnetic pulsation, could kill 100 % of these microbes, the physical form of which depended on the inner terrain of the patient.

Interestingly, although Pasteur was violently opposed to the theories of Bernard and Beauchamp initially, he admitted on his death bed:

"Bernhard was right . . . the trerrain is everything."

Because his original theories suited Big Pharma so well, he was very much pampered by them and later co-operated with them in such a way that he became the first corrupt scientist (11). He realized this finally before his death, hence the admission on his death bed.

According to one theory (11), environmental changes and other external toxins alter the cancer virus into cancer causing pleomorphs which disrupt cellular metabolism. These same external factors weaken the cell membranes, enabling the foreign organisms to enter the cell and, depending on the inner terrain, later appear as fungi, moulds or even bacteria. Once inside the cells, these microbes intercept cellular fuel (glucose) which they convert into energy by means of fermentation whereby acids (lactic acid) are produced. In the meantime, available glucose supplies are now diverted to the fermentation pathway, depriving the normal cells of much-needed glucose to produce energy. Hence the weakness of the cancer patient!

The acidic microbial products and a deficiency of intracellular oxygen produce the characteristic acidity in cancer cells first observed by Warburg.

Due to the general shortage of glucose created in this way, signals are sent to the insulin and glucose receptors on the cell membranes (of both normal and cancer cells) to increase activity and to bind more glucose in order to correct the deficiency. Since cancer cells have 15 times more glucose receptors than normal cells, they get the bulk of the additional glucose metabolized.

In Warburg's time and for many years subsequently, the acidity and oxygen deficiency in cancer cells was known and generally accepted, but no one understood why this happens. The abovementioned chain of events now, for the first time, explains this, at least partially.

In summary then, the cancer cell consists of a human cell that has been transformed as a result of membrane defects brought about by a deficiency of certain fatty acids and the activities of adaptable microbes which flourish because they are able to adapt themselves to the prevailing inner terrain circumstances. In addition, due to a lack of unadulterated w-6 fatty acids, oxygen transport into the cells has been reduced to critically low levels which further favor the anaerobic metabolism and acid production in cells (Brian Peskin, 2008. *The Hidden Story of Cancer*. Houston: Pinnacle Press).

Human cancers are mostly created by humans themselves through contact with a self-created environment heavily laden with industrial toxins, microbes and nutrients and nutrient deficiencies that alter healthy metabolic patterns. Most people get cancer because of the things they have taken into their bodies, of which the diet is the most important source. The wrong foods create an internal terrain which allows the body to be filled with cancer-causing toxins and micro-organisms. Smoking and air pollution are good examples of the first, while fungus-laden foods such as peanuts are an example of the second.

The following are some examples of how we poison ourselves:

- We eat mainly junk food, processed food and fast food with very little nutritive value
- We smoke, and drink masses of alcohol
- Each year, in the US, half a billion kg of pesticides are sprayed on the crops we eat
- Much of our food is contaminated with yeasts, moulds, etc. as a result of the way it is stored
- Billions of tons of toxic waste are deposited in waste sites, in the air and in rivers
- We drink water that has been poisoned with chlorine and fluoride
- Millions of people have toxic mercury-filled root canals whence it seeps into our bodies
- Millions of people submit to X-ray poisoning and other medical procedures by doctors.

According to available evidence, it is necessary to distinguish between the primary cause and secondary causes of cancer. The primary cause of cancer is cellular membrane abnormalities caused *inter alia* by a deficiency of w-6 fatty acids which is the direct cause of intracellular oxygen deficiency. Under these conditions and because of the oxygen deficiency, the cells switch from the normal aerobic metabolic energy producing mechanisms (respiration) to anaerobic pathways (fermentation) with the increased production of lactic acid. This is the primary cause of cancer (O. Warburg, *The Journal of Cancer Research* 1925, 9, p 148). All other causes are secondary causes.

Severe trauma and stress are other possible secondary causes of cancer. Dr. R.G. Hamer is an oncologist who has studied the histories of 20 000 cancer patients. He found that a particular area in the brain is associated with each organ in the body. Emotional trauma affects the brain in such a manner that specific organs are affected, according to his theory. He was jailed for promoting this idea, which the medical establishment did not welcome at all. It would appear, according to Henderson (22), that many but not all cancers develop from emotional trauma and stress.

From my own experience I would agree with this, but would add that emotional stress is only a major cause in some cancers, but in most others it may be a contributory cause, which if not attended to may prevent successful treatment. In addition, the effects of emotional stress are only seen in a patient with a distorted inner terrain.

There can be no doubt any longer that heavy metals such as mercury, present in root canals, may be a major secondary cause of cancer, at least in some patients. The American Dental Association has done its utmost to suppress the idea, without much success, because there are now many prominent dentists who agree that mercury in root canals can be a major threat to health. The cancer patient should therefore take steps to remove this threat if present.

Cancers are therefore theoretically easy to prevent; in practice, though, this is a mammoth task due to lack of knowledge and especially of political will on the part of governments to enforce unpopular laws and regulations in democratic societies. This is clearly demonstrated by the recent refusal of the US government to enforce measures to combat global warming which are analogous to the measures required to introduce practical measures to reduce environmental cancer risk.

It is easy to define cancer, but it may not be so easy to pin down the real causes in practice, because there are so many potential secondary causes. The properties of all cells in the body are determined by nucleic acids (DNA) in the cell nucleus. These properties are passed on from generation to generation as the cells divide to form new daughter cells by the information contained in the DNA molecules, This information is in turn determined by the sequence and nature of the constituent nucleotides in the DNA. In simple terms, it may be stated that cancer is a disease in which some of the cells of the body in defined areas have undergone changes in their genetic material (DNA) such as to confer on them the properties or characteristic of cancer cells, including a diminished ability to respond to the normal control mechanisms of the body.

However, in addition to what has been said above, there are many other secondary causes that contribute to the process of carcinogenesis. One single truth about cancer that nobody disputes, is that cancer has multiple, interacting secondary causes and frequently there is a certain amount of synergism between the numerous factors that can cause cancer.

Some of the secondary causes of cancer

The following are some of the known secondary causes of cancer:

- Sunlight, chronic exposure to electromagnetic fields, geopathic stress, ionizing radiation (including X-rays), nuclear radiation, pesticide/herbicide residues, industrial toxins, chlorinated water, fluoridated water, tobacco and smoking, hormone therapies, drugs (eg certain antidepressants), cholesterol-lowering drugs eg statins, food additives, irradiated foods, mercury amalgams in teeth, dietary factors, prostaglandin E2 (derived from certain fatty acids present in animal products), excessive intake of sugar and refined foods, excessive intake of alcohol, excessive intake of iron, excessive intake of caffeine, chronic stress, depressed thyroid action, intestinal toxicity, parasites, viruses and other micro-organisms including pleomorphic organisms as discussed above, and oxygen deficiency.

There is scientific evidence that each of these factors may cause cancer in humans, thus establishing cancer as a truly multifactorial disease. However, not all of them need to be present to cause cancer.

This information is fairly easy to understand and to verify. What is not so easy to unravel, is just how this happens. The numerous toxins, free radicals, industrial toxins, food additives, radiation, viruses and other micro-organisms and other similar factors all play a role, although precisely how they do this is more difficult to understand. Viruses and certain pleomorphic micro-organisms may be of particular significance. One thing is reasonably clear: cellular acidity and lack of oxygen in cells, apart from the many other adverse effects it has on various biochemical systems, is certainly a major factor in the process of carcinogenesis. It may even be the trigger which initiates the carcinogenic effects of the various carcinogens listed above. Restoring intercellular acidity (which may be pH 6 or even lower in cancer cells) to 7.4 or higher and intracellular oxygen levels seem to be necessary steps in any cancer treatment programme. This can be achieved by means of diet, but then the orthodox medical establishment does not believe that diet is a factor in human carcinogenesis. Chronically elevated blood levels of glucose and insulin may be equally important secondary causes of cancer.

Summarizing then, it may be stated that cancer is primarily caused by an intracellular oxygen deficiency leading to increased intracellular acidity, which is exacerbated *inter alia* by an acidic diet that allows the body to be overwhelmed by certain micro-organisms (viruses, yeasts, fungi moulds and other pleomorphic organisms) which further cause the cells to become more acidic and anaerobic, *inter alia* because of the increased oxygen consumption by these organisms. This results in a shift in cancer cells towards fermentation as a means of energy production which requires less oxygen and also leads to lactic acid accumulation, which in turn further increases acidity. The theory is based on a study by Otto Warburg in 1966 which showed that cancer cells are largely anaerobic (reduced oxygen requirements), for which he was awarded a Nobel Prize. Warburg showed that normal cells will become cancerous once the intra-cellular oxygen tension has declined by approximately 35 %. At one stage, this theory was disputed by some cancer specialists, but recently it has attracted increased attention by researchers. For normal cells to grow and replicate normally, sufficient oxygen inside the cells is critical. For a variety of reasons, the oxygen supply to some cells may be restricted. This may happen for example when oxygen supply through the cell membranes is restricted due to the presence of unnatural transfatty acids in the membrane structures and, according to Dr. Peskin, also when the correct mix of w-3 and w-6 fatty acids is not present in the cell membranes (B.S. Peskin. 2008. *The Hidden Story of Cancer*. Houston: Pinnacle Press). According to the Peskin theory, a relative deficiency of w-6 fatty acids (derivatives of linoleic acid) relative to w-3 acids (derivatives of linolenic acid) is the real cause of the disrupted cell membranes in cancer patients which disable cellular oxygenation. A decline of only 35 % of the oxygen tension inside a cell is sufficient to convert that cell irreversibly into a cancer cell. Greater cellular oxygen deprivation is directly correlated with worse prognosis, a shorter lifespan and greater risk of metastasis. This stresses the importance not only of supplementing with fish oil (w-3 fatty acids) but also of supplementing with a suitable source of w-6 fatty acids such as cold pressed sunflower oil. The important role of polyunsaturated fats in the process of cellular oxygenation was recognized many years ago by Dr. Budwig, and forms an integral part of the Budwig protocol for the treatment of cancer. She was the first to suggest that certain fatty acids in the cellular membranes act like little magnets which draw oxygen into cells This is discussed later in this book.

Oxygen levels inside cells may also be compromised when oxygen-consuming micro-organisms such as certain fungi are present. When the level of available oxygen in the cell falls below a certain critical level (35 % below normal), cells can no longer function normally and, in order to survive, the cells switch from the normal aerobic pathways (respiration) for the extraction of energy from fuel (glucose) which depend heavily on the presence of oxygen, to anaerobic pathways (fermentation) which require less oxygen. During fermentation, lactic acid is produced which lowers the intracellular pH (from perhaps 7.4 down to 6.5 or lower, even as low as 6.0 to 5.7) thereby destroying the normal function of the DNA/RNA system to control cell division. The result is that the cells begin to multiply in an uncontrolled manner (cancer cells). The lactic acid at the same time causes intense local pain and further inhibits normal cellular reactions by destroying critical enzymes. In this manner normal cells are converted into cancer cells and the cancer (in the case of solid cancers) appears as a rapidly growing outer cell mass with a core of dead cells. This scenario of the process of carcinogenesis (for which he was awarded two Nobel Prizes) was developed by Otto Warburg in Germany between 1920 and the 1960s.

In summary, the chain of events is as follows:

- Cell membranes become weakened as a result of many different environmental factors such as transfatty acids, carcinogens, free radicals, the wrong mix of membrane fatty acids, etc.
- This suppresses oxygen access to the cell, which increases pressure in the cell to switch towards a more anaerobic metabolic pattern which requires less oxygen for energy production
- This also enables microbes (viruses, pleomorphic micro-organisms) to enter the cells
- The population of pleomorphic organisms inside the cells intercepts the glucose entering the cells, thus further depriving the cells of glucose
- The micro-organisms inside the cells now produce toxic, acidic mycotoxins, lactic acid and slime which further suppress normal cellular metabolism

- The metabolic products of the microbes and the accompanying lack of oxygen now strongly increase acidity inside the cells, which is what Warburg observed
- The cell's mitochondria (where the energy is produced by metabolism of glucose) are now deprived of oxygen and glucose, which is the cause of the low level of energy in cancer cells
- Signals are then sent to the insulin receptors on the cell membranes in an attempt to increase the glucose levels inside the cells
- More glucose now enters the cancer cells (about 15 times more than in normal cells), but most of the glucose is intercepted by the multiplying microbes inside the cells where the energy-producing mitochondria are increasingly swamped by masses of mycotoxins and other metabolic products of the microbes
- Normally energy is derived from glucose by first converting it into pyruvic acid which enters the mitochondria where it is converted into energy (ATP)
- In this manner, a normal cell (high energy levels, low acidity, no microbes) has been converted into a cancerous cell (low energy levels, high acidity, dense microbe population)
- The cells harbouring the microbes are sick, while the microbes thrive. This makes it very difficult to kill the microbes without also killing the cell.

This model of the process of carcinogenesis immediately suggests the following steps that should be part of the treatment:

- Kill the cancer cells without killing normal cells (many natural substances will do that, eg CsCl, laetrile, carrot and beet juice, the Brandt grape mush, hydrogen peroxide and many others)
- Kill the microbes inside the cells (eg methylsulfonylmethane (MSM) or DMSO, Robert Young protocol)
- Increase oxygen supply to the cells (eg hydrogen peroxide, ozone therapy, w-6 fatty acids)
- Neutralize excess acidity in cells (CsCl, diet, supplements)
- Increase the energy levels (ATP) in the cells (restore oxygen supply)
- Strengthen the immune system (eg the Gerson protocol)
- Ensure the correct mix of w-3 and w-6 fatty acids in the diet (see Peskin ref above).

We see therefore that acidity and intracellular oxygen levels in cells lie at the core of the problem. These are initially induced by the typical Western diet, certain micro-organisms and possibly other factors such as a lack of antioxidants and the incorrect mix of w-3 and w-6 fatty acids.

As the blood acidity increases as a result of diet and other factors, the body tries to protect itself by depositing the excess acid in the tissues in an attempt to prevent over-acidity of the blood.

By addressing the problem of intracellular acidity directly, CsCl is an ideal agent for treating cancer.

Supporting evidence

- The known fact that cancer cells are acidic (Warburg)
- The known fact that energy levels (ATP) in cancer cells are very low
- Dr. R. Young states in his book (13) that he observed, through a live blood microscope, how microbes bore through the cell membranes of normal cells
- Several scientists have independently identified pleomorphic microbes in cancer cells
- Dr. T. Lebedewa removed sections of a tumor under sterile conditions and then submerged it in a highly nutritious sterile medium. Within days she noticed microbes (trichomonads) in the culture.

Much evidence is also presented in a number of books dealing with the relationship between cancer and microbes (23); see (13) for more references.

More on the Warburg theory

The Warburg theory is the only cancer theory that has never been seriously questioned or disproved.

Many other cancer theories and myths have not survived in the sense that they were seriously challenged. The following are some examples:

Theory	Called into question
Fruits and veggies protect against cancer	*JAMA 2001*, 285:769, 799
Mammography detects initial cancer growth	*Int J Health Services 2001*, 31:605
Fiber protects against colon cancer	*Lancet 2000*, 356:1286

| w-3 oils alone will protect against cancer | JAMA 2006, 295:203 |
| Low fat diets protect against cancer | JAMA 2006, 295:629 |

According to Warburg, if the intracellular oxygen tension is reduced to the extent that the oxygen transfer enzymes are no longer saturated with oxygen, respiration can decrease irreversibly, thereby transferring normal cells into facultative anaerobes. Intracellular, just 35 % less oxygen than normal can bring this about. The important point is that this statement does not refer to blood oxygen levels (which may be raised *inter alia* by means of exercise) but that it specifically refers to intracellular oxygen levels which are determined by the state of the cell membranes which control the flow of oxygen to the intracellular compartment. Thus impaired transmembrane oxygen transfer may occur even in the presence of adequate blood oxygen levels. This is why professional athletes also get cancer.

Several articles in cancer journals have confirmed the relationship between reduced intracellular oxygen levels and cancer. One particularly interesting study showed significantly lower survival in cancer patients with a pO_2 < 10 mmHg compared to those with better oxygenated tumors with a pO_2 > 10 mmHg.

The important question then is: what are the conditions that cause cells to become oxygen deficient, and what dietary and lifestyle factors might cause this?

Peskin (see ref above) showed that the body requires certain fatty acids which play a role in promoting oxygen transfer across cell membranes. These polyunsaturated fatty acids (PUFA) are called essential fatty acids because the body cannot make them from other available compounds, so that they have to be present in the diet. There are 2essential fatty acids from which the body can manufacture all other polyunsaturated fatty acids. These are: linoleic acid, which is the parent substance of the w-6 series, and linolenic acid which is the parent substance of the w-3 series.

Campbell and his co-workers were the first to show that linoleic acid (the parent of the w-6 polyunsaturated fatty acids) has the unique property that it can associate with oxygen in the blood and then transfer it across cell membranes to the intracellular space, there to dissociate from the oxygen it carries at the prevailing oxygen pressure. In this manner it acts like a magnet pulling oxygen into cells (*Pediatrics* 1976, 57:489).

The other parent polyunsaturated fatty acids (linolenic acid) share this property with linoleic acid, but to a much lesser degree.

These workers found that these two essential fatty acids also affect the permeability of cell membranes, thus facilitating the oxygen transport function by increasing cellular oxygenation by up to 50% (*Pediatrics* 1976, 57:480). It is not clear at this stage why the w-6 linoleic acid is so much stronger than the w-3 linolenic acid with regard to the oxygen transport function, although both contain unconjugated double bonds with pi-electron systems which are assumed to be responsible for the reversible binding of oxygen.

What is clear, though—bearing the Warburg theory in mind—is that insufficient quantities of these essential fatty acids in the diet can reduce oxygen transport into cells sufficiently to cause cancer (*Townsend Letter* Aug-Sept, 2007, p 84).

There are also other sources in the medical literature which confirm the oxygenating capacity of these essential fatty acids (*Ibid.*)

Campbell *et al.*, also concluded that interference with oxygen transport into cells can occur at any cell membrane in any tissue. This allows us to conclude that this is the universal primary process by means of which normal cells are transformed into malignant cells, and therefore that all cancers occur by means of the same primary mechanism, as originally postulated by Warburg.

Moreover, a deficiency of these EPA can be responsible for the incorporation into cell membranes of non-oxygenating fatty acids that may be present, eg hydrogenated fats and transfats which occur in some margarine. In this manner the abovementioned primary process of carcinogenesis may be accelerated.

The fact that linoleic acid is a so much stronger oxygen transporter than linolenic acid also has other important implications. As suggested by Peskin (*Townsend Letter*, Aug-Sep. 2007, p 92) one of the most important causes of cancer is related to the consumption of adulterated polyunsaturated fatty acids (through chemical manipulation of food) in food. These "foreign" molecules are incorporated into cell membranes, thus effectively interfering with cellular oxygen transmission by the natural molecules, especially by linoleic acid.

There are several reasons why linoleic acid and other polyunsaturated fatty acids are degraded (adulterated) under the practical conditions in which our food is prepared and stored. Natural oils in prepared foods may turn rancid due to exposure to aerial oxygen, and this also happens to oils used in restaurants and commercial deep fryers (Peskin). Food processors attempt to stop this from happening for economic reasons, and in this process they do even more damage. They convert the offending polyunsaturated fatty acids (from their point of view) into more stable but biologically harmful derivatives in the form of transfatty acids and interesterified fats.

Peskin was the first to recognize this as one of the prime causes of cancer and the unstoppable cancer epidemic in the Western world.

> *The only solution to the problem is to reintroduce unadulterated linoleic acid-containing oils into our diets by way of dietary supplementation.*

This was not done in the past, for two reasons. The existing sources of linoleic acid (eg sunflower oil) contain largely adulterated linoleic acid due to chemical manipulation of the product to make it commercially more attractive and stable. The other, and perhaps more important, reason is that we all believed that the most important polyunsaturated fatty acids deficiency in the Western World is that of the w-3 fatty acids. Over a period of many years, we were led to believe that the w-3 oils in the form of fish oils are the principal polyunsaturated fatty acids that should be supplemented because of the apparent abundance of w-6 containing polyunsaturated fatty acids in our diet. It was not recognized that the apparent predominance of w-6 polyunsaturated fatty acids in our diet is largely an illusion due to the reasons given above (Peskin, *ibid*).

A study of the w-3:w-6 polyunsaturated fatty acids ratios in various tissues further confirms that the linoleic acid-containing w-6 polyunsaturated fatty acids are of much greater importance in the various tissues (see for example *J Mol Neurosc* 2001, 16: 159 and 215). The following table (adapted from *Townsend Letter*, Aug-Sept 2007) clearly demonstrates this fact.

Omega—6 : 3 ratios in body tissues

Organ	Parent w-6 (linoleic acid)	Parent w-3 (linolenic acid)	% of total body weight
Brain (nervous system)	1	1	3
Skin	1000	1	4
Other tissues	4	1	9
Adipose tissues (fat)	22	1	15-35
Muscles	6.5	1	60

The table clearly illustrates the predominance of parent w-6 polyunsaturated fatty acids over w-3 polyunsaturated fatty acids in virtually all body tissues, but especially in the skin.

Only in the brain and nerve tissue are they equally represented, while in most other tissues there are many more w-6 than w-3 acids. This is in direct contrast to current medical teaching.

The skin contains practically no w-3 fatty acids. It means that all the skin benefits previously associated with polyunsaturated fatty acids (w-3+w-6) supplementation were in fact due only to the unadulterated w-6 (linoleic acid) part of the supplement. This has important practical medical implications, especially for the treatment of skin cancers as we shall see later.

What happens to the various tissues if the required quantities of unadulterated w-6 acids are not supplied in the diet? The body simply uses other polyunsaturated fatty acids that are available to incorporate into the membranes. These may include the damaged w-6 polyunsaturated fatty acids which resulted from food manipulation (eg transfatty acids) or even non-essential fatty acids such as the w-9 fatty acids in olive oil. Since these substituted fatty acids cannot fulfill the essential task of the unadulterated w-6 fatty acids—particularly with respect to oxygen supply to the cells—the endresult will be lowered oxygen supply to the cells, which increases the possibility that the cells may become malignant, according to Warburg (*Cancer Res*1979, 39: 1726).

Such a shortage of vital w-6 linoleic acid also has other implications. The body will then prioritize supplies in such a manner that the most vital organs (brain, lungs, kidneys, heart) are first supplied, with the result that other organs such as the prostate gland and breast receive even less of the available w-6 acid. The oxygen deficiency in these cells is consequently aggravated, resulting in an increased possibility of cancer. These organs have a high fat content, indicating an increased requirement of linoleic acid. It is therefore not surprising that cancers in these organs are amongst the most prevalent in the world

What is the main function of w-3 polyunsaturated fatty acids (fish oil) in the Body?

This question is relevant to the present discussion of w-3 vs w-6 supplementation. Studies have revealed that the major metabolic route of the w-3 acids in the body is that of energy supply to the cells via the process of beta-oxidation (*Lipids* 2002, 37,12:1113) and not for incorporation into cell membranes and tissue structure (*Lipids* 2002, 37:1123). These studies have also revealed that if large amounts of the w-3 acids are supplied by way of supplementation, they may nonetheless be incorporated into cell membranes with possible adverse consequences.

The current teaching that we require large amounts of w-3 acids such as DHA and EPA is therefore called into question by Peskin. Most of these compounds are used for energy production, less than 1 % being converted into structural derivatives. From the nutritional point of view, food sources rich in w-3 fatty acids (fish oil, flaxseed oil, sea food) can therefore overload the body, with possible harmful consequences. Such an abnormal supply of w-3 fatty acids can cause an abnormal pattern of essential fatty acids to be incorporated in the cell membranes, which may *inter alia* influence the fluidity of the membranes and consequently also trans-membrane transport of nutrients. The skin is one organ that may suffer grave consequences as a result of a distorted supply of w-3 and w-6 fatty acids. We have seen that there are virtually no w-3 fatty acids in the skin normally. It is quite possible that in the presence of too little w-6 acids and too much w-3 acids, the excessive quantities of the latter may be deposited in the cells, with predictable consequences for cellular oxygen supply and therefore cancer development.

In spite of all this information, nutritionists and medical doctors continue to advocate supplementation with excessive quantities of w-3 acids and very low quantities of unadulterated true w-6 fatty acids. Collectively this may be responsible for the marked increase of skin cancers and various other skin conditions in Western populations.

How much parent w-6 fatty acids are we consuming and how much do we need?

This question has recently been addressed by Peskin (*Townsend Letter*, Aug-Sept 2007, 89). Most scientists, nutritionists and medical doctors teach that we consume up to 30 times more w-6 than w-3 polyunsaturated fatty acids, and on the basis of this they advocate supplementation with excessive quantities of w-3 acids in the form of fish oil supplements. This assumption is wrong for two reasons. Firstly, w-3 polyunsaturated fatty acids are present in conservable quantities in many of our foods (eg meat, walnuts, avocados, etc.) which affect the abovementioned ratios. Many of these foods affect the ratios in prepared foods such as hamburger steaks and eggs in which the ratios are typically 2:1 to 10:1 in favor of w-6.

Such calculations are, however, further misleading because they contain a large percentage of adulterated w-6s with little or no oxygenating capacity. For example, as stated by Peskin (*ibid*), margarine and most supermarket cooking oils (olive oil excluded) have very little or no oxygenating ability.

This can be recognized from the fact that they are resistant to oxidation and do not become rancid even when exposed to aerial oxygen for a very long time. This is very much in favor with the manufacturers because of increased stability, shelf life and appearance, but ensures that these products have very little nutritional value. At the same time, they may contribute significantly to the rapidly increasing cancer mortality.

It is a tragic fact of life that commercial interests always enjoy preference over health concerns in such matters. For this reason, common oils available to the public continue to be adulterated in many ways, including hydrogenation, addition of preservatives and other chemical manipulations which reduce the nutritional value and cellular oxygenating capacity of the products.

Governments, who spend billions of dollars on cancer research in the futile search for a chemical weapon that will kill cancer cells, will do well to consider these facts and rather devote a small percentage of that wasted money to the development of unadulterated foods.

As far as dietary oils and fats are concerned, we need products that contain the correct ratio of unadulterated organically produced oils in which there are an optimal ratio of w-6:w-3 oils, bearing in mind that the body requires significantly less parent w-3 than w-6 oils.

What is the ideal ratio?

According to Peskin, the ideal ratio is one in which w-6:w-3 unadulterated oils are in a proportion of 1.1 up to 2.5:1 in favor of parent organic unadulterated w-6. With this ratio of oils, Peskin uses 3g of the composite oil mix per 70kg body weight daily. Details of how this formula was calculated are available at *www.BrianPeskin.com* (Go to "EFA Report").

This formula significantly reduces tumor growth in mice. The formula has also been successfully tested in numerous human cancer patients. For details, go to the following sites: http://brianpeskin.com/studies-experiments/macphailcasestudy-1.pdf http://brianpeskin.com/studies-experiments/mouse-experiment.pdf.

Some of the properties of cancer cells

What then are the typical properties of cancer cells that make them so dangerous? The following are some examples of the typical behavior of most cancer cells:

- *The capacity to proliferate in an uncontrolled manner.* Normal cells which form a part of the body as a unit are under some restraint on their growth so as to keep them functioning as part of the whole organism. Also, some normal cells die naturally as a means of tissue renewal. The phenomenon is called apoptosis or programmed cell death. Apoptosis is a genetically controlled process whereby cells commit suicide. Cancer cells no longer have this restraint. One of the goals of cancer therapy is therefore centered on methods that will induce the process of apoptosis, thus normalizing the cell population. Some natural agents that are known to induce apoptosis in cell culture of cancer cells are DMSO, quercetin and Vitamin D3.
- *The capacity to infiltrate neighboring cells* and thereby to continue uncontrolled growth elsewhere in the body, thus forming metastases. In order to achieve this, the cancer cells produce increased quantities of certain enzymes (eg hyaluronidase and collagenase) by means of which the surrounding normal tissues are broken down, thus facilitating spreading of the cancer cells.
- *The capacity to extract increased amounts* of critical nutrients from the circulation, thus depriving the normal cells of vital nutritional elements required for growth.
- *Many cancer cells may develop alternative metabolic pathways* by means of which they enable themselves to compete more effectively with normal cells for nutrients. For example, many cancer cells

have developed the capacity to extract energy from carbohydrates through a process of fermentation by means of which they require less oxygen and produce metabolites (eg lactic acid and increased acidity) which suppress the growth of normal cells.
- Cancer cells develop these properties during the course of several pre-cancerous steps before they become fully autonomous.

These different properties of cancer cells give us the possibility of different angles of attack, by means of which we might treat cancer selectively, and form the basis of many natural cancer treatments.

The structure, size and growth of a tumor

A tumor consists mostly of healthy cells. Therefore it is wrong to consider tumor size as an indicator of success of treatment or otherwise. Since a cancer cell is undifferentiated; it can neither differentiate into different tissues like normal cells nor have any other function. This can be readily seen on biopsies prepared from cancerous tissues.

A tumor is our body's emergency defensive response to abnormal cells that are out of control. We often see tumors that are "encapsulated". This is the body's attempt to isolate the tumor in order to prevent its spreading and thus to limit the damage.

Cancer is not a disease; it is simply a symptom of a disease. The actual disease entity consists of a mass of normal cells that have lost the capacity to respond to the body's normal regulatory mechanisms.

Only a small percentage of cells in a tumor are cancerous, therefore killing off the cancerous cells in a particular lump of cancerous tissue will not necessarily shrink the tumor. Eventually the body will get rid of the dead cancer cells, but this may take a long time. However, some alternative treatments do shrink some tumors fairly rapidly (which may in itself cause practical problems) but it is wrong to equate the amount of shrinkage quantitatively with successful treatment in all cases. The tumor size has little to do with therapeutic effect. Conventional chemotherapy does shrink some tumors, but these patients just go on to die in any case. Many of the reported "successful" clinical trials by conventional doctors using conventional methods used tumor size as a criterion of successful treatment, with results that are entirely misleading.

This view of a tumor and its structure allows us to understand that biopsies will promote the spreading of cancer cells. Cutting into a tumor will cause bleeding and since the cancer cells sit loosely amongst a mass of normal cells, they can be released into the bloodstream when a biopsy is performed.

The majority of cancer deaths come as a result of cancer-induced malnutrition and infections by bacteria, viruses and fungi—that flourish as a result of a suppressed immune system. This results partly from the systemic weakening as a result of the cancer, and partly because of the toxicity and negative side-effects of conventional treatments, notably chemotherapy. In this regard it is interesting to note that conventional chemotherapy also destroys the capacity of the intestinal mucosal cells to absorb nutrients, thus indirectly contributing to the malnutrition seen in many cancer patients.

An understanding of some cancer statistics is necessary in order to get a better overall view of what happens in the cancer patient. In spite of huge amounts of money spent on cancer, there are approximately 600,000 cancer deaths in the USA every year, and that figure is increasing every year. Modern medicine has therefore little to offer most cancer patients, especially in the case of cancer patients with metastases. This compels us to rethink the problem starting right at the core, and that is why Einstein said:

> "... the level of thinking that caused the problem cannot be used to solve it."

This is the reason why we should now take a new look at the cancer problem and in particular seriously consider what natural medicine has to offer.

Solid cancers (eg breast cancer) cannot usually be diagnosed before the tumor burden in the patient reaches at least 10^{10} malignant cells. A tumor burden of 10^{13} is usually lethal. Cancer kinetics describes the process by which the cancer burden increases in time. It is critically important in predicting prognosis and especially to monitor efficacy of treatment. The "doubling time" is a parameter that can be calculated from cancer kinetics measurements. The doubling time on the one hand tells us something about the virulence of the cancer (and thus patient prognosis). On the other hand it indicates the likelihood that the cancer will respond to chemotherapy treatment, especially IPT.

It is usually assumed that a solid cancer that has reached the stage of clinical detestability (approx 1cm diameter) has already undergone 30 doublings, thereby reaching a mass of 10^9 cells. Only 10 further doublings are required to reach a mass of 1kg, which is usually lethal. (Cecil's *Textbook of Medicine*, 18th Ed, Philadelphia, USA: Saunders). During the subclinical phase of the disease (before the patient becomes aware of the presence of the disease), the tumor mass consists of normal cells and cancerous cells which are very similar in appearance under the microscope, as previously explained. At this stage the cancer cells are rapidly dividing and therefore highly susceptible to chemotherapy and IPT because of the rapidly dividing cells. Unfortunately, during this stage the patient is usually not aware of the disease. Once the cancer has spread (metastasized), the cell population becomes more heterogeneous, with some cells even in a resting state at any particular time. These cells have a longer doubling time and therefore are less susceptible to chemotherapy or IPT.

For any therapy to be successful, the rate at which cancer cells are killed must exceed the rate at which new cancer cells develop. This means that in the case of conventional chemotherapy (usually given every few weeks) the treatment at any time must kill more cancer cells than the number that developed since the previous treatment some weeks earlier. In this regard, the prognosis with IPT is much more favorable, since the treatment is given at least once a week or even more frequently. This leaves much less time for new cancer cells to develop.

Pharmacokinetic considerations also show why surgical removal of solid tumors is likely to be much less successful on its own than if the procedure is followed by chemotherapy or, better still, IPT, unless all of the cancer burden is removed by the procedure and no metastasis had occurred before the operation. If some cancer cells (eg 1000) had metastasized before and during the operation, the time before the critical mass of $10exp13$ is reached depends entirely upon the rate of multiplication or doubling time of the cancer cells, and may be anything from 3 to 7 years. The doubling time of the cancer cells may be determined from a biopsy sample. Patients with a doubling time of 60 days or shorter need immediate and very aggressive treatment such as IPT and CsCl/DMSO. At the same time, it is necessary to determine the percentage of the cancer cells in the S-phase (or growth phase) which is when the cancer cells are killed by chemotherapy. If only 8 % of the cancer cells are in the S-phase, it means that conventional chemotherapy will only kill 8 % of the cancer cells with each monthly application of the drug, with 92 % of the cancer cells remaining and ready to grow. The chances of the patient surviving therefore now depend on the rate at which the cancer cells grow. For further information on the pharmacokinetics of cancer cell growth, see the book by Hauser and Hauser previously referred to.

An important consideration is that IPT recruits more cells out of the rest phase into the growth phase, thus increasing the toxicity of the anticancer drugs used, which also increases the chances of patient survival.

Some practical examples of how clinical manifestation of cancer depends upon cancer doubling time:

EXAMPLE 1: The patient has metastatic cancer with a doubling time of 60 days, according to the pathology report. If a 1cm nodule (10^{10} cells) is detected, it is easy to show that the cancer will reach a mass of 10^{13} in just 7 months' time and the lethal tumor burden in 2 years. It is, however, doubtful that any cancer is entirely localized so that more cancer cells may be present than assumed in the abovementioned example.

> *The important conclusion to be reached from these figures is that by the time a cancer is detected, it is well on its way to killing the patient and immediate urgent action is required.*

Elsewhere in this book we present an example of a scenario where 99 % of the tumor burden had been removed by surgery, leaving 1 million cancer cells that may continue to grow. If the doubling time of this particular cancer is 20 days, then 20 days after surgery, the cancer burden will be 2 million cells and 4 million cells 40 days later, etc. Within a year a positive mammogram will be detected in this patient even though surgery had removed more than 99 % of the cancer burden initially. The role that the immune system might play in this example has not been considered, but it is unlikely to be significant with such a high cancer burden.

Another important consideration to bear in mind is that after every treatment, in the case of high-dose conventional chemotherapy, regrowth of the cancer cells takes place. This means that the total cancer burden is more slowly reduced than might be expected from the example above. It also means that if treatment is prematurely terminated (which is often necessary because of toxicity in this type of medication); ultimately complete regrowth of cancer cells will occur, sufficiently to kill the patient.

The abovementioned examples show that a total cancer cure can only be achieved when the total kill from all the therapies including the immune system has eliminated the last cancer cell, because a single cancer cell has the capacity to regrow to a symptomatic tumor that can kill the host.

The immune system is important when small numbers of cancer cells are involved, such as in the beginning of a tumor. Later on, when a heavy cancer burden is present, the immune system is not capable of controlling the cancer on its own, and we have to rely on appropriate therapies.

This is one reason why the cancer status of patients should be regularly checked by means of the appropriate cancer markers as discussed in this book.

From the discussion above and from the cancer pharmacokinetics as presented in the book by Hauser and Hauser, it is clear why conventional chemotherapy does not work. In summary, it may be said that one of the most important reasons is that conventional chemotherapy is non-selective and does nothing to correct the underlying biochemical abnormalities in the patient. The drugs have to be administered far apart in time (once every few weeks because of toxic side-effects), thus creating favorable conditions for the cancer cells to regrow after each treatment. This also encourages the development of resistant cancer cells.

IPT overcomes some of these effects in addition to the fact that 3-4 different drugs may be used simultaneously, which minimizes the chances of the cancer cells becoming drug resistant.

Due to the absence of toxic side effects, immune stimulants and other treatments can be given to the IPT patient between treatments, eg 1-2 days preceding and 1-2 days following treatments. A wide variety of immune stimulants that can be used in this manner is now available. These include herbs, many Nutraceutical (eg Vitamin C) and many of the Stage IV and Stage III treatments discussed in this book. In this manner, the chances of remission and hopefully ultimate complete cure are greatly enhanced.

As a final thought, it is important to understand that subjective clinical improvement should not be used as an indicator of patient progress. Often patients appear and actually feel much better or even well, but they still retain cancer cells that in time may regrow. Feeling and looking good are poor indicators of the presence or absence of cancer. It is vital to continue treatment until objective parameters, such as the various cancer tests discussed in this book, indicate the absence of cancer and then to continue with these tests at least once every 6-12 months for a few years.

Please note that in the previous discussion of the pharmacokinetics of cancer and cancer drugs, the drastic changes to the various parameters that are likely to result from increased tissue oxygenation, have not been taken into consideration. The reason is that this type of information is not yet available.

Blood coagulation induces new cancerous growth (angiogenesis)

The process of blood clotting (intended to prevent bleeding) starts with the formation of a white thrombus (formed by the accumulation of blood platelets) followed by the formation of many interlocking strands of fibrin (formed from the precursor fibrinogen, a blood protein produced in the liver). The resulting network prevents further leakage of blood and red blood cells. If the body forms too much fibrin, excessive clotting will occur, which may be harmful. The process by means of which blood clots are dissolved is called fibrinolysis. For normal health, a balance between clotting and fibrinolysis must be maintained.

Several studies have reported reduced fibrinolysis in human patients with cancer which results in the formation of a fibrin stroma surrounding the tumor, as may be readily seen in patients with prostate cancer.

This formation of a stroma in and around a tumor appears to be an important mechanism by means of which cancers protect themselves against the immune system and anti-tumor drugs. *In vitro* and *in vivo* studies have shown that suppressing the formation of blood clots by means of warfarin (an anti-clotting drug) prevents the formation of a the red part or fibrin part of a clot and thereby increases the efficacy of anticancer drugs, thus increasing patient survival. Increased survival has also been demonstrated in cancer patients treated with dipyridamole, which prevents platelet white thrombus formation.

The fibrin coat that tumors form around themselves protects them against the immune system because the protective layer consists of host proteins and therefore appears as "self" to the immune system.

Fibrinolysis is reduced in cancer patients, but it still exists and research has revealed that fibrin degradation products and the accompanying inflammation play an important role in the formation and extension of the vascular system to feed the growing cancer. Obviously then, cancer growth can be inhibited by suppressing fibrin formation or by stimulating fibrinolysis. For this reason, blood tests to measure coagulation parameters and to control these if necessary should form part of cancer treatment programmes. At the same time, by suppressing angiogenesis (formation of new blood vessels), metastasis is reduced. Common tests that can be routinely done include platelet aggregation, blood fibrinogen levels, clotting time and others.

The increased coagulability of blood in cancer patients has been widely described in the cancer literature, but this knowledge is seldom utilized by oncologists in their treatment programmes.

Increased blood coagulability is also one of the unfavorable side effects of conventional high-dose chemotherapy, but not of IPT.

There are many different natural products that can be used to prevent blood coagulation in cancer patients. These include garlic, bromelain, curcumin, cayenne pepper, codliver oil (to suppress fibrin formation and to stimulate fibrinolysis) and horse chestnut. Butchers Broom inhibits increased vascular permeability and grapeseed extract, tocotrienols and ginger reduce platelet aggregation.

The drug Coumadin is also often used in cancer patients. When used in conjunction with conventional high-dose chemotherapy, promising results have been reported. It is also sometimes used in conjunction with IPT.

Heavy metals and blood clotting

Excessive blood clotting with all the abovementioned consequences for the cancer patient may be caused by many factors in the Western lifestyle and diet. These include certain fats, and sugar or a high carbohydrate diet. A low carb, high protein diet rich in vegetables has a favorable effect on blood clotting.

Heavy metal toxicity is a frequently overlooked cause of increased blood coagulation. One study found that mercury caused a 56 fold increase in the rate of thrombin formation in platelets (Hauser and Hauser). It is *inter alia* for this reason that many authors advise their patients to lower the level of heavy metals in their bodies by means of chelation therapy. This therapy is readily available in South Africa (details available from Fortifood at www.fortifood.co.za

Pain control in the cancer patient: the dangers of narcotics

Pain is often a major problem in cancer patients. It is customary to use pain-killing narcotics like morphine and pethidine to deal with the problem. There are many reasons why this is an extremely bad policy. Some of the reasons for this are, according to Dr. Hauser:

- Narcotics strongly suppress the immune system
- Narcotics stimulate the growth of implanted tumors and therefore also possibly metastases
- Narcotics increase the incidence of infections, which is a serious matter in cancer patients
- Narcotics cause the spleen and thymus to atrophy.

As a result of this and other reasons, Dr. Hauser states in his book (*ibid*, p 236):

"Nothing will send a cancer patient quicker to his grave than narcotics."

When severe pain is a problem, the best policy to control the pain may be summarized as follows according to various authors:

- Control the cancer as soon as possible by means of IPT or any one of the other Stage IV cancer treatments discussed in this book
- Use anti-inflammatory medications (eg ibuprofen, voltaren) to partly control the pain in the meantime
- Immediately supplement with 4g of a 1:1 mix of unadulterated w-3 and w-6 oils.

Glucose intolerance and cancer risk

We have frequently referred to the fact that sugar is bad for cancer patients. A more correct statement would be that raised blood sugar levels (accompanied by disproportionately raised insulin levels) are bad for cancer patients, meaning that glucose intolerance is bad for cancer patients. This is indeed one of the earliest metabolic abnormalities in cancer patients, which has been known for a long time. It also offers a therapeutic opportunity which is seldom taken advantage of.

The most widely used test to detect glucose abnormalities is the glucose tolerance test. In this test, a glucose load is given to the patient (70-100g of glucose in solution) after an overnight fast, and blood glucose levels are then determined every 30 minutes for the following 3-6 hours. Glucose intolerance is diagnosed if blood glucose levels rise above 8.9mmol/L and diabetes if levels exceed 10.6 any time during the test. Different labs and health specialists may have different critical values. According to one system, glucose intolerance is diagnosed if the following values are observed at any time during the test:

- fasting glucose levels above 6.7mmol/L fasting glucose levels below 3.9mmol/L glucose levels rise more than 50 % of initial value glucose levels rise above 7.8 glucose levels drop below 3.9 glucose levels fail to increase more than 20 % symptoms are present

The following criteria are also used to diagnose glucose intolerance:

	Normal	Abnormal	Pathological
2 h Value	6.7	6.8-7.8	7.8
Maximal Value	8.9	9.0-10.0	10.0

Various authors have reported a significantly increased incidence of glucose intolerance and diabetes in cancer patients.

From all the studies reported in this regard, it is clear that the driving force behind this is insulin.

One reason for the high cancer incidence in the West is the sugar content of the diet and specifically also of commercial food products. Manufacturers are aware of the fact that the word "sugar" on their labels is a non-seller. They therefore often use other sources of sugar or include what amounts to sugar under different names such as: cane sugar, dextrose, barley malt, fruit juice, glucose, honey, fructose, maltose, molasses, sucrose, rice syrup, corn syrup, high fructose corn syrup, lactose, milk sugar, and naturally sweetened. All of these are suspect and you should avoid them.

The stages of cancer

Depending on the severity, type and distribution of the disease, cancer has been classified differently by different authors into various stages (Stage I, II, III and IV). According to one widely used alternative classification, the various stages of cancer are defined as follows:

Stage IV: Advanced cancer patients, eg those whose cancer has spread throughout the body (bones, lungs, liver, pancreas, brain). These include:

- Patients with fast growing cancers (eg pancreas cancer)
- Patients with high fatality cancers (eg pancreas, lung, multiple myeloma, squamous cell carcinoma, melanoma)
- Any type of bone cancer including estrogenic sarcoma
- Patients with a history of extensive conventional chemotherapy and/or radiotherapy
- Any swelling or inflammation of a solid tumor that could cause blockage of the circulation at critical sites (eg in the brain)
- Patients with an estimated one year or less to live
- Any other situation where orthodox medicine rates it as Stage IV

The Stage IV patient generally has less than a year to live and should therefore be treated with the strongest possible Stage IV treatments (discussed later). In general such treatment should not rely on restoration of the immune system only, because of the limited time available. This provision illustrates an important difference between alternative cancer treatments and conventional cancer treatments: orthodox treatments must be carefully controlled because of the significant number of *normal* cells killed by the treatment (eg chemotherapy). This means that even though the patient is in a very critical condition, the dose of the drug (eg chemo) cannot be increased according to the condition of the patient. On the other hand, alternative

Stage IV treatments, because they target cancer cells (eg the CsCl/DMSO treatment) and do no harm to normal cells, *can be used in much higher doses if required*. The only reason why the level of such treatments has to be limited in some cases is because of the debris caused by the mass of dead cancer cells that the body has to eliminate.

It is important to appreciate the difference between a Stage III and Stage IV treatment. The Stage IV cancer patient has a short time to live and therefore any treatment that relies *inter alia* on restoration of the immune system (which is of necessity a time-consuming process) is of little use to the Stage IV patient. The focus of treatment in Stage IV patients must therefore be first and foremost to kill the cancer cells and therefore to save the patient's life and buy time necessary to restore all the other distorted systems in the patient, including a severely damaged immune system, which in many cases is the result of prior chemotherapy treatment.

The Stage III patient, on the other hand, is still in reasonably good health and has a year or more to live. The focus of treatment in these patients must therefore be (in addition to killing the cancer cells) to restore the immune system, repair organ damage (liver, kidneys), kill the fungi associated with cancer and especially to restore the inner terrain to a more healthy state, including a proper balance of w-3 and w-6 fatty acids as discussed elsewhere in this book. All of these will buy time for the patient. It is therefore wrong to think of a Stage III treatment as "weaker" in the sense that it might just as well have been replaced by the "stronger" Stage IV treatment. These two treatments simply serve different purposes in different situations. In many cases, after the cancer cells have been controlled by a Stage IV protocol (eg IPT and/or CsCl/DMSO), the follow-up treatment during remission should be one of the Stage III protocols (laetrile therapy and/or the Budwig protocol). From the discussion above, it is clear that it is futile to use more than one Stage III treatment or to use excessive quantities of a particular Stage III protocol when a powerful Stage IV is indicated.

There are a few Type III and Type IV treatments that have been found to yield best results. The following is a list of the most widely used Stage IV treatments:

- Insulin (DMSO) Potentiation Therapy (+)
- The CsCl/DMSO protocol (*)
- Supplementation with unadulterated w-6 fatty acids
- Hydrazine sulphate for cachectic patients (*)
- High dose and/or intravenous Vitamin C therapy (+)

- Ozone therapy (+)
- The Bill Henderson-Budwig Protocol (*)
- The Bob Beck (BB) protocol (electro medicine) (*, +)
- The Robert Barefoot Calcium Protocol (*)
- The Cancer Diet (*).

Code: * = active telephone support from an expert must be available
       + = preferably done at a clinic.

Some of the effects of these treatments

Depending on the severity of the disease, treatments selected will generally include killing of cancer cells, building the immune system and alkalinizing the cancer cells of the body as a whole, which amounts to altering the inner environment to be less favorable for cancer cells.

The key part of any initial protocol is to kill cancer cells, but the other effects may also be included in the treatment. For example, the CsCl/DMSO protocol (used in critically ill preterminal cancer patients) is a superb cancer killer, but it does not stimulate the immune system. In these patients, there is no time to attend to the immune system in the first place. Afterwards, when most of the cancer cells have been killed, provision should be made to build the immune system. In general and where possible, patients should be treated under medical supervision (eg at a clinic), but where this is not possible, patients can follow some of the protocols at home, but active telephone support should be available at all times. For example, the CsCl/DMSO protocol illustrated in this book is one of the most powerful cancer treatments available and can be administered at home by the patient and/or family with the aid of active telephone support by a professional.

The powerful Stage IV treatments vreferred to above should never be combined, because the mass of dead cancer cells created in this manner may exceed the body's ability to dispose of them safely, creating an overload of toxic material that may harm the kidneys and liver. Generally, the various Stage IV protocols as such have been worked out with this danger in mind, with the dosage levels of the active ingredients (eg cesium in CsCl/DMSO protocol) gradually increasing with time. This delicate balance must not be tampered with.

However, some other non-Stage IV treatments can be added to the basic protocol chosen for specific additional effects (eg to improve immunity in the case of patients previously treated by means of chemotherapy).

Such combinations should, however, be judiciously done and only under professional guidance.

Those treatments that can be safely carried out at home with active telephone support (eg CsCl/DMSO) should preferably be used in this manner, for obvious reasons including the assistance and comfort provided by family and friends. Other treatments (eg ozone therapy) must be undertaken in a clinic.

Examples of where a Stage IV treatment is necessary

- Cancer patients with fast growing tumors (eg pancreas cancer)
- Cancer patients with high-fatality tumors (eg lung cancer)
- Cancer patients with widely disseminated metastases where the cancer has spread throughout the body (lungs, liver, pancreas, brain, bones)
- Any type of bone cancer
- Patients who have previously had extensive radiation and/or chemotherapy
- Where swelling or inflammation of a tumor could cause blockages of key fluids (eg brain cancer, colon cancer).
- Patients who have less than one year to live
- Any patient rated as Stage IV by orthodox medicine

It is important to note that conventional treatments may sometimes cause such heavy damage to the immune system and other vital organs that these patients will die regardless of whether all cancer cells are killed using alternative methods. In such patients, the survival rate is obviously 0 %. In others, where less damage has been caused, a survival rate of up to 50 % may be possible if appropriate alternative methods are used (24).

Stage III: Typical treatments

Kelley Metabolic Diet, Essiac tea, Gerson protocol, etc. More than one such treatment may be combined.

The patient may well wonder why we sometimes use the "weaker" Stage III treatments; why not go directly to the strongest Stage IV treatments such as IPT or CsCl. One reason is that with the stronger treatment, too many dead cells accumulate which may cause pressure increases (eg in brain cancer patients). It is also important to realize that while Stage III treatments are sometimes necessary, several of them combined will not be sufficient for a terminal Stage IV patient.

Suggested treatments for the various other stages

Before embarking on any cancer treatment programme, it is necessary to consider if your programme includes the following:

- A colon cleanse (for details see the book by Jon Barron ([25](#)))
- A liver cleanse ([26](#)). Regardless of which liver flush you choose, it is always good policy to include lemon juice in pure water. This at the same time allows you to drink the necessary amount of water.
- Have you made provision to restore the immune system at the appropriate stage? This is discussed elsewhere in this book.
- Coffee enemas
- Restoration of the proper mix of w-3 and w-6 polyunsaturated fatty acids in the diet (see above for details).

Some of the Stage III treatments are either not "strong" enough (do not kill cancer cells fast enough, or they are based on immune restoration which takes a long time and may therefore not be suitable for the seriously ill patient). They have the advantage that they do not kill the cancer cells fast enough to create inflammation and tissue swelling, which may be a problem in some cancers (eg brain cancer). Here are some examples of Stage III cancer treatment methods. Choose only *one* of the following treatments (these are the stronger Stage III treatments discussed later in this book):

- *Budwig flaxseed and cottage cheese protocol.* Depends on a combination of polyunsaturated fatty acids (w-3, w-6) and sulphur-containing proteins (cottage cheese).
- *Brandt Grape Cure protocol* using high doses of carrot juice/ beet juice. This is one of the well-proven alternative treatments. It has been used since 1920. You should include the fiber in the vegetables, Choose a juicer or food processor that retains the fiber. Do not use both grapes and vegetables. Be very careful not to add any other items to this proto-col. The Brandt Cure is discussed in more detail elsewhere in this book.

- *The Gerson diet* using high doses of carrot juice combined with certain supplements (eg iodides, niacin, etc.) and liver cleansing by means of coffee enemas.

The following are two of the "weaker" Stage III treatments

- *Robert Barefoot Calcium protocol.* Depends on the use of high doses of coral calcium to alkalinize the body.
- *Robert Barefoot CsCl protocol.* Depends on the combined use of CsCl and coral calcium. Entirely different from the powerful CsCl/DMSO protocol listed above as a Stage IV cancer treatment.

Do not use these protocols at the same time, but note that if you choose the Barefoot CsCl protocol, it can only be used for 30 days. Thereafter you may continue with the Barefoot Calcium protocol.

Some of the abovementioned protocols may be judiciously combined since they do not generally create massive amounts of dead cancer cells.

It should be noted that the laetrile protocol and the Kelley Metabolic treatment, which are two excellent treatments, have been omitted from the list above. The reason is that both these methods rely heavily on building the immune system, which is a slow process and therefore perhaps not suitable for the Stage III cancer patient. If this is not a consideration, then these treatments should be seriously considered in all patients in whom overload with dead cancer cells is not a problem. In practice, however, very few such patients are seen, because the vast majority of cancer patients seen by alternative practitioners have been pre-treated unsuccessfully by means of conventional methods. These patients generally do not have much time to live. Therefore, cancer patients who have not had a significant number of orthodox treatments and who do not have a particularly dangerous type of cancer can usually have either or both the Kelley and laetrile treatments. Also, such patients can have any one or more of the other Stage III treatments listed above.

Unlike Stage IV treatments, the Stage III treatments listed above can be combined, and in fact should be combined.

Curing Stages I, II and III cancer is generally easy if the patient stays on the cancer diet (see later) and uses one or more of the Stage III protocols listed above. No cancer can ever be cured unless the body is alkalinized. It is for this reason that the diet is so important and why orthodox treatments so often fail.

The treatments for Stage 1 are generally based on various fruit and plant juices and need not be discussed here since they are available elsewhere (24).

Understanding the four phases of treating cancer

Before discussing this topic, it is necessary for us to briefly review the pharmacokinetics of cancer. The science of pharmacokinetics (a word with Greek origins) describes the changes in time of drug concentrations or, in this case, the mass of cancer cells. It is vital in understanding how a cancer grows and allows us insight into what might be the best therapeutic approach. The reader should also recall what was previously said about cancer pharmacokinetics.

Phase 1—Buying time

In the case of many cancers and especially in the case of fast growing cancers, the patient usually has limited time available to institute whatever treatment programme has been decided on. Conventional treatments may have put the patient into temporary "remission" (meaning that the symptoms are reduced). This does not mean that the patient has been permanently cured, because even if the treatment has killed every cancer cell in the body (which none of the conventional treatments can do), the original cause of the disease has not been removed and therefore the cancer may return. Such remission treatments must at least involve the following steps:

- Restoring the proper w-3:w-6 fatty acid balance as previously discussed in all patients and regardless of whatever other treatment methods are selected
- Killing of all the remaining cancer cells
- Rebuilding the immune system
- Provision of critical nutrients to assist in the healing process

- Repairing the electrical balance in the cells (eg by means of the Budwig diet).

In order to do all these things, the patient needs time, which may be a critical factor since many patients who come for alternative treatment have been unsuccessfully treated with conventional methods (especially chemotherapy) and they often have only weeks or months to live. There are fortunately methods available to "buy time". For this purpose, high-dose Vitamin C therapy including intravenous Vitamin C therapy is the best (see "Vitamin C Therapy").

Phase 2—Killing the remaining cancer cells

Every cancer patient in remission should at least have one course of a strong Stage IV treatment (eg IPT) even if the main treatment (which put the patient into remission) was based on one of these protocols. It is preferred to use a protocol for remission treatment that differs from the one used in the main treatment. In most cases, however, the main treatment was one of the conventional methods and in such a case the IPT or CsCl/DMSO protocol is suggested for remission treatment (see later).

Phase 3—Stopping the spread

There are two main treatments (in addition to the main treatment protocol) that will stop the spread of the cancer. These are:

- Increasing the alkalinity inside the cancer cells systemically. This is a very important problem which is discussed in greater detail elsewhere in this book (see the CsCl/DMSO protocol and the Cancer Diet). The growth of cancer cells and pathogenic micro-organisms is suppressed by an alkaline environment (pH above 7.6)
- Increasing the oxygen content of the tissues. Cancer cells—as Warburg has shown—are anaerobic, meaning that they grow best in an oxygen poor environment, while normal cells grow best in an oxygen rich environment. Oxygen levels in the body can be raised by means of taking food grade hydrogen peroxide (12 drops of 35 % food grade hydrogen peroxide in half a glass of water daily) or by means of the deuterium based Cell Food. Ozonated water can also be used for this purpose. These methods will not necessarily restore

normal oxygen levels inside cells. This is best achieved by means of oral supplementation with the correct w-6:w-3 mix of essential fatty acids.

Phase 4—Making sure

The first three phases will suppress all symptoms of cancer, but it cannot be assumed that the danger is now over. There may be various reasons for this. The original problem which caused the cancer in the first place may still be there (low oxygen levels inside cells), or the cancer has returned because the patient returned to his/her old lifestyle. There may also be other reasons such as distorted hormonal balances and mercury-laden root canals in the case of breast cancer patients. The treatment that the patient had been receiving might have been terminated too soon. For example, in the case of the CsCl/DMSO protocol, the patient may have reached his/her "cesium limit" before the cancer was totally gone. In such cases treatment must continue for at least another year, preferably using a different treatment from the one used initially.

Remission

The crucial point to understand is that cancer treatment does not stop once the outward signs of cancer have disappeared. The disappearance of detectable signs of cancer does not mean that the patient is permanently healed. It only means that you have won the first round! Treatment must therefore continue for at least one year. There are two rules that apply in this situation.

- First, no sequence of alternative cancer treatments (including the ones while you are in remission) should last for less than 12 months, excluding cesium based protocols with due regard to the associated limitations.
- Secondly, many Stage IV cancer protocols, although they are powerful cancer killers, are not necessarily designed to build the immune system. This is what remission treatment is all about: it should concentrate on restoring your immune system to prevent any further cancerous growths. This is of particular importance if the patient had been previously treated by means of conventional methods (especially chemotherapy). Remember, the main reason why you developed cancer in the first place was a weak immune system and low oxygen levels inside cells. If these are not corrected, the cancer may return at any time.

The Bill Henderson Protocol (based on the Budwig diet) is the treatment of choice for use during the remission period (unless it was used as the main primary treatment). The Budwig diet during the remission period generally uses 4-6 tablespoons of liquid refrigerated flaxseed oil combined with cottage cheese (8 tablespoons as explained in the section on the Budwig Diet). This is used for two periods of 6 months each.

Thereafter the dose of flaxseed oil can be reduced to 2 tablespoonfuls daily for another 2 years.

Do not mix the components of the Budwig protocol and then leave it standing in the refrigerator. The mixture has to be consumed immediately after mixing.

Laetrile therapy is also a key treatment for use during remission and to kill lingering remains of cancer cells. It is very suitable for this purpose because it acts slowly (suitable for prolonged use) and it kills cancer cells safely and effectively. It does not work fast enough for the initial treatment. It is also ideal as a remission treatment because it is able to reach cancer cells that are inaccessible to other treatments.

It is generally inadvisable to combine laetrile and cottage cheese because of possible absorption problems. *They should therefore not be taken within 90 minutes of each other.*

The diet, supplements and proteolytic enzymes (Kelley protocol) during remission should be given as part of the laetrile diet (see later).

The suggested treatments during remission are therefore as follows:

- Make sure that the proper mix of w-3 and w-6 fatty acids is provided in the diet
- Remove toxic heavy metals (mercury amalgams from root canals, do chelation therapy). Note that root canals are safe havens for many types of microbes. Cleaning out these root canals is, however, a tricky business: it has to be carefully done by an experienced dentist to prevent further systemic pollution by the heavy metals and micro-organisms being removed. There are claims that the Bob Beck protocol and soaking the affected teeth in your mouth with a 3 % medical grade hydrogen peroxide solution are also effective (39). Since the cancer-causing microbes can also hide in the stomach lining and the lymph system, the safest way of removing all the hidden microbes is by way of the Bob Beck protocol
- Bill Henderson (Budwig) protocol plus laetrile for 6 months
- Repeat the Bill Henderson (Budwig) protocol for a second 6 month period.

These precautions are especially necessary if the patient had previously been on chemotherapy.

The Bob Beck protocol should be considered to kill cancer-causing micro-organisms (see later). It is the only proven method to completely rid the body of cancer-causing microbes, but finding the right equipment may be a problem.

- Determine how much cancer is left in your body using *inter alia* the Navarro or AMAS techniques discussed elsewhere in this book.
- Supercharge your immune system as indicated above. The objective of this is to kill any remaining cancer cells that may be hiding in places difficult to access.
- Follow a diet and lifestyle that will not once again put you at risk of the cancer returning.
- For a year or more after the remission treatment programme has been concluded, the patient should continue with an easy to follow Stage III protocol such as the Budwig diet or laetrile therapy. Up to 50% less of the ingredients in each protocol may be used.

Laetrile therapy is the treatment of choice to kill lingering cancer cells safely and effectively, but it is not a fast acting therapy. It is the perfect therapy for remission treatment. However, do not combine laetrile with cottage cheese, at least not within 90 minutes of each other. Also make sure to supplement with proteolytic enzymes (Kelley protocol). For the diet while on remission, see Laetrile Protocol.

Additional supplements which may be considered:

- Inositol hexaphosphate (IP6)
- Glyconutrients (Aloe Immune with advanced Ambrotose)
- Moducare (a sterol and sterolin supplement)
- A good multinutrient supplement that *inter alia* supplies all the vital minerals (Fortifood).

Methylating supplements are very important at this stage. They supply vital I-carbon fragments (methyl groups) that are necessary intermediates in the process of rebuilding your body, including much needed DNA molecules required to build new tissues. Betaine (trimethyl glycine) (Fortifood) and MSM/DMSO are vitally important. Note that some of the best and most powerful cancer treatments (eg the CsCl/DMSO protocol) are very effective cancer killers but they do very little to rebuild the immune system and other damaged tissues. This aspect is therefore something you should pay special attention to during your remission treatment (see later).

Building the immune system: Preventing the return of the cancer

The immune system is a collection of cells (immune cells), chemical messengers and other proteins that are interrelated and work together to protect the body against foreign invaders (potentially harmful microbes, bacteria, viruses, fungi). The leucocytes (white blood cells) are the most important immune cells. These consist of two main groups of immune cells: the polymorphonuclear leukocytes (also called granulocytes because they appear to contain granules) which are able to digest microbes by phagocytosis, by "eating" or swallowing them. The granulocytes are further subdivided into neutrophils, eosinophils and basophils, each with different properties and functions.

The second group of leukocytes is the mononuclear leukocytes which include the monocytes and lymphocytes. Monocytes ingest dead or damaged cells, also through the process of phagocytosis, and in so doing provide immunological defense against many infectious organisms. Monocytes migrate into tissues and then become macrophages, which also ingest and destroy foreign invaders.

Lymphocytes are mononuclear leukocytes which *inter alia* produce antibodies against viruses and bacteria. The lymphocytes in turn are subdivided into B-cells (mainly responsible for antibody production), T-cells which are of special importance in fighting viruses, and Natural Killer Cells (NKC)

Note that building the immune system only becomes part of an overall cancer treatment programme at a certain stage. Patients who have only a few months to live, should concentrate on killing the cancer cells first. They can take immunity building products concurrently in so far as these do not interfere with the main treatment, which should be aimed at killing cancer cells. Also note that although there are many different immune system cells, only a few are of direct importance to the cancer patient. The main type of cancer killing white blood cell is the natural killer cells. Other cells that play a role are the macro-phages (that "eat" cancer cells). These are all T-cells. The B-cells also play a role though they work more indirectly.

Note that stimulating the immune system will almost ensure that your cancer will not recur after initial successful treatment. If you do not attend to your immune system, there is a significant chance that your cancer may recur months or years afterwards. Remember that one of the most important effects of conventional chemotherapy is that it destroys the immune system. Therefore, if you are unfortunate enough to have had one or more courses of chemo, you should pay special attention to your immune system.

The full treatment of the cancer patient is not limited to killing the cancer cells. That is only part of the full protocol, which should also provide for the following:

- Stimulation of the immune system with specific vitamins and minerals. Nutrients for the immune system include trace minerals (eg those present in Cell Food and in a good multinutrient supplement (Fortifood).
- Glyconutrients
- Treatment of systemic acidity (eg with coral calcium supplements)
- Remove all invading micro-organisms (fungi, viruses, pleomorphic organisms) these interfere with the immune system. There are drugs and natural products available for this.
- Heavy metals such as mercury, lead, aluminum, etc. in the body are another major source of compounds that suppress the immune system and should be removed as soon as possible. Chelating agents are used for this purpose, such as intravenous administration of drugs (EDTA), parenteral treatment (DMSA) and others. Every cancer patient should go on a course of chelation therapy at a clinic. Typically such a course runs over a period of 10 weeks and includes EDTA as and DMSA. Different drugs are used to remove different toxic metals. One great advantage of such a course is that at the end of the course the patient will know exactly how much of the heavy metals are still left in his/her body and whether further treatment is required.
- The treatment should include removal of dental amalgams from root canals. This operation must be carried out by a dentist experienced in the removal of dental amalgams to prevent flooding the circulation with mercury and micro-organisms liberated from the root canal. It is also a good idea to take high levels of chelating agents before

the operation. There are cases on record where cancer patients have improved by simply having the root canals cleared. The root canals are a safe haven for various micro-organisms which not only may play a role in cancer development, but which suppress immune function. By removing them, the immune system is "freed up", so to speak.
- Washing your mouth with 3 % food grade hydrogen peroxide may also help.
- Methylating agents are key supplements for the immune system. They are required for the synthesis of nucleic acids and also for key neuro-transmitters and numerous other molecules.
- Betaine and MSM (methylsulfonylmethane) are examples of methylating agents.
- When you reach this stage in your treatment programme, the problem is no longer to kill massive numbers of cancer cells but rather to concentrate on removing the lingering number of cancer cells that may still be hiding somewhere, and to make sure that the cancer never returns. For this purpose it is necessary to determine how much cancer your have left (discussed elsewhere) and to ensure that the immune system is restored.
- It is also necessary to attend to any leftover cancer cells which are still likely to be in the body. The restoration of the immune system should take care of that but just to make sure, a cancer protocol different from the one used in the initial treatment should be used.
- Rebuild your normal cells to improve general health and to ensure that the body develops resistance to possible future cancerous growths.
- Permanently follow a diet that will alter your inner milieu in such a manner that the cancer cannot return. This must include the proper mix of w-3 and w-6 fatty acids in the diet.

In addition to what has been said above, attention should also be devoted to what is particularly bad and particularly good for the immune system.

What is bad for the immune system?

- Obesity depresses immune response (T-cell production and mobility of macrophages).
- Cadmium (a toxic metal that occurs in tobacco smoke) suppresses anti-body production by the B-cells.

- Lead, also a heavy metal, suppresses T—and B-cell responses. It is produced in internal combustion engines.
- Mercury (*inter alia* from dental amalgams) reduces the number and response of T-cells.
- Industrial pesticides suppress immune function.

What is good for the immune system?

- The pancreatic enzymes trypsin, bromelain and chymotrypsin are amongst the foremost immunity building molecules. They do not directly stimulate immune cells but enhance their effectiveness by removing debris and the protein layers covering the cancer cells, thus permitting these enzymes to fulfill their proteolytic proclivities and opening the way for the immune cells to do the killing. Other pancreatic enzymes (lipases, amylases) also improve immune function by assisting in the process of digestion.
- Supplements: many nutrients are known to stimulate immune function. Amongst these zinc, Vitamin C, manganese, magnesium, selenium, Vitamin A and many of the B vitamins are prominent. There are many other natural products that have a stimulatory effect on the immune system, such as quercetin, selenium, turmeric, Echinacea, garlic, golden seal, etc.
- A raw food cancer diet, as discussed in this book, is a great stimulator of the immune system.
- Bromelain (a proteolytic enzyme that occurs in pineapples), has yielded outstanding results in the treatment of cancer patients (presumably because of its proteolytic action). Papain is a similar enzyme that occurs in paw-paws. All of the abovementioned enzymes should be taken in fairly high doses (500-1000mg) and with food, if it is the intention of improving digestion and promoting absorption, but on an empty stomach in cancer treatment
- Aloe Vera promotes the immune response to antigens (including cancer cells) in the body. Although not a specific stand-alone for the treatment of cancer, it is a valuable supporting treatment of cancer. Certain fractions in the plant have impressive anticancer properties. It promotes the growth of new, healthy cells and reduces the overall viral load in cancer patients, thereby supporting the body in its fight against cancer.

- Aloe Vera improves intracellular communication amongst cells of the immune system, which is a prerequisite for a vigorous immune response. This communication is achieved by means of simple sugars on the cell surfaces which, by forming access keys on the cell surfaces, either lock or unlock the required functions on the adjoining cell surfaces. There are eight simple sugars that make up this communication network.
- Some researchers (eg in Uganda) have obtained remarkable results in the treatment of AIDS and cancer with Aloe Vera.
- Properly prepared Aloe Vera extracts are the best source of these sugars (Fortifood). Further information is available on the Internet.
- Beta-1.3DGlucan. This is probably the best single immune booster available (22). It is marketed by the company Transfer Point in South Carolina, USA and for this reason will probably be pricy for the South African consumer. The product has been tested at various universities and has been found superior to all similar products tested. Its out-standing features include:

  > It doubles the effectiveness of the immune system, mainly by increasing the effectiveness of the neutrophils immune cells;
  > The product attaches a receptor to these cells, enabling them to recognize cancer cells and kill them. In this manner anti-cancer cells are added to the other cancer-killing cells of the immune system such as natural killer cells, macrophages and lymphocytes.

Many research papers on Beta-1.3DGlucan have appeared (27). Details are also available on Internet.

Different types of cancer

Cancers are classified on the basis of the primary cell types from which they evolved and their subsequent behavior patterns. On the basis of such a classification, more than 200 different kinds of cancer have been described. They all have the general properties of cancers described above, although some may retain some of the properties of the normal cells from which they developed. The term "benign tumor" is used to describe a steadily expanding mass of cells that does not infiltrate the surrounding tissues and also never metastasized to different other locations. They are generally relatively harmless, but may exert local pressure effects in susceptible organs such as the brain. Their surgical removal is generally advisable.

- A malignant tumor is the opposite of a benign tumor and is generally known as a "cancer".
- Malignant tumors are usually classified into 3 main categories: carcinomas, sarcomas and miscellaneous others. The suffix "-oma" literally means "tumor of" and usually indicates a benign tumor. Likewise a fibroma is a benign tumor of fibrous connective tissue. Lipomas, neuromas and chondromas are benign tumors of fat, neural tissue and cartilage respectively. An adenoma is a benign tumor of a gland. Benign tumors, as the name signifies, are generally slow growing tumors which do not have the potential of spreading (metastasis) that malignant tumors have.
- The suffixes—carcinoma,—sarcoma and—blastoma signify malignant tumors, eg lung carcinoma signifies a tumor of lung epithelial origin. Adenocarcinoma of the breast signifies a malignant glandular epithelial tumor of the breast.
- *Carcinomas*: these arise from cells of any covering membrane which may be external, as in the skin, or internal such as the epithelial

linings of the gastro-intestinal system, the breast, the lungs and other structures with membranes. Carcinomas represent a common type of cancer because the covering epithelial layers in many organs are the first to be exposed to environmental carcinogens. More than 90 % of all cancers are carcinomas. Adenocarcinoma are tumors that have arisen from some glandular structure and they may have retained some of the features of the original glandular structures from which they evolved, while anaplastic carcinomas are so primitive that they have not retained such glandular resemblances. A squamous cell epithelioma has retained the microscopic features of the squamous cells of the membranes from which they evolved.
- Sarcomas (which represent less than 5 % of all cancers) are tumors that evolved from supporting tissues such as the skeleton (estrogenic sarcoma), or the cartilage (chondrosarcoma). Such tumors may also evolve from the muscles (myosarcoma), fibrous tissues and other similar supporting tissues.
- The third group of cancers arises neither from covering epithelial structures nor from supporting tissues. They usually arise from highly specialized cells often associated with structures that have highly specific functions.
- Leukemias form in the blood and bone marrow and the abnormal white blood cells produced appear in the blood circulation, creating problems in the spleen and other tissues. Leukemias are therefore not solid tumors.
- Lymphomas are cancers of the lymph glands which act as filters in the lymph. The lymph glands are concentrated mostly in the neck, groin, armpits, and the centre of the chest and around the intestines. Lymphomas are usually made up of abnormal lymphocytes (white blood cells) that congregate in lymph glands to produce solid masses. Hodgkin's disease and non-Hodgkin's lymphomas are the most prevalent types in the Western World.
- Myelomas are rare tumors that arise in the antibody-producing plasma cells or haemopoietic (blood forming) cells in various tissues in the bone marrow.
- The majority of cancers have their origins in altered stem cells. Such altered stem cells will develop into malignant cells when given the appropriate environment (inner terrain). Thus giving the stem cells to an environment which encourages them to differentiate into normal cells would be one way of approaching the cancer problem.

Substrates such as DMSO, Vitamin D, quercetin, diadzein and butyrate are known to encourage this.
- Finally the concept of apoptosis (programmed cell death) is a natural, genetically-determined process by means of which "old" cells are killed and removed so that they can make way for young cells. A typical feature of cancer cells is that they have lost the capacity of apoptosis and therefore keep on growing. There are known natural substances like DMSO, genistein, quercetin, hydrogen peroxide, ozone and retinoic acid that induce apoptosis in human cancer cells in a dose-dependent manner.

The classification of the various types of cancer is available in medical textbooks and a short summary is also available (28).

From a practical point of view, it is important to know where the cancer is, how much of it there is and where it is spreading to. These are important considerations in determining a strategy to proceed in a particular case. When the cancer is in multiple locations, it is important to treat the cancer which holds the greatest danger first. Generally, lung cancer receives first priority due to the dangers of congestion. Pancreatic cancer is another type of fast-growing cancer which is almost always given top priority. Brain cancer is dangerous if there are signs of swelling and inflammation. This is something the attending oncologist and surgeon have to decide. In addition to its location, the type of cancer is another factor that determines its immediate priority.

Conventional medical treatment of cancer

The most important orthodox treatments of cancer are: surgery, radiotherapy, and chemotherapy and hormone treatment. Each one of these has been shown to have limited success in the case of specific cancers, but the overall combined effect on cancer mortality in the population is extremely disappointing; it has been claimed by various authors to be no better than 3 % overall survival.

> *The reason for this is the false perception that the cancer problem can be solved by killing the cancer cells.*

Thus we have witnessed the relentless hunt for the "magic bullet" that will kill cancer cells selectively. This idea also lies at the core of the thinking behind President Nixon's 1971 declaration of war on cancer. It was largely a failure, in the same way as the war on AIDS has been largely unsuccessful. In both cases the research was based on finding methods to kill the invading organism without addressing the question of why the disease developed in the first place and considering the fact that even if we kill all the cancer cells without killing the normal cells (which is very difficult), the original cause of the disease still remains in place. Therefore the cancer will surely return, no matter how effectively we kill the cancer cells, unless the patient's immune system is strong enough to take over control and the biochemical terrain is made unfriendly for the cancer cells to grow.

The statistics tell us that if a solid tumor is found early and removed, it will recur only in 50 % of cases. In other words, you have a 50 % chance that you will be back where you started before the operation. But in the meantime you have significantly increased the chances of spreading the tumor. (The 50 % chance of success in such cases relies on the lingering strength of the immune system still present. This is often not the case after the immune system has been severely damaged as a result of conventional treatment methods, especially conventional chemotherapy).

Finding the original cause and removing it is the only way forward which directs attention towards the patient's own defense mechanisms, which is very much in line with Pasteur's statement on his deathbed that:

> *"The patient is more important than the invader."*

In the light of this approach to the disease, the limited success that has been documented for each of these methods can only be ascribed to "spontaneous" recovery (see later) or to the fact that the particular treatment was instigated at a stage of the disease when the patient's reserve restorative capacity was adequate to enable the patient to overcome the disease after the burden of the cancerous cells had been reduced.

Overall, today's conventional methods will go down in history as crude and inhumane, much in the same way as we think today about medical treatments in the earlier centuries. Surgery is generally the smallest of the three evils, with less destruction of the immune system and other metabolic damage.

The treatment of cancer by means of surgery

The first reaction to the appearance of a cancerous growth is to remove it. If the tumor is still localized (Stages I, II and some Stage III cancers) such treatment is usually effective, at least on a temporary basis. The likelihood that the cancer has already spread to distant sites (metastases) by the time surgery is performed, is highly significant and also likely. The following example illustrates this fact in the case of breast cancer. The number of cancer cells in an average tumor detected by means of mammography is 600 million, and by the time the patient can feel the tumor, it has increased to 45 billion. The first line of treatment is usually surgery. Thereafter oncologists often recommend radiotherapy in an attempt to reduce the risk of recurrence of the tumor in the breast area. While this may be achieved to some extent, it does nothing to reduce the risk of spreading to more distant sites such as the bones, brain and lungs, which is usually what kills the breast cancer patient. Further follow-up treatment with combination chemotherapy may kill 98-99 % of the metastasized cells, but never 100 %. If only 1 % of the cancer cells remain, it still means that 450 million cancer cells are present and ready to multiply as soon as conditions permit. The growth of these cells is now greatly facilitated by the fact that the immune sys-tem has been weakened by chemotherapy and other treatments. This is serious, since the patient developed cancer in the first place as a result of a relatively weak immune system and the cancer-promoting biochemical milieu in the patient's body resulting from prevailing nutritional and lifestyle conditions and pre-treatment by immunity-destroying conventional treatments.

A vigorously active immune system is our only method of destroying every single cancer cell, since the cells and other molecules of the immune system pervade all organs and spaces meticulously.

This example illustrates why conventional methods may bring temporary relief—especially in the case of surgery—but the real long-term prognosis of patients treated with conventional methods is not good, and explains why the actual long-term survival rate of such patients may be as low as 5 % or less. The only hope for the cancer patient who has been treated by means of surgery is that the patient's immune system will be active enough to mop up remaining malignant cells, and also that the patient has altered his lifestyle and diet to such an extent that the biochemical milieu is now less favorable for cancer cells to grow. The chances of this happening are not good, because the very fact that the patient developed cancer in the first place, points to a weak immune system and faulty lifestyle.

Surgery does, however, have some advantages: it reduces the load of cancer cells in the body, increasing the chances that your immune system may be able to deal with the problem successfully.

Clearly then, boosting your immune system in every possible way must be a cornerstone in your cancer treatment and prevention programme.

The scenario above suggests that it is not a good policy to rely on the possibility of a reasonably active immune system remaining after conventional treatment, because all the conventional methods, including surgery but especially chemo, ultimately weaken the immune system significantly.

> *Clearly, steps should be taken to actively support the immune system and to restore tissue and metabolic damage that have resulted from conventional treatment methods. This is why it is so important to sensibly combine conventional treatment with suitable alternative methods, as discussed later in this book.*

In summary, surgery may be effective, at least during the early stages, in the case of a variety of solid cancers including breast, stomach, small and large intestines, muscle, bone, brain, ovary, testes, kidneys, uterus and bladder. In all these conditions, appropriate surgical procedures may bring relief, although such relief often does not mean permanent cure. It is indicated in cases where it may provide relief of particularly distressing symptoms. It is also of special value as an adjunct to alleviate pressure in certain anatomical regions (eg the brain) following treatment with alternative methods which may kill large numbers of cancer cells. Surgery should always be preceded by critical dietary and lifestyle adjustments, and other measures to improve immune function and biochemical terrain as discussed in this book.

Surgery removes cancerous tissue as well as normal tissue, lymphatic tissue and other systems vital to the patient's ability to fight cancer.

An article in the *New England Journal of Medicine* reported that women who had had their entire breast removed (radical mastectomy) did not live longer than those who opted for the less invasive lumpectomy (removal of cancerous lump) (see *http://www.alternativecancer.us*, p 11). Nonetheless, radical mastectomies are still performed.

This reminds one of the fact that there is now overwhelming evidence that conventional chemotherapy is not effective and very damaging to the patient, yet chemotherapy is still used daily by hundreds or maybe thousands of oncologists.

The treatment of cancer by radiotherapy

All forms of high energy rays used in medicine are dangerous in the sense that they may not only kill cancer cells but also normal cells, in addition to causing cancer in normal tissues.

The use of high energy radiation used in medicine depends on the fact that these rays damage dividing cells more than normal cells. They also damage the ground substance (intercellular cement) that surrounds all the cells in the whole field that is irradiated. In this manner scarred cells are left that form a much more resistant local environment for the tumor cells that have survived the treatment, thus suppressing infiltration of the surrounding normal tissues. As in the case of chemotherapy, it is the most malignant and fast growing cancers that respond best to radiation.

Radiation therapy has all the disadvantages of other conventional treatment methods, including an increased tendency for cancer cells to disseminate and especially also having harmful effects on the immune system. It is often used as an adjunct to surgery or chemo, but the overall effects as far as permanent cure rates are concerned are disappointing, as in the case of the other conventional methods, unless appropriate steps are taken to correct the patient's diet and to improve immune function. It may be of great value when used in conjunction with certain alternative methods (see later).

Like chemotherapy, radiotherapy increases the risk of secondary cancers, for example the risk of developing respiratory cancer is increased 2.7 times and the risk of female genital cancers of the uterus and ovaries increased 2.4 times after radiotherapy (29).

Radiotherapy (by means of implanting radiation seeds in the prostate gland) is routinely given for the treatment of the early stages of prostate cancer. This procedure hastens the development of advanced prostate cancer. The doubling time of prostate cancer cells is a reliable indicator of the status of the disease. Normally the doubling time of prostate cancer cells is up to 4 years, but after radiotherapy treatment the doubling time may decrease to 1-2 months, indicating a significantly increased growth rate. The five times doubling time for untreated prostate cancer cells may be as long as 20 years, but after radiotherapy this decreases to 6 months, indicating the greatly accelerated growth of the cancer cells. Despite these facts and perhaps because they are unaware of them, urologists send thousands of patients with suspected prostate cancer (mostly on the basis of prostate specific antigen determinations and physical examination) for radiotherapy. According to medical statistics about 30-40 % of men in their 50s have signs of prostate cancer, but of these only about 8 % will ever feel the effects of the disease in their lifetime and less than 3 % will die of it (30, 31).

The decrease in serum prostate specific antigen values seen after radiation therapy does not necessarily indicate permanent improvement of the patient. While 50 % of radiation patients may experience a decrease in prostate specific antigen values, only 20 % of these have sustained decrease, meaning that only 10 % of all radiation patients have a sustained decline in prostate specific antigen values. More significantly, it means that 90 % of radiation patients will have cancer cells that (as a result of radiation) now double 40 times faster than normal prostate cancer cells. It also means that a man who initially had a 92 % likelihood of having no ill-effects from latent cancer (revealed by prostate specific antigen measurements), now (as a result of surgery and/or radiation treatment) is likely to become incontinent and impotent, and also has to deal with a more rapidly growing cancer.

These studies should warn us to be very careful how we deal with suspected prostate cancer, and the patient should discuss this carefully with his physician.

The treatment of cancer by means of chemotherapy

It is crucial to note that when we refer to "chemotherapy" in the following pages, the reference is to conventional high-dose chemo in which relatively high doses of a chemo drug are given once every 3-4 weeks. It should be clearly distinguished from IPT in which relatively small doses of more than one chemo drug are given after co-administration of insulin to reduce blood sugar levels. IPT has many advantages over conventional chemotherapy, as will be discussed later in this book.

The theoretical basis of chemotherapy rests on the fact that cancer cells differ from normal cells metabolically in such a manner that these differences can be exploited to develop drugs that will, ideally, selectively kill the cancer cells in the presence of normal cells. That ideal is difficult to realize due to the fact that the differences that do exist between normal cells and cancer cells are not large enough to allow for the development of radical cancer-killing drugs that will not also kill normal cells. The situation is somewhat analogous to the antibiotics that have been designed to kill bacteria, although these have been much more successful in achieving their goal, due to larger metabolic differences between bacteria and human cells. Some of the poison gases (eg mustard gas) were used as starting points for the development of chemotherapeutic agents, with limited success. Many different chemotherapeutic agents (including derivatives of mustard gas, vincristine, procarbazine and other synthetic compounds) are now in common use, with a certain degree of synergism between different compounds.

In summary, cancers that have proved most responsive to chemotherapy are certain leukemias, testicular cancer in men, Hodgkin's disease, some rare cancers of the head and neck, and some other cancers that are rare in adults. In these cases, conventional chemotherapy may be a viable option. In general, fast growing cancers respond better to treatment with chemotherapy. It would be misleading to state that chemotherapy offers a chemical cure for these cancers. Results are highly unpredictable and the side-effects may be severe in some patients—outweighing the benefits. A great disadvantage of the chemotherapeutic agents is that they may seriously damage the patient's immune system which, especially in the case of cancer, is a very serious matter.

It should be mentioned, however, that when combined with insulin (IPT) many of the inherent disadvantages of chemotherapy can be circumvented, since in combination with insulin these agents can be used at much lower dosage levels (eg 10 % of normal dosage levels). This is discussed in greater detail later in this book.

There is a wide variety of natural substances that have been shown to enhance the success rate of chemotherapy, although these do not have such a strong potentiating effect as insulin. The following are some of these substances: Vitamins E, C, and A, Coenzyme Q10, beta-carotene, glutathione, N-acetylcysteine, glutamine, selenium, genistein, diadzein, quercetin, melatonin, green tea, milk thistle and others (30).

Nutritional support is also crucially important before and after chemotherapy.

The difference between the optimistic assessments by many medical doctors and oncologists of conventional treatment methods, and the actual results seen in practice by the patients themselves is due to the fact that the results of clinical studies on the efficacy of these conventional treatment methods are usually based on "five year survival" rates and not on the actual survival rates of patients. There are few of us who have not lost one or more family members after chemotherapy treatment even though we were assured by the physician responsible for the management, that the treatment (chemo) holds a reasonable chance of success.

In evaluating success of treatment, it is important to note the difference between "survival time" and "five year survival time"

- "Survival time" is the time interval between the time when the diagnosis of cancer was first made in a patient and when that patient dies from the cancer diagnosed.
- "Five year survival time" is a time interval of five years from the time when the diagnosis of cancer was first made. If the patient is then still alive, he is considered cured. If, however, the patient dies after five years and one day, he will still be counted as cured for purposes of statistical analysis.

Although these two concepts may sound similar, they are in fact vastly different. Much false information is published on the basis of the five year survival rates, which is the norm used in the evaluation of most of the conventional methods. Many cancers such as breast and prostate cancers are slow growing and may in fact be present for many years before the patient dies.

The drugs used in chemotherapy are very toxic—they have to be to have any chance of killing the cancer cells. The main problem remains selectivity. The only selectivity that these drugs have is that they target fast-growing cells such as the cancer cells. But there are also many other fast-growing normal cells, such as those in the hair follicles and gastrointestinal tract. For this reason chemotherapy drugs are toxic for many of the normal cells in the patient. They are carcinogenic, as illustrated previously, destroy redblood cells, devastate the immune system and damage vital organs. All of these severely compromise the patient's chances of recovery. Evidence of all this is clearly visible in the patient undergoing chemotherapy. The patients' hair falls out; they are constantly nauseated, feel sick, vomit, have severe headaches and are constantly dizzy. Diarrhea, anemia, mouth sores, infections, nervous system problems, skin rashes, and lung problems are common. In addition, secondary cancers may occur (often several years after the treatment). The secondary malignancies caused by chemotherapy include leukemia, lymphoma and sarcoma (30).

Patients treated with chemotherapy for Hodgkin's disease are 14 times more likely to develop leukemia, according to cancer experts from 14 different centers involving 10,000 patients. (*J Natl Cancer Inst* 1995).

All of these are the reason why most patients die of the chemotherapy treatment before they die of the cancer.

One well known oncologist minimizes these chemotherapy side-effects by immediately following the chemotherapy up with high doses of nutrients including germanium sesquioxide, multinutrient supplement and other antioxidants, including high-dose Vitamin C given intravenously.

At the very best these treatments (chemo, radiotherapy and surgery) can buy a little time for the patient. In many cases these treatments shorten the patient's life. Autopsy studies have shown that cancer patients died as a result of conventional treatments before the cancer had a chance to kill them. One study showed that patients who underwent chemotherapy treatment were 14 times more likely to develop leukemia and 6 times more likely to develop cancers of the bones, joints and soft tissues than untreated patients. (*NCI Journal,* 1983, 87:10)

Recently, an important paper on the efficacy of chemotherapy in the treatment of various cancers has been published in a leading journal (Morgan, G. *et al., Clinical Oncology* (R Coll Radiol), 2004, 16:549). All the authors are leading oncologists at prestigious Australian cancer hospitals, while one of the authors is also a member of the official body that advises the Australian government on the efficacy and suitability of drugs to be listed on the National Benefits Schedule.

The carefully designed study was based on an analysis of the results of all the randomized, controlled clinical trials performed in Australia and the USA that reported a statistically significant increase in the 5-year survival due to the use of chemotherapy in adult malignancies. Survival data was drawn from the Australian cancer registries, the US National Cancer Institute's Surveillance and End Results (SEER) registry spanning the period January 1990 to January 2004.

Wherever data was uncertain, the authors deliberately erred on the side of overestimating the benefits of chemotherapy.

> *Even so, the study concluded that overall chemotherapy contributes just over 2 % to improved survival in cancer patients.*

Elsewhere in this book I present evidence gathered by other respectable authors and institutions that have conducted similar surveys in different parts of the world and which came up with very much the same result:

- A 3 % increased survival rate having been reported in one major European survey by Professor Abel in Germany (37).
- In the case of lung cancer, the Australian authors commented as follows:

"In lung cancer, the survival time has increased by only 2 months during the past 20 years and overall survival benefit of less than 5 % has been achieved in the adjuvant treatment of breast, colon and head and neck cancers."

Regarding newer and "improved" chemotherapy drugs, Morgan (1995) commented that despite the use of new and expensive single and combination drugs to improve response rates, there has been little impact from the use of newer regimens.

Yet despite the mounting evidence presented collectively by these studies, oncologists continue to present chemotherapy as a rational and promising approach to cancer treatment.

Two other things are remarkable about these studies. Firstly, apart from some attention attracted locally in Australia in connection with the Australian study, these studies attracted no or very little international attention. This demonstrates how tight the control is that the medical establishment and Big Pharma exerts on medical practice and also on the press, as discussed elsewhere in this book. Secondly, the true survival rate is actually much less than the 2 or 3 % mentioned above, since the cut-off point used in these studies was based on 5-year survival data. Elsewhere in this book I have shown how this practice leads to grossly exaggerated benefits for chemotherapy treatment, since 5-year survival rates are by no means the same as long-term survival rates, which after all is what interests the patient.

Moreover, the matter of relative risk as opposed to absolute risk is also relevant in this regard.

Yet if one disregards all the disadvantages associated with chemo, one can say that they are *in principle* the ideal drugs to kill cancer cells. Although it is by no means all that is required for the successful treatment of cancer, it is certainly a vital step in the process. IPT is a technique that helps to minimize many of the serious side effects of chemotherapy.

> *IPT helps to concentrate the drugs in the cancer cells (because of the increased number of insulin receptors in cancer cells) thus greatly increasing the efficacy of the treatment, which allows much lower doses to be used while at the same time reducing the toxicity to normal cells due to the lower doses of the drugs used.*

Another serious disadvantage is the fact that, as shown by Bjorksten, conventional high-dose chemotherapy destroys the immune system beyond the point of repair (Bjorksten, J. 1987. *Longevity*. Charleston, USA: JAB Publishing, p 22).

Due to the lower doses used, with IPT it is customary to use a combination of two or more drugs concurrently, which further increases the efficacy of the treatment, because the drugs are usually selected in such a manner that each drug kills cancer cells by a different mechanism. This also reduces the possibility of the cancer cells developing resistance to the drugs.

Although the cancers that respond to conventional chemotherapy have been listed in a well-known textbook of medicine (*Cecil's Textbook of Medicine*, 18th Ed), there are only about nine cancers listed amongst the hundreds of known cancers that kill mankind. The important epithelial cancers such as lung cancer, colon cancer, prostate cancer and many others are not amongst those listed. These are the cancers that kill 80-90 % of cancer patients. Amongst these cancers, 75-90 % show a partial response to treatment (remission), but in the case of most others, long term disease-free survival is either rare or minimal (eg 10 %, see ref 10).

There are many reasons why conventional chemotherapy has such a dismal record in the treatment of the vast majority of cancers. Here are some of them:

- Insufficient killing of cancer cells due to serious side-effects which limit amounts of drug that can be given
- Failure of sufficient quantities of the drug to reach the cancer site, including the brain
- Limitations due to drug toxicity
- Insufficient selectivity to kill cancer cells in the presence of normal cells
- Small fraction (S fraction) of cancer cells that is sensitive to the drugs.

There are many other reasons, some of which have been mentioned elsewhere in this book

IPT offers a solution to many of these problems. It is able to target the cancer cells in the presence of normal cells due to the preponderance of insulin receptors on cancer cells. Given in frequent low doses (1-2 times a week) as opposed to large doses given once a month in conventional chemotherapy, IPT is remarkably free of side effects and because of this, allows the simultaneous use of other natural anti-cancer treatments discussed in this book.

Damage done by conventional treatments

- *The immune system* is severely damaged. Unfortunately the immune system is the one deciding factor which determines whether the patient will ultimately be completely cured or not. The damage goes much beyond what may be seen by the superficial methods currently used by conventional medicine to monitor the immune function during treatment. For one thing, effective immunity depends not only on numbers of immune cells, but relies heavily on balance within the immune system, which is determined by the cytokine system. This is not measured in routine determinations used to monitor patient progress.
- *Invading organisms*: due to the weakened immune system and the prevailing acidic conditions, the body has been swamped by fungi, pleomorphic and other microbes. These further prevent recovery by weakening the immune system and robbing the body of vital nutrients.

- *The nature of the cancer cells* has been selectively altered as a result of conventional treatment (especially chemotherapy). This means that the cancer has been strengthened in its fight to survive and has become more difficult to eradicate.
- *Valuable time lost.* In the meantime, 2-5 years of valuable time has been lost during which time the patient's immune system might have been built up and the metabolic abnormalities induced by the cancer and the patient's wrong lifestyle might have been corrected, with more than 90 % certainty of recovery (32).
- Although the primary cancer may have been superficially "controlled" by conventional treatment, the *cancer has now spread to other vital organs* and sites, although this may not be visibly present. These are the cancers that will ultimately kill the patient.
- *The acidic conditions* and lack of oxygen in all the cells of the body and which represent one of the primary causes of the original cancer have been acerbated as a result of the treatment. No cancer can ever be cured unless the overwhelming acidity and oxygen deficiency in the cells have first been corrected. Sometimes the body will be able to make these corrections on its own, but mostly it must be corrected as part of the treatment.
- *Cachexia*: the non-cancerous cells have been starved of nutrients (especially glucose) due to the voracious appetite of the fast-growing cancer cells. These now rob the body further of essential nutrients, leading to widespread tissue and weight loss. This will only be manifested later.
- *The digestive tract* has been severely damaged; leading to poor absorption of vital nutrients, which further adds momentum to the process of cachexia. Chemotherapy is known to severely damage the gastrointestinal mucosae, to such an extent that absorption of vital nutrients is impaired.
- The patients have not been warned about *the vital role that diet plays* in connection with cancer. This further makes it virtually impossible for the patient to recover.
- No attention has been given to the crucial role of the w-3 and w-6 fatty acids and intracellular oxygen levels in the process of carcinogenesis.

Spontaneous regression of cancer

A closer look at this concept is necessary at this stage, since it may be related to the effectiveness of conventional treatment methods and much can be learned from this phenomenon. Sometimes a cancer patient may improve or even recover for no obvious reason. Such improvement may be temporary (remission) or it may be for longer periods (regression) or the patient may recover completely. It is certain that such fluctuations in the severity of the disease do occur, but the reasons for this have been uncertain in the past.

Available evidence suggests that there is nothing "spontaneous" about such unexplained fluctuations in disease severity. In all human beings, there is a delicate balance between developing cancer and not developing cancer, and in the cancer patient between progression and regression of the disease.

There can be little doubt that lifestyle factors and especially nutritional factors play a role in determining this balance at any moment in time, and that this balance is sensitively susceptible to changes in the patient's nutritional milieu and therefore his inner terrain where all diseases originate. This means that if we understand the precise nature of this relationship we may be able to sway the balance in any direction we desire. Even more importantly, we may devise new and more effective treatment methods on the basis of such information.

> *This is the core principle on which many of the alternative cancer treatments are based.*

Such "spontaneous" regressions have been described ranging from the unexplained reversal of early malignant changes to far advanced, near-terminal cancers. There is some evidence that such regressions and remissions are an ongoing process in all cancer patients and even in healthy individuals, or at least that they are more common than hitherto expected. Cameron and Pauling have presented some evidence that this may well be the case (28). For example, malignant changes in the cervix (revealed by means of the Pap test) occur in 15 % of women at some time during their lives, yet only 0.37 % ultimately die of cancer of the cervix. This means that cervical cancer is far more common than generally assumed, but that the disease develops to its final stages only in one out of 370 women.

It is known that women with deficient intakes of folic acid have a diminished resistance to the papilloma virus which is one of the secondary causes of cervical cancer. Folate deficiency has been shown to be a worse risk factor for cervical cancer than smoking. (*JAMA,* 1992, Jan 22) On the other hand, folic acid deficiency is widespread and probably one of the most common vitamin deficiencies and it is rapidly getting worse as our food supplies become progressively depleted due to the decreasing quality of our food (33). Moreover, the RDA value for folate has been reduced from 400mcg per day to a very low 200mcg in the USA in order to keep pace with the declining quality of the food. This has been shown to expose an increasing number of people to the risk of serious long-term deficiency (34). This step was taken under pressure from the food industry to make the low folate values in the food look better, and is a good example of how commercial interests take precedence over health matters. Folic acid stores in the body (in common with many other water soluble vitamins) are very low and we depend largely on our daily food supply for metabolic requirements.

Due to all the known factors that are responsible for the depleted level of nutrients in our food (34), there are large variations in the vitamin content of fruit and vegetables (35). Thus the folate levels in our daily food supply may be assumed to fluctuate widely around levels that are at best very low. In view of this, it seems likely that cancerous growths in the cervix come and go as nutritional levels of the critical nutrient (folate) rise and fall on a daily and, perhaps more importantly, on a seasonal basis. Only those cases with the more severe deficiencies may be assumed to persist for longer, of which some would eventually develop into the final stages of cervical cancer.

What other nutrients are involved in a similar manner in the replication of cancer viruses? Could the amino acid lysine be one? Lysine is known to inhibit the growth of the herpes virus. Could it not be that there exists a critical mix of nutrients (all present in less than optimal quantities, which is a typical feature of the modern diet) which at certain times promotes papilloma virus multiplication (and perhaps that of other cancer-causing viruses) while at others, nutritional circumstances change, inhibiting it?

Cameron and Pauling mention that in many European hospitals, autopsies (which are routinely done) reveal a remarkably high incidence of cancers that were never detected nor suspected in life (30). Invariably, therefore, the number of concealed cancers far exceeds the number of revealed cancers. For example, in the case of cancers of the thyroid, this ratio was as high as 30-40-fold.

Similarly, cancerous growths of the prostate seen at autopsies increase with age until at the age of 75, these are seen in every second male. Yet less than 5 % of male patients die of the disease.

Enquiries revealed that in South Africa surgeons have observed a similar trend, although the phenomenon seldomly enjoys attention in the medical press. Such cancers are usually small and do not appear to cause much harm. Do these cancers perhaps differ histological or otherwise from fully developed cancers? According to the abovementioned authors and my own enquiries, such differences do not appear to exist.

Do these dormant cancers remain static over long periods or do they come and go, and if so, why?

It seems reasonable to suggest that fluctuations in the immune system are responsible for periods of improved immunocompetence which coincide with periods of improved nutrition, these in turn coincide with periods of reduced and increased cancerous growths.

This view is strongly supported by the results of a study by Dr. Foster in Canada. He found that of 200 patients who had experienced "spontaneous" regression of their tumors, at least 87 % had made comprehensive dietary changes, mostly by switching to a diet less reliant on animal protein. In addition, 55 % had used a detoxification programme while 65 % had taken vitamin and mineral supplements (36). All these changes would have strengthened the immune system. Although Dr. Foster's work was done 17 years ago, and the substances and quantities used by the patients were not optimal for supporting the immune system (selenium, Vitamin E, and coenzyme Q10 were not supplemented), the results were nonetheless impressive. What is remarkable, though, is the fact that potassium, iodine and niacin were among the supplements used.

In view of the latest findings and evidence presented by Professor Peskin, it is now highly likely that the changing w-3:w-6 fatty acid ratios that accompany dietary fluctuations are also involved in the phenomenon of "spontaneous" regression of cancers. Unfortunately, no published experimental evidence in support of this is available at present.

These ideas require a rethink of the concept of "spontaneous regression" of cancer and even of the interpretation of some treatment results. Perhaps even some advanced cancers that have been "successfully" treated by means of surgery or other conventional methods disappeared, not primarily because of the treatment as such, but because of a major boost given by the treatment to the immune system. Of course, the surgical removal of a cancerous mass could have contributed to the result due to the removal of a large burden of cancer cells which may have been robbing healthy cells of vital nutrients. Cameron and Pauling point out that many surgeons can recall carrying out cancer operations that for technical reasons were less than satisfactory, only to find that such inadequately treated patients were still alive and well years later. Clearly, in addition to what the doctor does, the immune system and the other nutritional factors discussed above play a vital role. This indicates that preoperative fortification of the patient's immune system, which seldom receives attention from conventional doctors, may be an important factor which could determine the ultimate outcome of whatever treatment is chosen.

Alternative cancer treatments

I would like to make it clear that the various secondary cancer treatments that follow are not my inventions. In fact, some have been around for many years and numerous authors have included them in their books and publications, often in a somewhat modified form. In most cases, the methods have been named in honor of their original inventors. More and sometimes valuable additional information is available in the books that I have cited above (1), and also in the book by Peskin and Habib (*The Hidden Story of Cancer*, Houston: Pinnacle Press, 2008). As originally suggested by Warburg, the primary cause of all cancers is an intracellular deficiency of oxygen and all the other causes and treatments of cancer should therefore be classified as secondary.

Although there are many different secondary alternative treatment protocols, the basic philosophy which is shared by all may be summarized as follows:

- The patient is encouraged to accept at least part of the responsibility of dealing with the cancer. This includes the task of recovery and maintenance of health in future. It also encourages patients to study as much as possible on what cancer is and how it may be cured and prevented.
- It emphasizes the importance of diet as a causative and healing factor in cancer.
- It treats the patient in the first place rather than the cancer and recognizes that the patient can never be completely cured unless the causes of cancer are removed, which amounts to re-establishing a healthy inner terrain in the patient.
- It includes correction of various lifestyle factors that are usually not clearly linked to cancer (exercise, sleep, relaxation and emotional well-being) as contributory factors in cancer therapy.

- It seeks to repair the function of various organs and to restore abnormal metabolic patterns to normality, eg excessive acidity and oxygen levels in cells.
- It stresses the importance of removing metabolic and environmental poisons from the body as a prerequisite of a successful anticancer programme.

Alternative treatments depend largely on the use of natural compounds in the form of biological extracts and molecules which are known to affect metabolic pathways in cancer cells favorably. There is a strong difference of opinion on the treatment of cancer between the proponents of alternative cancer treatment (ACT) and conventional cancer treatment (CCT) as practiced by most members of the medical profession. These differences run so deep that compromise between the two sides sometimes seems impossible. The alternative cancer treatment side charges that orthodox medicine, perhaps for historical reasons, has been so infiltrated by commercial interests (Big Pharma) that they are no longer able to look objectively at alternative cancer treatment since this poses a serious threat to the interests of Big Pharma (3). This is undoubtedly the case to a certain extent, but does not mean that conventional methods are entirely without merit. On the other hand, the conventional cancer treatment side argues that the alternative side has very little solid published scientific evidence to support their claims, but fails to mention that this is partly due to the fact that health authorities, under pressure from Big Pharma, largely oppose such investigations by prohibiting trials with and even the use of alternative medicines, sometimes even with physical violence and confiscation of supplies of natural medicines. As with all major disputes, there is an element of truth on both sides. The extent to which health authorities suppress the investigation and even use of natural methods of cancer treatment is difficult to believe, yet much evidence in support of such claims has appeared in several books on the subject (see for example ref 1 and 3). There can be little doubt that health authorities such as the FDA, NCI, American Cancer Society and other similar organizations in the USA, as well as the Medicines Control Council (MCC) in South Africa, have been guilty of unfair prejudice against natural medicines in the past. Mainly as a result of this, there is a dearth of scientific publications to evaluate the merits of these compounds. On the other hand, there are thousands of personal reports on the Internet and elsewhere of cancer patients who had been successfully treated by alternative cancer treatment methods.

It has been claimed by the alternative cancer treatment side that:

"there are alternative cancer treatments that can provide a 97 % true cure rate on recently diagnosed cancer patients, and can even achieve a 50 % true cure rate on cancer patients given up on by orthodox medicine" (32).

This is a very strong statement for which, unfortunately, no or little direct published supporting scientific evidence is given—partly at least due to the reasons given above.

Since the 1990s there has been a steadily rising acceptance and use of alternative methods as a treatment option by the public and an increasing number of medical professionals. A study published as early as 1993 in the prestigious *New England Journal of Medicine* documented the extent of this shift in cancer medicine (*New Engl J Med* 1993, 328:246). The article reported that out of a total of 1539 Americans interviewed, 34 % had consulted at least one alternative practitioner, and that of these one third had consulted an alternative practitioner on average 19 times in that year. The study also reported that in the year 1990 Americans had made 425 million office visits to alternative practitioners, spending about $13.7 billion, of which $10.3 billion came out of their own pockets. The high level of spending out of their own pockets indicates dissatisfaction with official treatments (for which Medical Aids pay). According to another source (*Alt Med Dig* 1995, p 42), 41 % of people in the San Francisco area tried alternative medical treatment at least once in 1995, and 54 % said they were very satisfied with the results, while 80 % said they would do it again.

At least 10 % of all cancer patients in the USA (100,000 patients) were under alternative care in the 1990s and this figure is growing (Bulk, J., 1995. *Cancer and Natural Medicine*. Oregon: Medical Press). A similar trend exists in many other countries, including the UK, Germany, Holland, Poland and others.

These figures reflect the situation 17 years ago when the strong movement towards alternative treatments was gaining momentum. All indications are that at the present time the figures are very much higher.

In their book on alternative cancer treatment, Diamond, Cowden and Goldberg (69) list numerous patient success stories covering a wide range of different cancers. These include the most important types of cancer such as prostate, breast, bone, lung, pancreas and others. The interested reader with a particular problem might wish to read about the experience of other patients with problems similar to his/hers.

In selecting any treatment programme, it should be remembered that each patient and each cancer within that patient is unique and that treatment should always be individualized.

More detailed information on a large number of cancers with suggested treatments for each cancer is available in the Moss Reports (10). These sources are a gold mine of information on alternative treatments of cancer, which I would strongly recommend as essential reading for all cancer patients.

The following table lists the most important types of cancer with suggested alternative treatments to be included in the treatment programme based on cancer patient reports and other information.

Note: *In the treatment of all cancers, the patient should immediately be put on the cancer diet as discussed in this book. The patient should also immediately be given a supplement of w-3 and w-6 fatty acids regardless of any other treatment option that may be selected.*

Type of Cancer	Suggested treatment includes:
Bladder	Diet, CsCl/DMSO, Detox programme, Laetrile, Aloe Vera
Bone	Diet, CsCl/DMSO, germanium, DHEA, Barley green
Brain	Gerson, Budwig, pancreatic Enzymes
Breast	Surgery, IPT, CsCl/DMSO
Cervix	IPT
Colon	IPT Surgery
Hodgkins lymphoma	IPT
Kidney	IPT
Leukemia	IPT
Lung	IPT, CsCl/DMSO
Lymphocytic lymphoma	IPT
Lymphoma	IPT
Melanoma	Gerson
Non-Hodgkins lymphoma	IPT

Ovarian	IPT, CsCl/DMSO
Pancreas	Enzymes
Prostate	IPT
Testicular	IPT
Uterine	IPT
Skin cancers (various)	Gerson
Fast growing cancers (various)	IPT

You can obtain very good advice how best to manage your particular cancer by consulting the Moss Reports which present the best treatments for various cancers as listed by Dr. R. Moss (www.cancerdecisions). In this manner you may arrange to speak to Dr. Moss personally on your specific problem, which in my view you will find very rewarding.

Which way to go?

In deciding which strategy to choose, it is important to bear the principle of selectivity in mind. This is the all-important factor. Alternative treatments, by their very nature and design, target cancer cells but leave normal cells intact. Conventional anti-cancer drugs (eg chemotherapy drugs) kill all cells including the healthy cells, only they kill fast-growing normal cells as well as cancer cells faster than most other cells. Conventional cancer treatments can never really succeed, since they treat the cancer while ignoring the patient and in particular, the patient's diet and immune system. In this regard, alternative methods are clearly superior. However, conventional methods are useful in particular situations, eg where a large, well-defined tumor mass is life-threatening. In such a situation, removal of the tumor (eg by means of surgery) will relieve the patient of the mass of cancer cells, thus relieving the immune system of an unnecessary burden.

Clearly, in such cases, the initial treatment by means of surgery has to be followed up by alternative treatment aimed at strengthening the immune system to prevent the cancer from returning.

Many patients ask the critical question: should I go with orthodox treatment or alternative treatment? This is not a valid question. In the light of what was said before, it is clear that the answer to that question lies with the individual patient and the cancer. Whenever possible, we should make intelligent use of both disciplines as indicated by the condition of the patient.

In practice, by far the majority of patients seen by alternative practitioners are those that have been given up on by conventional medicine.

It is only after they have tried everything that conventional medicine has to offer (chemotherapy, surgery, radiotherapy, drugs, etc.) that they finally realize that they are not getting better. They then turn to alternative methods, often in desperation.

These patients then have no other option than to go with alternative medicine at this late stage, when curing the patient is very much more difficult than in the beginning when the patient was treated by conventional doctors.

Fortunately, we can now say that a growing number of progressive conventional doctors and alternative therapists are now learning to cooperate in a multidisciplinary context, much to the advantage of the patient who now gets the best of what each side has to offer. Already there are indications that patients who get the best of what everyone has to offer fare consistently better than those forced to choose one side or the other.

The information above summarizes in much abridged form the essential facts about the two treatment modalities that are available to the cancer patient. In many ways, the two systems hold directly opposite views, making it extremely difficult for the cancer patient to decide which system to follow. On the one hand the orthodox establishment has all the authority of government institutions like the ACA, many medical doctors and oncologists, and others to support it. This may include the patient's own medical doctor and oncologist. The patient has perhaps over the years built up a trust relationship with his doctor on the basis of previous health problems which were successfully treated by his doctor. This is the doctor who now advises his patient to follow his oncologist's advice to choose conventional high-dose chemotherapy as the first line of treatment. On the other hand, the patient has been hearing (perhaps from friends and relatives) very disturbing reports about the many people who have died after chemotherapy and/or orthodox treatment. What is most disturbing is that almost every cancer patient that the patient or his friends knew had died after unsuccessful medical treatment. The fact that anecdotal reports are seen in the popular press about miraculous cures of such patients after using natural (alternative) methods of treatment, further complicates matters. Of course, such anecdotal reports cannot be counted as scientific evidence of efficacy, but when exceedingly large numbers of such reports become available (eg on the Internet), the patient starts to doubt everything that he had previously heard of standard medical treatment of cancer.

It is against this awe-inspiring background that the patient must reach a decision which, to him or her, is a life and death decision.

Dr. Kehr, in the *Cancer Tutor* (32), suggests a logical approach to reaching a decision in this situation, which depends on the answers to some crucial questions:

> Will the treatment I have chosen be any better than a placebo, in other words will a person treated in this manner live longer, have a higher quality of life than someone treated with orthodox methods?
>
> **Answer:** There have been several major scientific studies that have addressed this question. Three of them concluded that a person who does nothing will have a better combination of longer life and higher quality of life than one treated with orthodox medicine (1).

The most extensive and convincing of these studies was done by Dr. Ulrich Abel of the Heidelberg/Mannheim Tumor Clinic in Germany. He did a comprehensive review and analysis of every major trial of chemotherapy ever done (37). To make sure he had reviewed every study on chemotherapy ever published, he sent letters to 350 medical centers around the world asking them to send him anything and everything they had ever published on the subject. In the course of this survey, which took several years, Abel reviewed thousands of articles, so at the end he was probably the man who knew more about chemotherapy than anyone else.

Abel concluded that the success rate of chemotherapy was appalling because:

> *"there was simply no scientific evidence available anywhere that chemotherapy can extend in any appreciable way the lives of patients suffering from the most common organic cancers."*

He goes on to stress that chemotherapy rarely improves the quality of life, describes chemotherapy as a scientific wasteland and states that 80 % of chemotherapy administered throughout the world is worthless. In spite of this, neither patient nor doctor is willing to give up on this futile exercise.

Even more surprising than the conclusion itself, is the fact that not a single mainstream medical journal or other publication has ever mentioned this study—it was effectively buried. It is incredible that the powers that be (Big Pharma and the opinion formers in the medical world) have said nothing and can so effectively bury anything that does not suit them.

There are other experts nowadays who would say that Abel's figure of 80 % is much too low and that the real figure is more likely to be close to 100 %, especially if you also consider the very poor quality of life of the chemotherapy and radiation patients.

There is no real evidence that orthodox treatment (chemotherapy, radiotherapy, surgery) can extend life at all, and if so, the effect is minimal and not worth the suffering (38). The orthodox establishment and their financial bosses use many "coverups" to create the impression that Nixon's "War on Cancer" is being won. The interested reader can read much more of this in the *Cancer Tutor* (24) and in the excellent book by Ty Bollinger (1).

In all fairness, we should now ask the same question as it applies to alternative treatment.

Firstly, alternative medicine uses natural products, so that in most treatments there are no significant side-effects: no loss of hair, no extra pain, any gastrointestinal upsets, any brain damage, etc.

The only possible side-effects in alternative medicine are the difficulties which accompany the massive change in diet. Wheat grass juice and carrot juice with beet juice do not taste nice, especially when one has to stay with this type of diet for long periods (months). But these are not really important if one considers the alternatives: death or a horrible tasting diet.

The question of whether or not such a treatment will really prolong life depends on how much effort the patient is prepared to put in and how well he/she has studied and prepared. If everything is done correctly (correct treatment or combination of treatments, correct diet, etc.) there can be no question that the patient's chances of recovery are better than 90 % is he/she had received no prior damaging conventional treatments. Even in the case of patients sent home to die after unsuccessful conventional treatment, they still have a 50 % chance of recovery (24).

This figure can be substantially improved if IPT forms part of the natural treatments selected. For a more detailed discussion of this important topic see *Insulin Potentiation Therapy* by Hauser and Hauser previously referred to.

The answer then to the question if a cancer patient will live longer on alternative treatment than on standard medical treatment or on no treatment, must therefore be a resounding "yes" with two provisos. Firstly, the patient must be very serious and committed to what he is doing and must pay strict attention to detail. Secondly, he must pay careful attention to his diet and be prepared to study. This is the only way in which the patient can become sufficiently motivated. Thirdly, the treatments selected should be started as early as possible (immediately after diagnosis and preferably before the patient has been subjected to destructive conventional treatments such as high-dose chemotherapy).

The cancer patient might also wish to know if alternative treatments can actually cure his cancer, meaning really cure it, not in the sense of 5-year survival rates as used by orthodox medicine. Again the answer has to be qualified: did the patient do his homework, did he choose the right treatment for his condition (and stage of cancer); did he adhere strictly to prescribed details and did he meticulously follow detail? Has he critically compared all the available alternative methods and are there good reasons to believe that the one selected is the best one for his condition? Has he carefully compared IPT with the other methods, and if so has he included IPT as one of the options available to him? Has he corrected the fatty acid imbalances in his diet? If so, then his chances of complete recovery are better than 90 % if his immune system and other organs have not been totally ruined by previous medical treatment. The better the condition of the patient at the beginning of the alternative treatment, the better the end results will be.

Later in this book I discuss IPT in greater detail and present evidence which shows that the best option for the advanced cancer patient in many cases appears to be to select IPT as the main treatment while using some of the other methods presented in this book as auxiliary treatment in so far as these are not contra-indicated in the case of patients using IPT.

Of course, patients on alternative therapy do die, because there are so many possible loopholes in executing the treatment protocols and because of the many imperfections of human nature (eg failure to fully understand the importance of detail in treatment and of diet). This much is absolutely sure: if the same patient had gone the orthodox way, he would also have died, but considerably sooner.

It is a sad fact of life that more than 95 % of cancer patients who go to alternative clinics do so after they had been given up on by conventional doctors, as in the case of Coretta King (wife of Martin Luther King) who died in Mexico while receiving alternative treatment. This was of course great news to the press, who unfortunately forgot to mention that conventional medicine had already given up on her and left her to die after poisoning her with chemotherapy. It is quite natural that she should have sought alternative medicine as a last resort. Unfortunately, as in many other similar cases, she was too late.

The message conveyed by the press was of course a very different one.

In spite of the cancer industry's very stringent measures to suppress the use of alternative methods, successes of alternative treatments do become more and more known, thanks largely to the Internet and the word-of-mouth grapevine.

The Cancer Industry has a ready-to-use plan to deal with this problem, and the usual response world-wide is by way of one of the following:

- The patients are said to have been cured as a result of the delayed action of one of the conventional treatments previously given to the patient (even if it took place months earlier).
- The evidence is disputed as unreliable, hearsay evidence or anecdotal evidence, no matter how many thousands of such reports are available.
- The patients are said to have undergone spontaneous remission and not improved as a result of the alternative treatment.
- The doctors who administered the treatment are punished by having their medical licenses withdrawn or even being jailed.
- Nothing is said and it is assumed that the problem will go away in time. The silence thus created allows many oncologists to say: "Well, since I haven't heard of the method, it is unproven and perhaps experimental." It also prevents the public in general from hearing too much.
- Some oncologists will not even look at the evidence or discuss alternative treatments. In this manner, alternative treatments are further denied access by the public.

Final advice on choosing a strategy

In his book *Cancer-free,* Bill Henderson (22) gives some general guidelines on choosing a strategy. I agree with some provisos which are included in the following summary:

- Remember that most cancers grow relatively slowly and that your cancer has been developing over years. The decision how to treat is therefore not an emergency decision that has to be taken in days.

You probably have weeks to decide. Pancreatic cancer, which is a known fast-growing cancer, is perhaps an exception.
- Killing the cancer cells must not be your first priority—restoring the inner milieu in which the cancer cells grow is the most important issue in most cases, excluding dire emergencies such as may occur in pancreatic cancer.
- Most alternative treatments can be evaluated in a matter of weeks. Even the strongest, such as IPT and the CsCl/DMSO protocol, should give a clear indication within weeks whether or not it is being successful in your case.
- Do not be misled by 5-year survival statistics that some doctors are so fond of using in support of their conventional treatments. These are meaningless.
- If you don't have time or energy to study your various options carefully, get someone else to do this for you, eg a good friend, your partner or your doctor if he is open-minded enough to look at all options.
- Avoid mainstream, large cancer institutions and hospitals. They have a dismal success rate and are prohibitively expensive.
- Consider IPT as a primary treatment by an experienced therapist and use the other therapies discussed in this book as supportive treatments.
- Pay careful attention to your diet, including the proper mix of w-3 and w-6 fatty acids as detailed in this book,

I include all this information here because it is important for the patient to make a choice as early as possible. Do not wait until you are at death's door before you realize what is happening. It may be too late. Choose the correct natural medicine protocols as soon as reasonably possible and do not persist with harmful conventional methods which may cause irreparable damage to your body's ability to heal.

There is little doubt that, using the correct alternative treatment or combination of treatments, more than 90 % of cancers can be cured if treated soon enough according to the literature.

The big problem that remains is that there is at present no reliable direct test that you can use to determine whether a particular treatment will work for you. In general, one can say that the correct use of IPT and CsCl/DMSO will work for many patients but not for all. For some patients it may be necessary to fall back on any one or more of the other important alternative protocols discussed in this book, but there is no way to predict which one will be the most suitable. The only options left are of an indirect nature. The first one is based on kinesiology, which tests the body's response to different treatments and for this purpose a test kit has been developed in America. For more details go to "Alternative Cancer Test Kit" (*http:// www.alternativecancer.us*). The test kit comes with illustrated instructions for testing your response to 12 alternative cancer treatments discussed or referred to in this book.

Another indirect method consists of listing on a daily basis some typical symptoms associated with cancer as shown in the following table:

Cancer Intensity Symptom Score
(14 days, period from . . . to . . .)

The intensity (on a 0-10 point score) is listed on the following symptoms (Daily totals indicate trend in the developing cancer)

Date	1	2	3	4	5	6	7	8	9	10	11	12	13	14
Clinical*														
Appetite														
Pain														
Energy														
Patient assessment**														
Daily total medication***														
Dosage****														

NOTE:
* General clinical assessment (0-10)
** How the patient feels (0-10)
*** Protocol
****Quantity of key ingredient of protocol administered daily

The daily total scores obtained in this manner allow the patient and his doctor to estimate whether or not he/she is losing or winning the war.

Do not believe your doctor or oncologist when they look at some X-ray or lab test and then say that you have 6 months to live. This in itself, apart from not being necessarily true, is a death sentence and extremely harmful to the patient. Remember that up to 50 % of such patients have been cured by alternative methods. The doctor or oncologist's pronouncement on your chances of living is based on his system of medicine. In most cases he is not qualified to tell you how long you might live under some other system of medicine.

It is important to realize that the doctor or oncologist is not lying to you when he makes such pronouncements. They are probably true if you limit yourself to his protocol.

Remember that nothing will cure your cancer if you keep on giving yourself cancer by eating processed foods, exposing your body to harmful chemicals (drugs, chemotherapy, cosmetics, pesticides, sunscreens, etc.) and persist with a wrong diet that *inter alia* does not provide the correct ratio of w-6:w-3 fatty acids.

No therapy in the world can compensate and reverse the collective powerful pro-cancer effects of these agents to which most people keep on exposing themselves.

As far as metastatic cancers go, a remark by Dr. R. Hauser (an internationally recognized authority on IPT) seems relevant. He states:

> *"I have never had or seen a documented case of a metastatic cancer go into complete remission without the use of some type of chemotherapy."*

In the context of what Dr. Hauser says in the rest of his book (previously referred to), it is obvious that the type of chemo he refers to is IPT and he cites many case histories, seen by himself as well as many other doctors, in support of such a statement.

Finally, never lose sight of the fact that curing cancer involves much more than killing cancer cells.

It also requires massive cleansing of the body (colon, liver, kidneys) and creating the conditions in your body that are unfavorable for the development of cancer cells (the "inner terrain").

In a later section of this book we discuss a number of the most important secondary cancer treatments. We also attempt to classify them according to the literature in order of efficacy for most cancers. These treatments are the aggressive cancer treatments, of which we rated IPT as the best overall treatment. It is necessary at this stage to point out that there are certain situations in which such aggressive treatment is immediately required. The following are some examples:

- Systemic swelling which may endanger the patient's life
- Aggressive tumors, eg pancreas tumor
- Gastrointestinal tumors which may cause obstruction
- Brain metastases
- Tumors involving the spinal chord
- Liver metastases
- Severe cachexia
- Lung tumors with breathing problems
- Severe pain.

These treatments should preferably be done under the guidance of an oncologist who will be able to locate the cancer and who is best qualified to decide whether or not there is a danger that massive and life-threatening occlusions may occur.

Combining orthodox and alternative treatments

Most cancer patients are treated by means of conventional methods first, following advice from their doctor or oncologist. During the course of treatment, it may become apparent that the conventional methods are not working. It may even be that the patient is told by his oncologist that nothing more can be done for him. It is at this stage that the patient, now desperate, starts to look beyond conventional treatments and starts to investigate alternative methods.

Thus a large group of critically ill cancer patients have in the past been grossly neglected by alternative physicians, often on the basis of arguments that prior treatment with conventional methods (such as chemotherapy) created too much interference and also may have damaged the patient's immune system too much for even proven effective alternative treatments to have any effect. This is a serious mistake. A good example is the successful use of the CsCl/DMSO protocol in combination with chemotherapy (IPT).

On the other hand, a strong case can now be made to adopt a more complementary approach by blending alternative and conventional therapies in an appropriate manner, regardless of the cancer status of the patient. There are also patients who do not wish to work exclusively with either disciplines, who may find it very beneficial to combine the two types of treatment. It makes perfect sense for patients undertaking complex and time consuming conventional treatments, such as bone marrow transplants, to also at the same time use an appropriate alternative technique. The same situation applies also in the case of patients with well-defined solid tumors where the surgical removal of the tumor mass will reduce the burden of cancer cells in the patient, thus creating a more favorable milieu for treatment by means of alternative methods.

IPT is an outstanding example of the successful combination of alternative cancer treatment and conventional cancer treatment. Based on available evidence, IPT is one of the first options that every cancer patient should consider in addition to correcting intracellular oxygen levels and proper fatty acid balance. With that statement in mind, the cancer patient will do well to consider the following additional combinations of conventional cancer treatment and alternative cancer treatment (in every case IPT must be seen as an important additional and/or alternative consideration).

The following are examples of the successful use of alternative and conventional methods in the treatment of various cancers:

Type of cancer	Conventional treatment	Alternative treatment
Breast	Chemotherapy, radiation, mastectomy	Comprehensive nutritional support, diet, immune support, stem cell replacement (I), CSCl/DMSO
Leukemia	Bone marrow transplant, chemotherapy, IPT	Lycopene, IPT, EXCl/DMSO, laetrile
Prostate	Radiotherapy, various	IPT, immune support (II), radiotherapy, CsCl/DMSO, Laetrile
Various	Chemotherapy	IPT, Vitamin C, Selenium, Vitamin E, Melatonin, Whey protein Stage IV protocol (II),

The cancer patient should always inform his doctor/oncologist of his decision to augment his conventional treatment with natural therapy. No patient should self-prescribe, and the patient should make sure that he understands and applies the restrictions that apply to alternative methods as discussed in this book. Certain therapies are contra-indicated in certain situations and in many cases supervision and close monitoring by a physician are vital.

Is my treatment working?

The Navarro Test

This is a critical matter with many cancer patients. The best way to answer this question is to determine the number of cancer cells left in your body by means of the Navarro or AMAS test discussed more fully elsewhere in this book.

Stage III treatments generally do not show results before 8 weeks. But if the number in the Navarro Test goes up with repeated tests before that time, it is usually a sign that you are not using the correct treatment. Immediately discuss the problem with a health professional with the necessary experience and make the necessary adjustments. Even with the strong Stage IV treatments, the time required to kill all the cancer cells may run into weeks, although, especially in the case of the CsCl/DMSO treatment, pain may disappear within days. Do these tests at least every two months.

Other analyses that may help you in assessing your progress include the following:

- *Blood analyses.* You should make an attempt to understand what the different compounds in your blood mean in terms of disease. It does not mean that you have to become a chemical pathologist, but understanding the rudiments of what your blood levels of, for example glucose, minerals, etc. mean in terms of disease, is not such a complicated matter.
- *Live blood cell analyses.* A phase contrast study of your blood may yield valuable information. This is done by placing a drop of blood under the lens of a high-powered microscope and the image is screened on a TV monitor. In this manner you will be able to see formations

and activity of the various cells floating around and in living color. You will need the aid of your health professional to point out any abnormalities and what these signify. Deficiencies and deformities of the cells may provide information on kidney and liver conditions and much more. Your health professional will be able to suggest the best lab to do the test. Do this test on a monthly basis to assess progress.

- *Liver function tests.* These are usually done as a panel of tests at chemical pathology labs and include determinations of bilirubin, alkaline phosphates, gamma glutamyl transferase, alanine aminotransferase, aspartate aminotransferase and lactate dehydrogenase.
- *Kidney function tests.* These are also done as a panel and include urea, uric acid, creatinine and protein.
- *Thyroid panel.* This includes T3, T4 and TSH. Both hyperactivity and hypoactivity of the thyroid may contribute too many diseases including cancer.
- *Natural killer cells activity.* This test is of special significance for the cancer patient and indicates the ability of your immune system to kill cancer cells. Do this test every 2 months.
- *The AMAS Test.* This is claimed to be one of the most sensitive tests for cancer. It can detect the presence of cancer nearly 2 years earlier than most other methods, with an accuracy of better than 99 %. It is especially useful to detect the recurrence of cancer for example following surgery.
- A test kit is available to doctors at Dr. Bogoch's Oncolab, 36 The Fenway, Boston MA, Tel USA (800) 922-8378. Your health professional will be able to advise you if there is a lab in your vicinity that can do the test. This test is relatively expensive and it may be desirable to do the Navarro Test instead which is much cheaper. This test works best for cancers during the initial stages and yields less reliable results on advanced cancers.

Cancer markers

These refer to a variety of standard lab tests designed to measure the level of certain cancer-specific proteins produced by certain cancers and which appear in the blood. These markers become elevated in the presence of certain tumors and may therefore be used to indicate the presence and amount of the particular cancer. Some of these tests are more reliable than others, and they should never be relied upon exclusively for diagnostic purposes. They are, however, useful as a guide to treatment.

The following are some cancer markers for a few of the more common types of cancer:

- CEA (carcinoembryonic antigen): used as a test for colon cancer
- CA 125: used as a test for ovarian cancer
- PSA (prostate specific antigen): for prostate cancer
- CA (carcinoma) 27.29: for breast cancer
- AFP (alpha-fetoprotein): for liver cancer.

You should note that while these tests give information on particular types of cancer, they are not very reliable. On the other hand, although the Navarro and AMAS tests give highly reliable information on the presence of cancer or not, they do so regardless of the type of cancer. These tests are discussed elsewhere in this book.

Warning about the diet and acidity

At all times, no matter what type of cancer or what stage of cancer we are dealing with, it should be stressed that the cancer diet is just as important as the treatment itself. Apart from other considerations, the diet ensures that the patient's body is alkalinized, without which no cancer can be permanently cured. This is also the reason why conventional treatment methods fail so often, because traditionally orthodox doctors do not pay attention to these factors.

How to balance foods to maintain alkalinity

Digested foods are metabolized ("burned") in the body leaving a residue which usually consists of an inorganic residue—also referred to as "ash". It is this ash that determines the effect of the particular food on systemic acidity. For example, when potassium citrate is metabolized in this manner, the citrate part of the molecule is metabolized to produce energy, while the potassium remains, which is an alkaline mineral. It therefore has an alkalinizing systemic effect. The same happens with derivatives of calcium and magnesium, which are also alkalinizing minerals. The "ash" may, however, also consist of other inorganic elements such as sulphur, phosphorus and chlorine, which are ultimately converted into acids (sulphuric acid, phosphoric acid and hydrochloric acid). These acids have an acidifying systemic effect. For this reason many animal products have an acidifying systemic effect. On the basis of this, we see that some foods may have an acidifying effect while others may have an alkalinizing effect, which may be either strong or weaker. The ultimate effect that the diet therefore has on systemic acidity or alkalinity depends on the composition and ratio of the different foods in the diet.

In order to be able to select an alkalinizing diet, it is important to balance the different foods selected in such a manner that the ultimate effect of the diet will be alkalinizing.

As pointed out before, normal body function and optimal health require adequate alkaline reserves (eg adequate reserves of the alkalinizing minerals calcium, magnesium, potassium) as well as the correct acidity in blood and tissues. The principal means of ensuring this is the proper dietary ratio of alkaline to acidic foods. Practical experience has shown that, in order to achieve this, the ratio must be at least 80 % to 20 %, or 4 parts of alkaline foods to 1 part of acid food. This will ensure that the growth of yeasts, moulds and other pathogenic organisms is suppressed. This ratio is heavily laden in favor of the alkaline foods because these micro-organisms (which are present in all cancer patients), when they grow, add their own acids to the acid side of the equation. This is of special importance in the cancer patient who already bears a heavy load of these organisms. In calculating this ratio, we should bear in mind and allow for the fact that foods may be either strongly or weakly acidifying or alkalinizing.

- Systemic acidity in the patient is often determined by means of litmus paper on the tongue (saliva). The reading should be in the vicinity of 7.4. Litmus is, however, not a very sensitive indicator of acidity, and therefore this is not a very reliable method. A much more reliable method is to measure the urinary pH 2 hours after a meal with a pH meter. Much can be learned about acidity in the body by repeated analysis of this nature which allows a trend to be discerned.
- In general, animal, dairy, processed and fermented foods, sugar, most grains and alcohol are acid forming. Buckwheat and millet are exceptions.
- In the process of sprouting, grains and seeds become alkalinizing, or more so if they are already alkalinizing.
- All vegetable juices are highly alkaline, especially those made from green vegetables and vegetable tops such as beet tops. All vegetable soups and broths, especially those made from cucumber, onion and garlic are strongly alkalinizing. Low sugar fruits (eg lemon, tomato and avocado) are also alkalinizing, in contrast to high sugar fruits such as grapes which acidify and encourage overgrowth by pathogenic micro-organisms.
- It is not possible to induce a condition of harmful excessive alkalinity by means of diet.

In the following table I have summarized, from various sources, the relative alkalinizing and acidifying potential of various foods. The symbol (-) is used to indicate relative acidity while (+) indicates relative alkalinity.

1. FOODS FREELY ALLOWED

Vegetables (permissible)

Brussels sprouts	-1.5	Garlic	+13.2
Asparagus	+1.2	Celery	+13.3
Architokes	+1.4	Barley grass	+28.0
Lettuce	+2.1	Soy sprouted	+29.0
Onion	+3.1	Alfalfa grass	+29.1
Cauliflower	+3.1	Cucumber fresh	+30.7
Cabbage	+3.1	Peas fresh	+5.1
Red Cabbage	+6.3	Leeks bulbs	+7.0
Water cress	+7.6	Spinach	+8.4 - +13.0
Beans (green)	+11.2		

Root vegetables (permissible)

Radish white	+3.1	Carrot	+9.5
Kohlrabi	+5.0	Beet red	+11.4
Horse radish	+6.8	Radish red	+16.5
Turnip	+7.9		

Fruits (permissible)

Limes	+8.0	Tomato	+13.6
Lemon fresh	+10.0	Avocado	+15.3

Grains (organic, non-stored) (permissible)

Buckwheat	+0.5	Lima beans	+11.8
Lentils	+0.7	Soy beans fresh	+12.0
Soy flour	+2.5	Millet	+.17
White beans	+12.0	Tofu	+3.2
Soy lecithin pure	+38.0		

Nuts (permissible)

Almonds	+3.6	Hazel nuts	-2.0
Brazil nuts	0.0		

Seeds (permissible)

Pumpkin seeds	-5.0	Sesame seeds	+1.2
Sunflower seeds	-5.4	Flax seed	-1.2

Oils (fresh, cold pressed) (permissible)

Olive oil	+1.0	Evening primrose	+4.1
Borage oil	+3.1	Fish Oil	+4.8
Flaxseed oil	+3.4		

2. FOODS NOT FREELY ALLOWED

Fish (eat sparingly)

Fresh water fish -11.3

Fruits (moderate)

Pineapple	-12.6	Raspberry	-5.2
Mandarin	-11.3	Plum yellow	-4.9
Banana (ripe)	-10.0	Dates	-4.7
Pear	-9.7	Cherry sweet	-3.7
Peach	-9.7	Grapefruit	-1.7
Apricot	-9.6	Watermelon	-1.0
Papaya	-9.2	Cocoanut fresh	+0.3
Orange	-9.2	Banana not ripe	+4.8
Mango	-8.7	Tangerine	-8.5
Gooseberry ripe	-7.7	Grape ripe	-7.0
Black currant	-6.1	Strawberry	-5.4
Blueberry	-5.3		

Non-stored grains (moderate)

Rice brown	-12.1	Wheat	-10.1

Nuts (moderate)

Walnuts -8.0

OILS (moderate)

Sunflower oil   -6.7

Root vegetables (limit)

Potatoes stored   +2.0

Animal protein (limit strictly)

Pork	-38	Eggs	-20
Veal	-34	Oysters	-5.2
Beef	-34	Liver	-3.0
Fish ocean	-20	Organ meats	-3.0
Chicken	-20		

Milk and milk products (limit)

Cheese hard	-18.0	Cream	-3.9
Cottage cheese (quark)	-17.0	Homogenized	-1.0

Bread, biscuits, stored grains (avoid strictly)

Bread white	-10.0	Bread whole grain	-4.5
Biscuit white	-7.0	Bread rye	-2.5
Bread whole meal	-6.5		

Nuts (avoid strictly)

Pistachios	-16.9	Cashews	-9.3
Peanuts	-12.9		

Fats (avoid strictly)

Margarine	-7.5	Butter (limit)	-3.9
Maize oil	-6.5		

Sweets (avoid strictly)

Artificial sweeteners	-27	Fructose	-9.5
Sugar white	-18	Honey	-7.7
Molasses	-14.7		

Beverages (avoid strictly)

Liquor	-35	Fruit juice natural	-9.0
Wine	-17	Fruit juice sweetened	-33
Beer	-26	Tea black	-27
Coffee	-25		

Condiments (avoid strictly)

Ketchup, Mayonnaise, Mustard   -12 to -19

NOTE:
1. When selecting food items, remember that information from this list only gives an indication of the effect of the particular food on systemic acidity. It does not give information on sugar content, which is another very important matter as discussed elsewhere in this book. When selecting foods from this list, you should also consider the sugar (glucose) content of the particular food. The best indicator of this is the glycemic index, as discussed earlier. Information on the glycemic indices of various foods is available on the Internet.
2. It is possible to check the acidity of your body by means of pH paper (available from your pharmacy). For best reliable results, do the saliva test in mid-afternoon and the urine test on a urine sample first thing in the morning.
3. In order to do the saliva test, fill your mouth with saliva at least 2 hours after eating and then swallow it, and repeat this step to ensure that the saliva is clean and free of food particles. Then repeat a third time, and then put some saliva onto pH paper.
4. Healthy saliva values fluctuate in the range pH 6.6-7.0 while the urinary pH values are always more acidic (6.0-6.8).

Understanding the phases of treating cancer

- In the case of many cancers, and especially in the case of fast-growing cancers, the patient usually has limited time available to institute whatever treatment programme has been decided upon. Conventional treatments may have put the patient into temporary remission (meaning that the symptoms are gone). This does not mean that the patient has been permanently cured, because even if the treatment has killed every cancer cell in the body (which none of the conventional treatments can do), the original cause of the disease has not been removed and therefore the cancer may return. Such remission treatment must at least involve the following steps: killing all the remaining cancer cells rebuilding the immune system provision of critical nutrients to assist in the healing process repairing the electrical balance in the cells (eg by means of the Budwig diet).

In order to do all these things, the patient needs time, which may be a critical factor since many patients who come for alternative treatment have been unsuccessfully treated with conventional methods (especially chemotherapy) and often have only weeks or months to live. There are fortunately methods available to "buy time". For this purpose, IPT and high-dose Vitamin C therapy, including intravenous Vitamin C therapy, are the best (see "Vitamin C Therapy"). It works within 8 weeks.

Some remarks on combinations of drugs and natural products

From a broader perspective, it is vitally important to consider some other complicating factors such as pregnancy and forbidden drug combinations, which will be discussed in greater detail later.

For now, it is necessary to realize that if you are on any prescription drugs or even over-the-counter everyday drugs such as aspirin, you must check with your doctor or pharmacist that the alternative cancer treatment protocol that you are on could not cause any complicating cross-reactions. Problems can occur when one drug negates or interferes with another or when one substance enhances the effects of another.

Such complications are possible with a variety of drugs, especially the drugs used for hypertension, heart medications, blood thinners and pain medications.

The interaction can also be of such a nature that the drugs interfere with the alternative medicine used. There is a particularly dangerous conflict that can be immediately fatal in the case of a combination of tranquillizers with hydrazine sulphate, which is used for the treatment of cachexia in cancer patients. Other forbidden combinations include blood thinners and proteolytic enzymes. Cancer patients are usually on a variety of prescription drugs, which makes it impossible to deal with possible harmful combinations in a comprehensive way. One way is to make sure that the other drugs that you are taking are really necessary and beneficial in your case.

A practical solution to the problem is to do your utmost to avoid possible conflicts by consulting with your doctor, pharmacist and specialists in the field of alternative medicine but at the same time to make sure that you are using the best possible alternative protocol for your condition. There is no other way to overcome your cancer problem.

A particularly interesting and also very effective combination is that of chemotherapy (also IPT) and the CsCl/DMSO protocol. According to one source (32), there seems to be some synergy between chemotherapy drugs and CsCl, and possibly with DMSO. While the CsCl/DMSO protocol generally causes temporary swelling and inflammation, it does not appear to be the case when the protocol is used with chemotherapy or IPT. Thus for those critically ill patients who have been treated with conventional chemotherapy and now wish to use some alternative method because of their steadily worsening condition, the CsCl/DMSO protocol appears to be an important option that could be considered.

Those contemplating chemotherapy should seriously consider IPT which is based on the combined use of chemotherapy drugs and insulin. This has many advantages. When used with insulin, the doses of the chemo drugs can be very much reduced (to about 10 % of the normal doses) thus reducing toxicity drastically and increasing the efficacy of the treatment. When used in conjunction with insulin, chemotherapy loses many of its disadvantages and becomes a valuable treatment option. The treatment must be done at a clinic, preferably under guidance of a medical doctor. There is no published evidence that indicates a harmful interaction when CsCl/DMSO is used in conjunction with IPT.

Nutrient supplements in combination with conventional cancer treatments

Evidence shows conclusively that, in the majority of cases, both the efficacy as well as safety of conventional treatments (chemotherapy and radiotherapy) can be significantly improved by the judicious combination with nutrients (mostly antioxidants). There are, however, some exceptions. These are relatively few if one considers the large number of proven cases where the concomitant use of anti-oxidants and either chemotherapy or radiotherapy provides very real advantages to the patient in terms of reduced toxicity and increased efficacy.

The following are some examples of potentially harmful combinations:

Harmful combinations (39)

- N-acetyl cysteine (NAC) with cisplatinum and Adriamycin. This combination offers little advantage; it is much better to use other antioxidants that have been shown to reduce the toxicity of these drugs.
- Melatonin should not be used in the treatment of patients with leukemia, lymphoma and Hodgkin's disease. In view of the effects of melatonin on the immune system and until more clinical information is available, this combination should only be used with careful monitoring of the patient or perhaps, better still, altogether discouraged.
- The use of isoflavones (diadzein and genistein, present in soy beans) in patients undergoing radiotherapy. The therapeutic effects of radiotherapy are dependent on the activity of the enzyme protein kinase. Isoflavones inhibit this enzyme and could therefore interfere with the efficacy of the treatment. It is advisable not to use soy products or isoflavones for one week before and during the period that the patient is being treated by means of radiotherapy.
- The use of tangretin (antioxidant bioflavonoid in citrus) in breast cancer patients undergoing treatment with Tamoxifen. Tangretin completely

blocks the action of Tamoxifen. Other plant bioflavonoids may have a similar effect. Whether or not Tamoxifen should be used at all in breast cancer patients is questionable (see discussion in this book).
- The use of beta-carotene in patients being treated with 5—fluorouracil: the nature of this interaction is not clear at present. It is therefore better to avoid this combination until more information is available

Advantageous combinations of nutrients with radiotherapy

- Cis-retinoic acid in the treatment of advanced cervical cancer ([40](#))
- Vitamin A (1, 5 m Iμ) in advanced cervical cancer: increased T-cell response and reduced relapse rate and toxicity ([41](#))
- Vitamin C (5000mg), different tumor types: improved response, fewer side-effects ([42](#))
- Selenium: animal studies show that selenium depletion reduces the lethal dose of radiation ([43](#))
- Co-enzyme Q10, small cell lung cancer: Q10 did not increase toxicity of radiation, but high doses did ([44](#))
- Melatonin (20mg): Glioblastoma (1 year): six out of fourteen patients alive after 1 year compared to one out of sixteen in control group; also fewer side-effects due to radiotherapy ([45](#)).

The dangers of swelling and inflammation

These dangers are inherent in the use of many of the more potent alternative treatments. Because cancer cells die as a result of the treatment (eg by CsCl/DMSO), they have to be disposed of by the body. Some may be digested and thus removed, while others are "eaten" by cells of the immune system. In most cases, however, these dead cancer cells are concentrated in certain areas of the body where there is simply too much debris for the surrounding cells to "eat". This places a burden on the liver, lymph system, kidneys and perhaps other organs. These accumulated dead cells may cause inflammation and swelling, which can be extremely dangerous, especially in the case of certain types of cancer such as lung and brain cancers, and in cancers of the digestive system. These masses of dead cells may restrict blood flow to certain critical areas, thus causing an immediate and serious threat. This is one of the reasons why treatment in such cases should preferably be carried out in a clinic under medical surveillance since dosage levels may have to be adapted.

This problem puts the seriously ill cancer patient in a paradoxical situation. If the patient opts not to use these alternative treatments, he/she will almost certainly die. But if he/she uses these alternative methods, the swelling/inflammation problem (in the case of certain cancers) arises and they may get worse before getting better. Typically, the swelling may block the movement of vital fluids (eg blood) or fecal matter in the case of colon cancer. Fortunately, there are methods with which to combat these complications.

There are a few alternative treatments that do not seem to make inflammation, congestion and swelling worse. The Bill Henderson protocol is one of them, and generally it can be said that treatments that work mainly through improving immune function will also not cause this problem. There are other methods that can be used to counter the problem.

One method is to use high concentrations of proteolytic enzymes (Vitalzyme) which is an excellent way of keeping inflammation and swelling down. Enzymes cannot be used in patients who are on blood thinners, as previously explained.

MSM and DMSO are generally the main supplements to keep inflammation and swelling down. Fortunately, DMSO is one of the main ingredients of the CsCl/DMSO protocol. In addition and as a safety measure, extra DMSO and/or MSM may be taken a few hours after each CsCl dose. Both DMSO and MSM are known to reduce inflammation, swelling and pain. The situation is particularly serious when it occurs in the brain, where the flow of blood may be blocked, and in the pancreas, where the flow of bile may be restricted.

Finally, the best way to control the problem of swelling is to use the right treatment for the particular situation. Swelling and inflammation are particularly dangerous in the case of cancers which are present in anatomically restricted areas such as the brain and gastrointestinal canal.

All Stage IV cancer patients will have some inflammation. This may be hazardous as discussed elsewhere depending on the location and type of cancer. Severe inflammation is usually accompanied by pain. Inflammation in the brain, pancreas and generally in the intestinal tract requires immediate medical attention and such patients should not be treated with CsCl or other strong Stage IV protocol until the swelling is under control.

How to read patient reports and testimonials

Since scientific research and clinical trials with alternative cancer methods are virtually banned by the health authorities in many countries, for reasons previously discussed, the alternative cancer treatment movement has to rely on personal reports and testimonials of patients' experience in the use of these methods. There are hundreds of these personal reports of successful treatment of a variety of cancers. The orthodox establishment scoffs at these and brushes them off as "anecdotal reports" which have no merit as scientific evidence of successful treatment. This may be the case if only a few isolated reports are available, but when hundreds of such reports become available on the Internet and elsewhere, the situation changes and compels us to look more seriously at the methods used.

We should, however, be careful in evaluating such individual reports. For example, the cure rate for a raw food diet in the treatment of a Stage IV cancer patient is about 15 %. Now one of the 15 % patients who had been cured by the diet puts a testimonial on the Internet reporting his successful cure and the report may be perfectly true. Another Stage IV patient, perhaps with the same type of cancer, reads this report and decides to use this method to treat his own cancer. He now only has a 15 % chance of success, although the other patient was in fact cured. But the second patient may not be so lucky, because of the low inherent cure rate of the method of only 15 %. There are many other Stage IV treatments with a much higher success rate.

Cure rates: the great deception factor

How is it possible that respected and experienced clinicians and scientists continue to promote conventional chemotherapy as a promising approach to cancer treatment when so much evidence to the contrary has now come to light?

The term "cure rate" means different things to different people. To the ordinary person the term "cured of cancer" simply implies that such a person will never ever again get cancer and that he/she will die of old age. Not so with the statisticians in charge of clinical trials reporting on the efficacy of conventional treatment methods. If you read the relevant literature of clinical trials sponsored by the American Cancer Society and other official bodies, you will often come across claims that a particular treatment resulted in a cure rate of 50 % or more. They define cure rate as the entirely misleading concept of "5-year cure rate". They monitor patients during a trial for 5 years and if a patient has lived that long, he/she is classed as "cured" for the purposes of the trial. If the patient dies after 5 years and one day, he/she is still classed as cured. Many cancers are slow growing and also cancers in elderly patients (eg prostate cancer patients) grow slowly. Such cancers will therefore have a high 5-year cure rate. Moreover, most orthodox treatments do have some effect on the number of cancer cells in the patient, and after such treatment the patient appears to be "cured" for a certain time after the treatment. In the meantime, however, the cancer is still there and growing, but in most cases it may take more than 5 years before this becomes apparent, especially in the elderly in whom many cancers grow more slowly than normal. This effect may be aggravated by the fact that such a patient, after a brush with cancer and death, has changed his lifestyle and perhaps even diet because so much is written in the popular press these days about the causes of cancer. All of this contributes to conveying an entirely false impression of the value of the orthodox treatment they have received. A grossly misleading impression is also created by the practice by the medical establishment of presenting the benefits of chemotherapy in statistical terms, which, while technically correct, create a grossly distorted view of chemotherapy and which are, moreover, seldom clearly understood by patients and even some doctors.

For example, the benefits of chemotherapy are often calculated in terms of "relative risk" rather than true risk, which give a true assessment of the likely impact on overall survival.

Typically, if as a result of treatment, the patient's risk declines from 4 % to 2 %, this can be expressed statistically as a decrease in relative risk of 50 %. The figure 50 % looks much better than the absolute risk percentages of 2 % or 4 %. It actually means a decline of 2 % in the absolute risk, which is what interests the patient, but does not look as impressive as the 50 % relative risk (Bucher, *BMJ*, 1994, 309:761).

One study showed that when physicians are given relative risk reduction figures for a chemotherapy regimen compared to another, they are more likely to recommend it to their patients than when they are given the identical statistical information expressed as an absolute risk figure. The implication is that the apparent gulf between the public perception of chemotherapy's effectiveness in clinical trials and its actual mediocre track record can largely be attributed to the practice of expressing clinical trial results in terms of relative rather than absolute risk. As an example, the authors of the abovementioned Australian study cite the treatment of breast cancer in Australia in 1998. Out of a total of newly diagnosed breast cancer cases, 4638 women were considered eligible for chemotherapy. Of these, only 164 (3.5%), were judged to have derived some survival benefit as a result of the treatment, and the extent of that benefit was not large, as shown above.

The authors also mention that the situation is not much improved by the use of newer chemotherapy drugs such as the taxanes and anthracyclines. These newer drugs raised the survival rate by an estimated additional 1 % at the expense of increased cardiac toxicity and nerve damage.

Another factor that is also used sometimes to make clinical studies with conventional drugs look better than they are, is to use so-called "surrogate end-points". In this method, some other endpoint than death (which is the only real endpoint that the cancer patient is interested in) is used to measure drug effect. Typical surrogate endpoints that have been used in the past are "progression free survival", "disease free survival" or "recurrence free survival". These are all relatively meaningless endpoints with little real significance which have been used to make chemotherapy trial results look better. Neither the patient nor his doctor should devote any significance to such trial results, since they reflect at best temporary lulls in the progression of the disease which do not last long. Then the cancer typically returns, often with a vengeance, and the overall result is that real patient survival time is not improved.

In view of the highly controversial nature of the findings of this study, which corroborate the findings of similar previous studies (such as those of Professor Abel at the Heidelberg Cancer Research Institute in Germany: Abel, U. 1990. *Chemotherapy of advanced epithelial Cancer*. Stuttgart: Hippocrates Verlag), one might have expected it to receive enormous international attention. Instead, media and medical attention has been largely limited to some reaction in Australia but none in the USA. Internationally it received no attention at all, meaning that it did not come to the attention of thousands of doctors, and their millions of patients, worldwide, to whom this information is of vital importance.

This is one method that conventional medicine uses to keep unwanted information away from the public. It is noteworthy that anything vaguely positive about the successes of conventional treatments generates widespread press coverage and enthusiastic comments by health officials, quite unwarrantedly. A typical example is the announcement by the National Cancer Institute that the number of annual cancer deaths had declined for the first time in 70 years. The news was hailed by the National Cancer Institute as a notable milestone. Such a comment was totally unwarranted in view of the fact that the total number of cancer deaths had declined from 557272 in 1993 to 556902 in 1994, a total of only 370, which, expressed as a percentage, amounted to a decline of 0.066 %, the significance of which is highly uncertain.

Another method consists of indulging in hair-splitting arguments about technicalities of the trial set-up which are of no real significance. Such trivial attempts to maintain the status of the chemotherapy drugs do nothing to restore these drugs to their previous pervasive popularity, but rather diminish it.

Choosing a treatment strategy: some general remarks

Before choosing a particular treatment plan, you need to know how the proposed protocol works. This is necessary in order to choose the right treatment for a given situation. Fortunately cancer cells are very different from normal cells in many respects. They are also fragile and easy to kill safely although not so easy to kill selectively. Many types of cancer can be treated identically but a few require special measures. Examples are brain cancer (because of the blood-brain barrier), bone and bone marrow cancer (because no blood vessels are in direct contact with the cancer cells) and leukemia (which originates in the bone marrow).

Most alternative treatment plans that kill cancer cells fall into several main categories

- *Those that improve oxygen supply in the cancer cells.* We have seen that the more oxygen deprived cancer cells become, the better they grow. As cancer cells get more and more oxygen, their spread slows. When the oxygen level inside the cancer cells gets above a certain level, they die. Several of the better treatment plans work by raising the oxygen levels inside cancer cells. There are several ways of achieving this. The chief method is by means of antioxidants (which free up oxygen molecules already present in the body), hydrogen peroxide, ozone and oxygen treatment which bring more oxygen molecules into the cancer cells. The most important of these are, however, certain polyunsaturated fatty acids (mainly w-6 linoleic acid) which have the property of transporting oxygen from the circulation across cell membranes to the interior of the cells. By raising the intracellular oxygen levels, these

essential fatty acids prevent the cells from becoming cancerous. This will be discussed in more detail elsewhere.
- *Those that increase the alkalinity inside the cancer cells.* As discussed previously, cancer cells are very acidic. If the alkalinity inside the cells is increased to pH 8.0 or above, the cells will die. Note that this statement applies to the alkalinity inside the cancer cells and not in the body in general. Administration of CsCl is by far the best way of achieving this (see the CsCl/DMSO protocol). CsCl not only stops the growth and spread of cancer cells immediately, but in many cases also stops the pain of cancer within a few days.
- *The third way of killing cancer cells is by means of certain nutrients.* There are many nutrients that promote growth in normal cells but which kill cancer cells. A good example is purple or red grapes that are used in the Brandt Grape Cure. These grapes and their seeds contain more than 10 different nutrients that kill cancer cells. The problem is getting enough of the cancer-killing nutrients inside the cancer cells, because the nutrients have to pass certain barrier membranes such as those in the gastrointestinal tract and blood-brain barrier. Colon cleanses and avoiding chlorine in drinking water are amongst the methods that will improve absorption. There are also other means of tricking the cancer cells into ingesting increased quantities of cancer-killing nutrients, of which short fasts is one of the best methods. In this case the cancer cells are "starved" (12 hours) so that they become less selective in assimilating nutrients. Another method is to attach the toxic molecules (for cancer cells) to other "carrier" molecules (which are acceptable to the cancer cells) so that the toxic molecules as it were, ride piggyback on these carriers into the cancer cells. Examples of such carrier molecules are DMSO and MSM.
- *A fourth method is to stop the spreading of the cancer cells.* This can be done by improving the connective tissue which fills the spaces between cells. It can be achieved *inter alia* by means of large doses of Vitamin C or by inhibiting glucose from getting into cancer cells (cancer cells are voracious sugar "eaters"). The theory is that if the cancer cannot spread when the existing cancer cells die, the cancer will disappear. The success rates of these last two methods are not as high as in the case of the first two. These methods should therefore preferably be used in conjunction with other methods that directly kill cancer cells, such as CsCl.

- The *fifth method is to improve the immune system*. To achieve this, special diets and supplements are used, especially those that increase the immune cells that are more directly involved in killing cancer cells such as the natural killer cells. With the special diets what you don't eat is just as important as what you do eat. These special diets (the macrobiotic, raw food, Gerson and other diets) will improve the immune system but they do not work fast enough in the case of severely ill cancer patients (Stage IV). For these patients, such diets should be used in conjunction with other methods that directly kill cancer cells such as CsCl. Also, such diets should be evaluated in the light of their glycemic load and influence on blood sugar levels and may have to be adapted accordingly
- I have previously referred to the fact that the vital enzymes are destroyed in natural raw foods by the process of cooking. The trend in alternative cancer treatments and diets is towards raw, organic food diets that limit meat and most dairy products. This is clearly of less importance to critically ill patients who have been given up on by orthodox medicine and who have only a short time to live; too short for improvements to the immune system to have any effect.
- *A sixth method of killing cancer cells is to starve them to death*. Here fortunately cancer cells have an Achilles heel in that they require massive amounts of glucose (15 times more than normal cells). One anti-cancer diet is based on the selection of foods that contain very little glucose and other simple sugars (32). On such a diet the cancer cells literally starve to death while the normal cells survive. This is the principle on which IPT is based (see later).

These are the most widely used principles on which alternative treatments are based, although they are by no means the only methods used.

To treat a patient with advanced cancer, you need to know several things:

- Has the patient been pre-treated by conventional means, and if so, which means?
- How far advanced is the cancer, meaning how much cancer is there?
- Where is the cancer located (pancreas, liver, brain, lungs, bone, etc.)?
- What type of cancer is it (fast-growing)?
- What are the various treatment options?

You need to know how fast the different treatments work. Obviously, for a patient with less than 4 months to live you would not use laetrile or a metabolic enzyme treatment based on improved immune function, as these methods work slowly.

You cannot simply use any Stage IV treatment for any patient. There are situations where this may be dangerous. The following are a few examples. If the cancer is located in an area where swelling due to the treatment may cause a dangerous situation to develop, there are several alternative cancer methods that may not be used even though the treatment as such would effectively kill the cancer cells. Brain cancer is a typical example. Although the CsCl/DMSO protocol will effectively kill the cancer cells, it has to be used carefully under expert supervision to prevent dangerous swelling in this sensitive area. References to specialists in the USA, Canada and Mexico who can be approached for advice and guidance are available (32).

Lung cancer is another example where congestion and swelling is almost always a serious problem no matter which other concerns there may be. Only very specific alternative cancer treatments have any chance of success in lung cancer patients that have to go on oxygen therapy.

Another critical issue is whether the patient is taking any prescription drugs including chemotherapy. These patients cannot be treated with certain alternative methods in which there is increased cellular absorption of the drugs (32).

Other examples of where alternative treatments may be less effective are those patients who cannot digest or absorb supplements and medicines.

There are, therefore, many issues that determine which alternative treatments can be used in a specific case and which cannot. Some of the critical issues that have to be considered include the following:

- Is the tumor situated in an anatomical region where dangerous occlusions may result from swelling and congestion following the killing of cancer cells?
- Can the patient absorb and digest supplements?
- Is the patient being treated with prescription drugs?

These are some of the questions that have to be considered, and although the list may sound formidable, in practice it is possible in most cases to design a treatment schedule around these problems with the help of a competent and experienced adviser.

It is advisable that every cancer patient who undergoes treatment at home should have a knowledgeable person available to guide and help him over the telephone if necessary. A Stage IV patient has a lot of cancer in his body, and any cancer treatment that will kill his cancer fast enough to save his life will create side-effects that may be scary but are not necessarily dangerous. For this reason it is necessary to have someone at the other end of the line who has experience of this and who can tell the patient what to expect and which adjustments to make if necessary. Telephone numbers of experts in the USA who perform this type of function are available (32).

Patients mostly obtain advice from the vendors that supply the products they intend to use. This is usually all that is necessary. In complicated cases, advice may be sought from internationally recognized specialists (11).

When more than one organ or tissue is affected, which one should be treated first?

When the cancer is in multiple locations (eg as a result of metastases), it is important to treat the cancer in the most dangerous location first.

- Generally, lung cancer is usually treated first due to the danger of congestion.
- Pancreatic cancer is another type of cancer which is always given top priority because it is so fast-growing.
- Brain cancer and squamous cell carcinoma are also usually accorded high priority. The former is potentially deadly if there is brain swelling, and the latter because of the manner and speed at which it spreads. The type (malignancy) of the cancer usually takes precedence over its location.

Before deciding on a treatment programme, it is essential to consult an oncologist who is qualified to identify the type and location of the cancer(s). The oncologist should also identify the most dangerous tumor(s) if there is more than one. You should make every effort in finding an oncologist who also under-stands the value of alternative cancer therapies.

You should personally devote much time and effort to studying everything that relates to your condition. Remember that Stage IV requires the most potent treatment available, or perhaps even more than one protocol. When combining different treatments, it is important to understand that there are warnings and possible conflicts that you should be aware of (see above). You should read and re-read this book several times, paying special attention to the sections that are of particular importance in your case. A typical example is that the use of more than 250mg of supplemental Vitamin C is forbidden if you are taking hydrazine sulphate for cachexia.

You should clearly distinguish between causes and symptoms. If you have removed a symptom, the original cause of the disease is still there. For example, when orthodox medicine uses radiotherapy to treat a cancerous growth in the breast (which is a symptom), the cancerous growth may recede but even if it temporarily disappears completely, the original cause of the cancer is still there and the cancer may therefore return at any time. And so it is with other orthodox treatments—they treat symptoms and do nothing about the causes. However, especially in the case of seriously ill patients, it may be necessary to treat the most threatening symptoms first in order to save the patient's life and then to attend to removing the causes.

Once the cancer has been cured, we need to think of the possible causes in any particular case.

The following possibilities should be considered: poor inner terrain (resulting *inter alia* from low quality food); lack of essential fatty acids, especially of unadulterated w-6 fatty acids; microbial infections and toxins, ineffective immune system, presence of toxic fatty acids such as the transfatty acids in margarine and many others. The inner terrain and the immune system should receive urgent and immediate attention after killing the cancer cells. While the treatment selected is killing cancer cells and therefore treating the symptoms, the diet treats the causes, *inter alia* by building up the immune system while not interfering with the treatment.

In this sense, we should perhaps talk of the short-term (cancer killing) phase of the treatment and the long-term treatment which restores the immune function and prevents the cancer from returning. We should always separate these two concepts in our minds.

A good rule of thumb regarding your diet after the cancer cells have been killed is to have 80 % of your diet in harmony with the cancer diet that helped cure you, while the other 20 % should be reasonable foods according to your taste, but should not include junk foods.

One of the greatest weaknesses of the orthodox treatments of cancer is that they only think in terms of killing the cancer cells and will even repeat certain treatments when the cancer cells flare up again, because no attention had been devoted to the diet and the immune system. In this manner, they may repeatedly suppress the cancer cells until the patient dies.

Ultimately, the actual healing treatment therefore resides in the diet.

Regardless of which treatment is selected, it seems wise to give the following to all cancer patients:

- Unadulterated w-6 and w-3 polyunsaturated fatty acids (see later for details)
- IPT(see later)
- A good multinutrient formula
- Oral Vitamin C (starting with 12g and gradually increasing the dose to bowel tolerance limit, which is usually in the vicinity or 16g daily.) Vitamin C is only given intravenously to those patients who cannot tolerate more than 10g orally daily.
- Nicotinic acid: 500mg 3x daily
- Selenium: 400-600mcg daily (taking into account the selenium in the multinutrient)
- Zinc: 30-60mg daily (taking into account the zinc present in the multinutrient)
- Essiac tea: 3-4 cups daily (not easy to obtain a good quality product)
- A daily supplement of 4g of a 1:2 mix of w-3:w-6 fatty acids.

The spiritual aspect

Many cancer patients who have been through the horrors of chemotherapy and radiation are in such pain and so miserable and without hope that they have lost the will and hope to live. This is when strong support by family and friends is required. Without strong encouragement, which should be genuine and fact-based, there is little chance that the patient will be able to face the stringent requirements of alternative treatment and the diet that goes with it.

Family and friends should help the patient to be as comfortable and relaxed as possible and he/she should be constantly reminded of others who have been successfully treated in the same way and also that those around him/her want him/her to beat the cancer. Considerable time and effort should be spent to improve the patient's mental condition. This should include, if possible, arrangements to get the patient out of the house and in a different environment, at least once every day or two. Also, the patient should do mild exercises, even if it is only lifting a book up and down. He/she should also devote time to spirituality daily and be induced to forgive others. This whole exercise must, however, not create the impression that he is being prepared for death. The word death and the possibility that he/she might die should never be mentioned.

The cancer diet

There are many different cancer diets, which differ substantially in many crucial points. For example, some strictly forbid meat while others allow meat. Some are based on fruit and vegetable juices (to which I will refer as the "general cancer diet") which others say are strongly contra-indicated due to the high glucose content which stimulates insulin production (Hauser diet). It is extremely difficult to say which is correct and which not—probably all of them have some merit in certain situations. In what follows, I have given two main versions. The first allows fruit and fruit juices (the general cancer diet) which I have qualified by introducing the glycemic index to identify the permissible items. The second one is the Hauser diet which strictly forbids fruit and fruit juices, but allows animal products (poultry, fish).

It should be emphasized right at the onset that the cancer diet is the most important part of any treatment programme. The inner terrain of the patient is controlled by the diet and it is this inner terrain that allows a cancerous growth to grow or otherwise.

This is reminiscent of what Pasteur said on his deathbed:

> *"The patient is more important than the invader."*

- The main objectives of the cancer diet are to prepare the patient so that he/she can best deal with the invader (cancer). Here are some of the more important objectives: to promote detoxification and to limit the intake of toxins to optimize blood sugar and insulin levels to suppress blood coagulation to stimulate immunity and prevent intake of immune suppressive compounds to suppress anaerobic metabolism and limit lactic acid production to enhance aerobic metabolism to provide natural cancer-fighting substances to optimize hormone activity to eliminate carcinogens to help starve the cancer by limiting access to glucose to provide the correct mix of w-3:w-6 fatty acids as discussed before.

It is important to realize in connection with diet that what you are not allowed to eat is just as important as what you must eat.

Forbidden foods

Here is a short list of forbidden items which are more or less part of all cancer diets:

- Do not use tobacco in any form, severely limit alcohol and caffeine (one drink a day and one cup of either coffee or tea is maximum), absolutely no recreational drugs and sodas (diet or otherwise).
- No processed food of any kind; no restaurant food. If it is not entirely natural, don't eat it. These are all non-foods.
- No animal protein of any kind (in some diets) during the first 2 weeks (meat, fish, chicken, seafood, eggs, shellfish). Later, when your cancer is under control, you will be allowed small portions of fish or chicken not more than once or twice a week. In the Hauser diet you are allowed more meat.
- Sugar in any form is absolutely forbidden. This includes sugar-rich fruit juices as well as all other high GI foods. Avoid high GI fruits such as ripe bananas.
- All products that contain gluten (cereal, pasta, bread). Sprouted seeds are an important source of gluten-free foods.
- Dairy products such as milk, cheese, and butter are forbidden (in some diets) or limited. These products are strongly mucoid and acid-forming. Yoghurt and cottage cheese are permitted in both the Budwig diet and the general diet.
- Avoid all commercially stored grains. While many fresh grains are good food, the commercially stored variety is not. Stored grains begin to ferment after a few months under most conditions. In this way they become full of mycotoxins and pathogenic yeasts and moulds. There is even a published study which showed a positive correlation between oesophageal cancer and stored grains (46).
- Avoid all products containing yeast (bread, muffins, pies, cakes, beer, etc.). The grains in bread usually contain yeast, moulds and

mycotoxins, and the moisture content of the finished products aggravates this. These products may be the cause of many cancers
- Avoid condiments (mustard, ketchup, soy sauce, mayonnaise, salad dressings, horse radish, etc.). They are acid and mucoid-forming.
- Avoid malt products such as beer and malted cereals.
- Avoid alcohol in any form.
- Avoid caffeine in any form.
- Avoid peanuts and peanut products. Peanuts contain 26 carcinogenic fungi.
- Avoid maize and maize products. They also contain a heavy load of carcinogenic fungi. Maize has been correlated with certain cancers in clinical studies.
- Do not combine high protein foods with high carbohydrate foods in one meal.
- Never eat rancid oils, seeds or nuts.
- Include some fat in the diet to feed the normal cells. Olive oil on salads is a good choice. Butter is acceptable, provided it is free of hormones and toxins.

Foods that are permitted

In the same vein, we might summarize here the groups of foods that are permitted:

- Raw, whole vegetables and juices prepared from them in those diets which allow juices. Try to obtain organic vegetables, especially the green and colored varieties. Those that cannot be eaten raw, such as green beans and asparagus, may be lightly steamed.
- Sprouted seeds, including breads prepared from them.
- Use olive or flaxseed oil instead of butter on your sprouted seed bread.
- Cereals prepared from unstored millet, quinoa, buckwheat and other non-gluten cereals. Use almond milk on these cereals instead of milk or soya milk. Avoid commercial almond and soya milk which contain sugar. Unstored brown rice may also be included in this list.
- Fruit: only berries, pineapple, apples and limited amounts of paw-paw. Limit other fruits (bananas) to one a day. No fruit juices, but limited quantities of diluted (50 %) fruit juices are permitted.
- All yellow and dark green vegetables.

- High carbohydrate vegetables (eg beet, potato, yam, sweet potato, pumpkin) can be eaten in moderation but seriously ill Stage IV cancer patients should avoid them for the first 8 weeks during treatment.
- Fresh water fish (fresh) is permitted because it is anti-fungal. Avoid fish that smells.
- Drink lots of clean, filtered water. It has been suggested that the reason certain people who live in mountainous regions grow so old (120 years is not unusual) is because of the mineral-rich mountain water.
- Tomato, lemon and lime may be eaten freely.
- Proteins: the best protein sources are lentils, avocado, raw seeds (sesame, sunflower, pumpkin, flax), raw nuts (almond and hazelnut). Soaking seeds, nuts, legumes and grains for 12-24 hours before eating releases enzyme inhibitors (which may cause indigestion and stomach discomfort), partially digests protein and allows these foods to be digested with much less demand on the body's enzyme reserves.

Special therapeutic functions of foods

- *Foods that improve immune function.* Many nutrients can produce pharmacological changes in immune function. The most important of these are: protein, arginine, glutamine, w-3 and w-6 fatty acids, iron, zinc, and certain B vitamins, Vitamins A, C and E.
- *Foods that have an effect on blood coagulation.* There are many different foods that influence thinning of the blood. Such foods may assist the body in its fight against cancer by reducing coagulopathy which *inter alia* suppresses metastases. These are generally to be found amongst the vegetables and in foods that are rich in fatty acids (eg fish, oil). Important examples are garlic, onions, avocados, broccoli, Brussels sprouts, cabbage and cauliflower

Other foods are known to increase blood thickening and are therefore to be avoided. These are mainly the hydrogenated oil (margarine), fried foods, gravies, mayonnaise, packaged foods and certain vegetable oils such as corn oil, and chemically treated sunflower oil. From this perspective, fish and codliver oil are extremely beneficial in limited amounts. The ratio of w-6 to w-3 fatty acids is an all-important consideration. For example, in grain-fed beef this ratio is only 1:20, whereas in animals that graze on grass the ratio is 1:3, which is much nearer to the desired level of 1:2. For further information on w-3:w-6 ratios see the discussion of sunflower oil

- *Foods that suppress anaerobic metabolism.* Anaerobic metabolism (fermentation) and aerobic metabolism have been discussed in some detail in this book. As pointed out, anaerobic metabolism can cause the body to become too acidic due *inter alia* to the lactic acid produced. Vegetables are highly recommended in most diets, but if too much high-sugar veggies and fruits are consumed, elevated insulin levels which are favorable for the development of cancer may result. Cancer patients should regularly do blood analyses to check for lactic acid production as well as insulin levels and blood pH to determine to what extent the patient's diet is contributing to this aspect of cancer. The patient's diet should emphasize foods that inhibit anaerobic metabolism such as low-sugar food items. It is also important to note that certain bioflavonoid (eg quercetin) inhibit anaerobic metabolism. Other important sources of bioflavonoid are berries (especially dark blue berries), citrus fruits (especially the white rinds), green tea, onions and parsley.
- *Foods that enhance aerobic metabolism.* As previously discussed, oxygen is good for normal cells but bad for cancer cells. The mitochondria are the energy-producing structures in cells where fuel (glucose) is burned (in normal cells) to produce energy. For oxygen (which is required for aerobic respiration) to freely move in (and carbon dioxide out of) the mitochondria, it is necessary for the membranes of these cells to remain fluid, pliable and permeable. Saturated fats decrease (while certain unsaturated fats increase) the permeability of these membranes, thus suppressing oxygenation and promoting anaerobic conditions in the mitochondria. Unadulterated w-6 oils (sunflower oil) are particularly effective in promoting intracellular oxygenation.

Many nutritional products are known to increase aerobic metabolism. These include thiamine, riboflavin, coenzyme Q10, gingko biloba and ginseng.

- *Foods that promote detoxification.* The primary organs that promote detoxification are the liver, kidney and skin. Foods and liquids that promote effective defecation and urination should therefore receive prime attention by the cancer patient. The following are examples:

- High fiber foods, especially fresh vegetables
- Onions and garlic
- Yoghurt
- Purified water.

- *Foods that provide anti-cancer compounds.* The anti-cancer compounds in certain foods may provide valuable support in the cancer treatment programme selected. The following are a few examples:

  - Carotenoid rich and colorful foods (carrots, beets, spinach, tomatoes, berries)
  - Members of the cabbage family
  - Cold water fish and fish oil supplements (in limited amounts)
  - Members of the allium family (onions, garlic)
  - Quercetin supplements
  - Members of the bean family (soy and other legumes) which provide proteases
  - Kelp
  - Yoghurt
  - Green tea (contains powerful antioxidant catechins).

- *Foods that affect hormones.* Estradiol is one of the oestrogens with strong cancer-promoting properties. Improving your hormonal status, from the point of view of cancer, means lowering your oestrogen levels and oestrogen-binding capacity. High levels of Estradiol in the blood have been linked to increased breast cancer risk.

Soy is a typical food that will reduce the effects of Estradiol. One daily serving of soy may decrease the risk of certain cancers by 40 % and the cancer incidence in the soy eating countries (China, Japan) is significantly lower than in Western countries. Soy beans contain phytoestrogens (plant oestrogens) which oppose the effects of the strong cancer-promoting oestrogens such as Estradiol. Many food sources of soy are available on the market (soy milk, soy protein, etc.) but make sure the product you select does not contain any sugars, and limit intake of soy-containing foods to sensible amounts.

The Hauser diet

- (Hauser, RA and Hauser, MA. 2002. *Treating Cancer with Insulin Potentiation Therapy*. Oak Park, Ill: Beulah Land Press). It is interesting to compare the abovementioned guidelines with those given by Dr. Hauser (*Ibid.*, p 293), many of which are similar in many respects but significantly different in others from those given above. The following are the most important points of the Hauser diet: eliminate sugar and sugar substitutes or anything that may be converted into glucose use only chemical-, hormone—, and preservative-free foods eat organic foods as much as possible eat food that is fresh carbs are the enemy (do not eat more than 60 g of complex carbs per day) do not consume an inordinate amount of soy natural fats and oils are friendly protein is very important strictly avoid all junk food or foods that contain additives, colorants, preservatives and other chemical substances increase consumption of vegetables, especially those with a GI below 60 increase consumption of good fats (olive oil, flaxseed oil, codliver oil, unadulterated sunflower oil, etc.).

Fruits are very high in carbs and should be avoided in general. Fruit and vegetable juices are not in the Hauser diet, because of their high sugar content. The Hauser diet strongly promotes soy, which may make up 25-50 % of the diet. These are obtained from such sources as tempeh, tofu, miso, soy milk, soy protein isolates and whole soy beans. The reasons why soy is important to the cancer patient are given by Dr. Hauser:

- It stabilizes blood sugar and insulin levels
- It is an excellent protein source
- It contains soy isoflavones including genistein and diadzein which are phytoestrogens that suppress cancer by opposing excessive oestrogen activity
- It provides lignans, also with anti-oestrogen activity
- It inhibits new blood vessel formation
- It decreases cancer cell adhesiveness and therefore metastases
- It blocks Estradiol binding to oestrogen receptors, thereby inhibiting cancer cell proliferation in oestrogen positive breast cancer cells.

The Hauser diet food pyramid gives the relative proportions of food components in the cancer diet for the critically ill cancer patient. These are as follows:

Hauser diet	Comments
Total protein: 45 %	Up to 50 % of this preferably in the form of so products
Carbs: 30 %	Select complex carbs with a GI below 60. Less than 60g carbs daily.
Fat and oils: 25 %	Mainly as olive, flaxseed, cold pressed sunflower and fish oils
Fruits and whol grains: 0-2 servings	Perhaps up to 4 servings if you select low sugar and low GI fruits

Note: Remember that your blood biochemistry and cancer status are more important than the absolute quantities of the different foods consumed. Therefore closely monitor changes in glucose-insulin tolerance as well as the cancer markers selected (eg AMAS test). Depending on the results of these tests and especially when your cancer goes into remission, these guidelines may be somewhat relaxed in consultation with your doctor.

The Hauser diet is less strict than other cancer diets with respect to certain food items that are forbidden in other cancer diets. The following items are allowed in the Hauser diet:

- Organic meats: fish, pork, beef, lamb, venison
- Dairy products: organic milk, cheese, yoghurt, butter
- Eggs: organic free range eggs
- Nuts and nut butters: preferably raw. Avoid rancid products
- Soy products (unsweetened soy milk, also when fortified with protein and calcium), tofu, tempeh, soy protein shakes
- Vegetables: preferably dark, deeply colored, fresh veggies. Limit intake of maize products, white potatoes, carrots and beets to two servings per week.
- Fruit: limit to one serving per day. Berries are preferred. Limit bananas and oranges to two servings a week and avoid over-ripe bananas. Avoid all fruit juices except immediately following IPT to restore blood sugar levels.

The following food items are prohibited in the Hauser diet:

- Avoid all grains and flours except soy flour. One or two servings per week are permitted of brown rice, millet and quinoa.
- Avoid all breads.
- Pasta: avoid all pastas. High protein lentil pasta once or twice a week is permitted.
- Beans: limit all beans (except soy) to 1-2 servings per week
- Avoid all sugars and artificial sweeteners.

These principles are extremely important for the cancer patient, and adhering to them will also prevent you from getting cancer in the first place.

Note that as it stands the diet is extremely strict. It may be relaxed somewhat in consultation with your doctor when blood analyses confirm that your cancer is in remission. Consult the book by R. and M. Hauser referred to above for more detailed information.

If cancer cells receive the nutrients which they require, they are very difficult to kill, which is the reason they will "steal" so many nutrients from normal cells to the detriment of the patient. There are cases on record where patients have cured their cancer simply by making a massive change in their diet. On the other hand, many alternative cancer treatments have failed simply because the patients did not appreciate the importance of diet. We see, therefore, that the diet either interferes with, or supports the treatment.

It is, however, very difficult for a person used to a typical destructive Western diet to suddenly switch to a strict cancer diet, especially bearing in mind that the person will perhaps have to live for months or years on the cancer diet. It is therefore permissible to modify the cancer diet for a transition period of one month to facilitate a process upon which his life depends. This can be done by allowing a few low glucose items during this period such as pineapples, avocados, celery, spinach, etc.

Ideally, the cancer diet should provide more fat (25-30 %), fewer carbs (30-40 % complex carbs) and more protein (25-30 %) than the diet advocated by most dieticians. Select only food items (especially the carbs) with a glycemic index (GI) lower than 60. Lists of the GI indices of foods are available on the Internet.

The principle is to eliminate all foods with a GI index of more than 60, and to replace some of the carbs. It is also important to supplement with essential fatty acids using more or less equal quantities of w-3 (fish oil) and w-6 fatty acids (sunflower oil, unadulterated and cold pressed). A good level of supplementation is 3g daily of each.

Metabolic typing and the cancer diet

Even the utmost dietary refinements are of little value if we treat all people in the same way, because we are not all the same, metabolically speaking, and therefore also in the dietary sense.

The previous section gives general outlines of what the cancer patient should eat and what not. Within these dietary guidelines, many different food combinations are possible, not all of which will be equally acceptable or beneficial to all people. This has led to the recognition of at least 2 different types of people: the slow reacting Type A (parasympathetic) person and the fast reacting Type B (sympathetic) person. But experience has also shown that everyone has some Type A and some Type B characteristics. In spite of this, it is possible to distinguish between the predominantly Type A or predominantly Type B patient by means of certain personality traits and even with the aid of certain blood determinations. In the Yin and Yang types recognized by traditional Chinese medicine, Yin roughly corresponds to the Type A or parasympathetic type and Yang with the sympathetic nervous system dominant type. Such a distinction assumes added significance if we are dealing with sick people such as cancer patients.

It has also been documented that the Type B patients feel quite well on a low protein diet while the Type A person requires a higher intake of protein. These limitations are not so sharp in practice because, as we have said, most people are of the mixed A and B types, but in any particular patient either the A or B characteristics may be dominant. It is therefore of some importance to be able to recognize these and to consider them when selecting foods from the list above for cancer patients.

General dietary guidelines for Type A and Type B patients

Ideal for the Type A patient:

- Low carbohydrate foods with limited fiber content. In these patients, high intake of dietary fiber may cause fermentation in the gastro-intestinal system
- Increased dietary protein intake including some meat
- These patients should restrict salads, fruit and raw food.
- These patients can handle apples, bananas, beetroot, celery better than stone fruit and berries.

Ideal for the Type B patient:

- Higher intake of carbohydrates with a relatively high fiber content
- Limited protein intake as proteins are not as readily digested by these patients, leading to the production of toxic by-products
- The best protein sources for these patients are yoghurt and cottage cheese.
- Meat should be avoided or strictly limited. The differences between the two types of people (A and B) go beyond dietary differences. They include differences with respect to climatic preferences, physical activity, temperature preferences and psychosomatic traits. The following table lists these in such a manner that you can use the information to determine whether your are predominantly Type A or B. Allot yourself points on a scale from 0 to 10 for the following preferences:

Type A	Type B
Do you prefer warm weather: (A)	Or are you more comfortable in a cold and windy climate (B)?
Are you uncomfortable in draughts and more comfortable in warm clothes (A)	Or do you prefer lighter clothing (B)?
Do you rarely perspire and if so then only to a limited degree (A)	Or much more pronounced (B)?
After physical exertion, do you perspire readily (A)	Or less readily (B)?
Do you prefer physical activity (A)	Or do you prefer to work reclined (B)?
Do you enjoy warm water baths and do you enjoy staying as long as possible in the hot water (A)	Or do you become uncomfortable after a while (B)?
Do you feel uncomfortable with flatulence after large quantities of fruits and salads (A)	Or do you quickly reach decisions without considering the consequences (B)?
Totals	
The following are some other characteristics of Types A and B:	
A	B
Diet carnivorous	Vegetarian
Diseases: hypertension, diabetes	Hypertension diabetes, high blood glucose
Preferences: meaty, fatty foods	Sweet fruits, dislike fatty foods

Supplements: K, Mg, Mn, Cr, B1	Ca, P, Vit A, E, B5, Biotin, Inositol
Requirements: Vit B2, D, B3, Biotin, PABA	Choline, bioflavonoids, niacinamide, folic acid.

The cancer patient will do well to use the information above to determine his/her dominant metabolic type and to take this into account in selecting foods from the abovementioned list.

Distressing symptoms that may accompany a change of diet

The above information implies that the cancer patient must be prepared to make radical changes to his customary diet, which he has been used to for so many years but which is probably the reason he now has cancer. Many alternative treatments (eg carrot and grape based protocols) have a strong cleansing effect by dissolving toxic deposits. The patient must therefore be prepared for some strong reactions from his body, many of which can be quite unpleasant. Also, the bowel movements may be foul smelling and in addition the person's body may also give off unpleasant odors. The patient may also suffer from diarrhea or constipation, which has to be treated symptomatically. These symptoms are a sign that the treatment is working, and distressing and unpleasant as they may be, the patient just has to live with them if he wants to get rid of his cancer. Fortunately, these symptoms become less severe after a few weeks.

Many alternative treatments rely heavily on a particular "cancer diet" or a "juice fast".

Several alternative treatments use a juice fast (which may last from 3-6 weeks) as a cancer diet. A true cancer diet, however, provides more and better balanced nutrition than any particular juice fast on its own, which should only be used for a limited time. For example, the Brandt Grape Cure uses a juice fast of nothing but grapes. Alternatively, as in the Gerson diet, carrot or beet juice is used. The theory behind such a juice fast is that the body (i.e. the cancer cells) is offered nothing but the particular juice. For example, in the Brandt Grape Cure, the body (and cancer cells) has access only to the juice or mush from red, black or blue grapes. These grapes are known to contain several cancer-killing compounds such as resveratrol. Thus, during this treatment the body has access only to a food source that is rich in cancer-killing nutrients. In addition, the glucose present in grape mush helps to carry these cancer-killing nutrients into the cancer cells.

Killing the cancer cells by means of whatever treatment protocol is decided on, whilst at the same time feeding them by means of a wrong diet, is a futile exercise.

Such a juice fast should not exceed 6 weeks without a break and the patient should be aware that nutritional deficiencies may develop during such a fast because these juices—while rich in cancer-killing compounds—do not necessarily provide overall balanced nutrition. It is a good policy to be on the lookout for deficiency symptoms and to do blood analyses from time to time to check for adequate levels of critical nutrients (eg magnesium).

Because our typical Western diet is so full of cancer-causing junk food, the cancer diet severely restricts what you are allowed to eat. Conversely, do not eat what you are not specifically allowed to eat. Also beware of the foods that you crave for. Most of the time, people crave foods they are allergic to and those are often the very cancer-causing foods you need to avoid. This calls for a special effort on your part. According to the *Cancer Tutor* (32), fungi create food cravings because a fungus needs certain foods which it can only get from the patient. The patient, then, being deprived of the specific food, is stimulated to eat more of that food and in this manner a craving is created and the fungi are fed.

Not all cancer diets are the same. In some diets certain food items are forbidden for specific reasons.

In those diets which depend heavily on increasing systemic alkalinity, almost all fruits are forbidden, because these contain varying concentrations of acidifying glucose, and because cancer cells need large amounts of glucose. In other diets, on the contrary, fruit-derived glucose is a necessary part of the treatment, the reason being that the glucose is necessary to carry other cancer-killing compounds in the fruit into the cancer cells. A good example of where this principle is applied is to be found in the book by R.O. Young. The cancer diet, given below, resembles Dr. Young's diet (13).

The different food categories in the cancer diet (generally applicable)

The following food categories play a role in the cancer diet:

- Foods that contain cancer-killing nutrients stop the spread of cancer or in some other way helps in the treatment of cancer (eg red and purple grapes with skins and seeds as in the Brandt Grape diet),

strawberries with seeds, red raspberries with seeds, broccoli, carrots, pineapples, almonds, etc.
- Foods that cause cancer such as many commercial processed foods, margarine (because of the transfatty acids and other unnatural fatty acids), commercial sunflower oil, chemical additives to foods eg NutraSweet, MSG, etc.)
- Compounds that interfere with alternative treatments such as chlorine (eg in drinking water), fluoride (eg in toothpaste), alcohol, etc.
- Foods that feed and strengthen cancer cells and the microbes in the body (refined foods, refined sugar)
- Foods that damage the immune system and divert immune cells away from cancer cells (eg processed products).

You should also notice that the cooking and pasteurization of foods and especially of vegetables destroy many important enzymes and other susceptible compounds such as certain vitamins. Such foods are far less effective in treating cancer. Hence the fact that so many cancer diets are based on raw foods and juices. Thus, although carrot juice and beets are ingredients of many cancer diets, when these foods are cooked they are much less effective in the treatment of cancer.

For these reasons the foods in the ideal cancer diet should all be in the first category above ("foods that contain cancer-killing nutrients"). Every time you eat a food that is not in this category, you are interfering with your cancer treatment.

Foods in more than one category

Some diets, however, contain foods that are in more than one category. For example, the glucose present in grapes may be contra-indicated in many diets because it feeds the cancer cells which have a voracious appetite for glucose. However, in the Brandt Grape protocol, nothing but grapes is permitted and it is an excellent cancer treatment. In this case the glucose serves to convey the other cancer-killing compounds in grapes into the cancer cells. Thus grapes and other glucose rich foods should not be allowed in any other protocol where it will do more harm (by feeding the cancer cells) than good (killing the cancer cells).

Juices vs whole foods. When fiber is important, whole raw vegetables (mushed) are preferred to juices. When you juice, you also discard many nutrients that may be important. Also, mushes of whole fruits and vegetables are more easily digested and therefore provide more nutrients. But the fruits or vegetables used to prepare the mushes must be of the low GI variety (GI value preferably below 55-60).

Not all fruits and vegetables are the same as components of the anti-cancer diet. Some vegetables and fruits do not contribute significantly to the anti-cancer activity of the food.

Note that the word "fast" means something different from its usual meaning in alternative cancer terminology.

In alternative medicine it does not mean the total exclusion of food. First of all, it always implies that the patient can drink unlimited quantities of water as well as ingesting limited amounts of specified foods according to the particular protocol. For example, in the Brandt Grape Cure, which is called a "juice fast", the patient is allowed fairly large amounts of grapes in the form of a mush in addition to unlimited amounts of water.

The typical cancer diet consists largely of raw vegetables and greens including sprouts and juiced grasses.

However, the terminally ill and weak patient may not be able to digest these foods. Therefore special provision has to be made for such patients.

Diet for very weak and terminally ill patients

The following foods are used for such patients:

- Organic beef broth is essential
- At a slightly later stage, the patient may consider the Gerson diet because cooked foods are much easier to digest
- A well-balanced multinutrient supplement, preferably in liquid form
- Barley powder (5g or more daily).

Warning

You should strictly avoid chlorine, fluoride and other chemicals. It is extremely important to understand that tap water may contain all of these toxins and therefore no food product that has been made with tap water must be used, nor must tap water be used as such in the patient's diet. Once in contact with tap water, a product remains toxic although tap water as such may no longer be present in the product. For example, bottled grape juice must be avoided because during the preparation the chlorine in tap water reacts with the important anti-cancer phytonutrients in the juice to convert them into toxic, chlorinated compounds. Once chlorinated, the process and therefore the toxicity cannot be reversed. This example illustrates how meticulously careful the cancer patient must be in general about what he puts into his mouth.

The critical components of the diet

Vegetables. These should be organic. Green vegetables, grasses (juiced if possible) and sprouts are the foundation of the cancer diet. These products provide the fiber, enzymes, vitamins, minerals and many other nutrients that are required by the healthy cells in the cancer patient. These items are an absolute must for the cancer patient. Some of these should be in the form of whole foods to provide the necessary fiber which is critical for the patient. If the patient is in a very weak condition, some of these whole foods may be presented in a lightly cooked form. Juices should be drunk immediately after preparation. Take these in the form of vegetables/salads/juiced grasses and sprouts for breakfast, lunch and dinner. Many of these can be mixed into salads.

The following are allowed vegetables according to Dr. Young (13):

- *List A (known anti-cancer foods) a*sparagus, broccoli, beets, cabbage, carrots cauliflower, peppers, kale, parsley wheat grass, barley grass, sprouted grains and beans garlic, onion as much as desired to improve taste.

These items should preferably but not necessarily be juiced.

- *LIST B (other permitted foods) c*elery, cucumbers, egg-fruit (brinjals) squash green beans and peas spinach, collards • lettuce, radishes, Swiss chard, sea vegetables.

Notes:
1. *Sprouts* sourced from healthfood stores may be heavily contaminated with micro-organisms. Wash carefully but preferably prepare them yourself.
2. In general only whole *nuts* are permissible, especially almonds and macadamias, because they both contain laetrile. Walnuts are also permissible—they contain omega-3 fatty acids. Peanuts and cashews are not allowed since they are heavily contaminated with fungi. Walnuts, of course, are part of the Budwig diet
3. High quality *protein* may be somewhat of a problem with such plant-based diets. This is best included by means of legumes and certain sprouted seeds such as beans or peas.
4. *Soya* in all forms should be preferably avoided, according to this diet but not in the Hauser diet.

5. *Whole grains* are only included on a limited scale to avoid serious weight loss, but avoid commercially stored grains because they are heavily contaminated with micro-organisms. In cases of severe weight loss, consider the hydrazine cachexia plan presented in the CsCl/DMSO protocol. Maize, rice, and potatoes should be avoided because of the way they are handled commercially. A small portion of boiled potato fresh from your own garden is allowed
6. *Yeast products.* Avoid all products made from yeast such as all types of bread and beer.
7. *Animal products.* Meat, fish, poultry, eggs and dairy products should in general all be avoided or strictly limited for many different reasons. The only exceptions are a small amount of fresh water fish eaten alone (if the patient cannot eat beans and other legumes), yoghurt and cottage cheese as in the Budwig diet. In general, anything that comes from an animal is forbidden or should be strictly limited in this diet but not in the Hauser diet.
8. *Sweeteners.* All man-made sweeteners are forbidden. Use only the natural products Stevia or Xylitol.
9. *Sugar and refined grains* are all strictly forbidden, without exception. These products feed the invading fungi and also feed the cancer cells. Sugars not only deplete the body of key nutrients but also increase acidity. Honey is also disallowed because of its sugar content.
10. *Fruits, dried fruits and fruit juices.* The only fruits allowed in this diet are unsweetened lime, lemon and avocados.
11. *Chlorella and Spirulina.* Some experts allow this, but others disagree. I see nothing wrong with sensible amounts of both.
12. *SALT.* You must clearly distinguish between refined salt, which is mainly sodium chloride, and solar dried sea water salt which is a mixture of a variety of different salts (including magnesium). Refined kiln-dried sodium chloride (commercial "salt") with added anti-caking agents is a major cause of cancer, because together with the wrong fats (too much adulterated omega-6, too little omega-3, margarine) it causes the red blood cells in the blood to form stacks in which they stick together (called rouleaux), which interferes with their vital function of delivering oxygen to the cells. These clumped together bundles cannot pass freely through the smaller arterioles and capillaries, meaning that certain areas in the body get no or very little oxygen, which creates the conditions for them to become anaerobic (oxygen free) and therefore cancerous. Natural sea salt, on the contrary, has a mineral content which is very similar to that of blood and therefore much healthier. As a cancer patient you may use limited quantities of natural sea salt (47).
13. *Bad fats and oils.* Partially hydrogenated fats (meaning margarine) may be one of the main causes of cancer. The transfatty acids in these products are

incorporated in the cell walls, partly replacing cholesterol, making the cell stickier and less rigid (39). This may *inter alia* also interfere with the cell's oxygen exchange mechanism, further promoting anaerobic conditions inside cells and therefore cancer. Certain polyunsaturated oils (mainly those sold in supermarkets, eg commercial sunflower oil) have much the same effect. They should therefore also be avoided. Unadulterated sunflower oil (eg not hydrogenated, heated, or otherwise chemically treated to improve appearance) is a very important part of the cancer diet (see above), because according to Peskin, it promotes cellular oxidation as noted previously. A rule of thumb is to avoid all commercially manipulated and heated oils.

14. *Herbs and spices.* Most herbs and spices are acceptable in moderate quantities, but black pepper (which is a principal cause of acid reflux) should be avoided by the cancer patient because it is also highly acidic. Turmeric, which contains curcumin, is a potent anti-cancer food and is therefore acceptable.

15. *Restaurant, junk food and condiments.* Virtually all restaurant foods and condiments are absolutely forbidden and no compromise is possible. There is a long list of foods that should be avoided. The most important ones are any refined or processed food that contains sugar, refined carbohydrates, margarine, MSG, coloring, any additive, refined flour. Foods marketed as "no-transfatty acids" (eg the new generation of margarines) are not necessarily healthy: they have also been processed. Other obvious items to be avoided by the cancer patient are alcohol, smoking, caffeine as a food (it restricts blood vessels and oxygen supply to the cells), peanuts (because of fungi), maize and rice (because of the way they are stored), and cashews (high level of fungi). Also avoid oranges, tangerines and dried fruits and do not microwave your food, which, in any case, should be eaten raw as much as possible.

Warning

One danger of being on a juice fast or other diet high in raw plant food and juices is the possibility that one may be ingesting excessive quantities of Vitamin K. Vitamin K is needed for blood clotting and taking too much of the vitamin may cause blood clotting problems. Fortunately, not all vegetables are high in Vitamin K, so that it is possible to limit only those vegetables that are high in the vitamin whilst retaining the others. The following vegetables are high in Vitamin K: lettuce, cabbage, spinach, broccoli, Brussel sprouts, endive, turnip greens and green scallion. These items should make up no more than 30-35 % of the diet. When such a diet is followed for a long period (more than 40 days) it may be advisable to check blood clotting tendencies by means of appropriate blood tests. It is best not to try and balance an increased clotting tendency by means of blood thinner drugs and/or proteolytic enzymes which are blood thinners. It is best to use both in moderation where indicated

Excessive quantities of Vitamin K every day may cause blood clots to form, especially in the heart, lungs and brain. This may happen if the patient consumes large quantities of green, leafy vegetables which are rich in Vitamin K over long periods. It is essential for the cancer patient to use moderation and variety in selecting his diet.

The cancer patient and liver function

Compromised liver function is one of the earliest manifestations of impending cancer, and poor liver function is one of the risk factors for cancer. Dr. Gerson states that even before the symptoms of cancer appear, evidence of liver damage is present in many patients and as the cancer progresses, this becomes worse. The reason is that the liver is one of the most important outlets of toxins in the body. This is of special importance when, because of treatment, large quantities of toxins are released into the circulation which collect in the liver where they are processed (detoxified) before elimination. Liver function is therefore a critical issue (which is often neglected) in the cancer patient. Some alternative cancer protocols assist in supporting liver function as part of the treatment (barley greens, grape cure), but in others provision must be made to support liver function. One of the best known natural products used for this purpose is Milk Thistle.

Several alternative treatments devote special attention to liver function, eg the Gerson therapy which uses coffee enemas for this purpose. Coffee enemas open the bile duct of the liver, thereby promoting excretion of toxins to the colon for elimination.

There are many other things that the patient can do to support liver function. These include drinking more water, increasing the fiber content of the diet and exercising more. The lymph flow also relieves the toxic burden in the liver, and this can be promoted by means of exercise, especially the muscles of the arms and legs (47).

Many toxins that reach the liver come from the colon which means that at the beginning of any cancer protocol there must be a colon cleanse. More details of this are available elsewhere in this book and on the Internet.

Overview of treatment protocols of some types of cancer

Lung cancer (and emphysema)

Note: lung cancer is not a type of cancer that you should try to cure quickly. Treatment should be methodical but sustained. This means that you should not add other treatments in addition to those described below.

Because of the danger of congestion, treatment must include provision to deal with this problem. It is easy to kill the cancer cells in the lungs, but getting rid of the debris from the dead cancer cells without causing congestion is the problem. The resulting inflammation and swelling are mainly responsible for the congestion and inflammation. Moreover, the cancer itself can also cause congestion, aggravating the problem.

The other factors that can contribute to inflammation and congestion are obviously also important to consider in this situation. The following are some examples of complicating conditions:

- Any factor that may form excessive fluids inside or outside of the lungs
- Any factor that suppresses alveolar function (the alveoli are the structures in the lungs where the exchange of gases occurs)
- Other diseases that may cause inflammation and swelling (eg pneumonia).

Therefore, treating advanced lung cancer is a delicate matter best left in the hands of a health professional with experience. Success of treatment also depends on how far advanced the condition is. By the time the patient has been put on an oxygen mask, the condition is already far advanced and the prospects of suitable alternative treatment less favorable. The main reasons are that alternative treatments require time (2-3 weeks) before effects are seen and the patient may not have that much time available. As previously pointed out, alternative treatments may cause further inflammation and swelling, thus making matters worse when there is little time left.

It is therefore necessary to act as quickly as possible and to try and anticipate these problems and choose a treatment protocol that causes as little as possible inflammation and swelling. Unfortunately, although there are many protocols that will do this, they do not act fast enough. The immune-building treatments may be indicated if there is enough time left. Moreover, the treatment selected will also depend on whether you are dealing only with lung cancer or whether emphysema is also present.

For those patients who do not also have emphysema, a possible choice is the Bill Henderson protocol which largely depends on the Budwig Diet. The Bill Henderson treatment is a very gentle Stage IV treatment which does not increase lung congestion.

When used under medical supervision, IPT is the preferred treatment, but all patients should also receive a w-6 fatty acid supplement (unadulterated sunflower oil) to improve cellular oxygenation as suggested by the work of Peskin and Warburg previously referred to. This is important in all cancer patients, but it assumes special significance in the case of lung cancer patients where oxygen delivery to the tissues may be compromised.

The third option is the CsCl/DMSO protocol, which is a powerful Stage IV treatment that works quickly but which may cause congestion. The method can, however, be adapted to minimize this problem, *inter alia* by reducing dosage levels. The great advantage of this method is that it works quickly. Anyone contemplating it should consult a vendor with experience in this field. I recommend the Life Extension Foundation in America (for details see Essence of Life on the Internet).

Required additional treatments regardless of primary protocol

- Methylsulfonylmethane (MSM). This is compulsory treatment for lung cancer patients, regardless of whatever main treatment has been selected. MSM is a useful supplement in many different conditions, but it is especially valuable for lung cancer patients. It concentrates in the lungs (hence the bad breath that it causes) and is well known to reduce inflammation and swelling, also in other conditions. It also increases the oxygen level in the blood, amongst other things.

High doses are necessary. For example, an 80kg patient should take 10-20g a day, but the dosage should be gradually built up from 3g a day and increased by 3g per day.

All cancer patients should always pay meticulous attention to diet, and the cancer diet described in this book is a good starting point. However (according to the *Cancer Tutor*), in the case of lung cancer patients, it may be advantageous to substitute the Brandt Grape Cure for the cancer diet portion of the Bill Henderson protocol because of the excellent detoxifying properties of the Grape Diet.

- *The Overnight Cure for Cancer* (OCC). This is an experimental procedure (not yet widely used) which was developed by Webster Kehr and which may be resorted to as an emergency measure when all else fails. It does not cause inflammation and may reduce congestion. It is a perfectly safe procedure if the patient follows the safety warnings carefully. It has the advantage that it can be given safely to a patient who is in a coma because the main ingredients can be given either externally (DMSO) or by means of a feeding tube (MSM). Details are available elsewhere in this book.
- *Enzymes*. All lung cancer patients should take two enzyme supplements. The first is Vitalzyme (or Wobenzyme) to prevent inflammation and thus help to avoid congestion. Both enzymes are blood thinners and should therefore only be taken in moderate doses (eg 12 tablets per day of Vitalzyme for the first two weeks and then 6 per day for longer periods). These enzymes should never be taken with any anti-coagulant drugs; if you are on such drugs, you should inform your doctor. Barley powder is an alternative rich source of enzymes which could be taken instead of these two enzymes. Enzymes are necessary because they remove the protective protein coating around the cancer cells, which allows the immune system better access to the cancer cells.
- *Oxygen*. In order to raise the oxygen content of the blood. This is of special importance to the lung cancer patient because of the compromised oxygen absorption in the diseased lungs. Use a product such as CellFood (20 drops in water, twice a day) or, preferably, hydrogen peroxide therapy as discussed elsewhere in this book. In addition, a source of unadulterated w-6 fatty acids should be included to improve intracellular oxygenation.

- *Fungi.* Lung cancer is often the result of smoking. This is usually accompanied by a heavy load of fungi from the heavily infected tobacco leaves. Therefore, apart from treating the patient with antifungal agents such as SpectraZyme, caprylic acid, undecenylic acid and olive leaf extract as discussed elsewhere in this book, the patient should also be treated with agents that remove fungal toxins such as MycoDetox I and MycoDetox II (24).

Warning
Do not give large doses of Vitamin C as an additional treatment to lung cancer patients, as it can kill cancer cells, resulting in an excess of dead cells in the lung cancer patient who already has large numbers of dead cancer cells to cope with as a result of other treatment(s).

All cancer patients should receive a fatty acid supplement containing the correct proportions of unadulterated w-3 and w-6 fatty acids.

Emphysema

This is a very difficult condition to treat. The main problem here is a lack of oxygen in the tissues and treatment with oxygen-enhancing compounds is indicated. It results from the destruction (mostly by smoking and other chemical fumes) of the alveoli (air sacks) in the lungs. The patient finds it increasingly difficult to breathe due to loss of elasticity in the lung tissues until a wheelchair and supplemental oxygen become a necessity. Reduced tissue levels of oxygen force the heart to pump more forcefully, which in turn may result in elevated blood pressure. Conventional medicine has very little to offer the patient other than the wheelchair and supplemental oxygen.

Hydrogen peroxide for lung cancer and emphysema patients

Hydrogen peroxide is the first product to consider. It can be administered either orally or intravenously. Both can be used by the patient with emphysema, but the intravenous route is much preferred.

As a first step, dilute 40ml of medicinal grade 35 % hydrogen peroxide in 5 liters of chlorine-free pure water. Use this solution in a vaporizer to improve night-time breathing

Intravenous hydrogen peroxide given in a clinic has other more lasting effects as it has the ability to cleanse the inner lining of the lungs, thereby at least partly restoring the ability to breathe. Within minutes after administering the hydrogen peroxide intravenously, the liberated oxygen starts to clear membrane linings of the alveoli. According to Dr. Farr, the patient then begins to cough, thereby expelling the accumulated material in the lungs. The process can be controlled to avoid excessive coughing simply by decreasing or increasing the flow of hydrogen peroxide.

As the lung surfaces are being cleared in this manner and the accompanying bacterial infections are being cleared, the patient regains the ability to breathe more normally. According to the website "Educate Yourself" (Dr. Farr), reports have been received from patients who improved so much that a wheelchair and supplemental oxygen were no longer necessary.

This treatment must, however, be done at a clinic by an experienced health professional, because these patients are often on a variety of drugs which might cross-react with the peroxide. For example, the blood pressure may decline too much. There are also numerous other possible interactions that cannot be foreseen. Hence the desirability of having good medical supervision is recommended.

Moreover, a patient being treated with intravenous peroxide as described above is likely to experience additional congestion of the lungs due to the load of liberated toxins before there is permanent improvement.

Intravenous hydrogen peroxide is usually done by infusing a 0.375 % solution of medicinal hydrogen peroxide in a 500ml bottle, 1-3 times a week, each treatment lasting 1-3 hours. It is essential that the treatment is done in a clinic under medical supervision.

Hydrogen peroxide works not only by supplying oxygen to the tissues, but also by stimulating the immune system and the system of antioxidant enzymes including glutathione peroxidase, superoxide dismutase and catalase. The usual provision to increase intracellular oxygen as explained previously is always indicated when oxygen is administered.

Additional supplements

These are substances that will deliver additional amounts of singlet oxygen to the lungs in addition to that provided by the peroxide:

- DMSO and MSM
- Alpha lipoic acid
- CellFood
- Glutathione inhalation.

Details are available elsewhere in this book.

If the emphysema patient cannot arrange intravenous hydrogen peroxide treatment at a clinic as outlined above, the next best option is intravenous Ozone treatment which delivers controlled quantities of ozone gas from an ozone generator directly into the bloodstream and which can be done at home (see Ozone treatment discussion elsewhere in this book).

Ozone is only dangerous when mixed with nitrogen (when toxic nitrogen oxides may be formed), but pure medicinal ozone introduced directly into the arteries without contact with nitrogen is not dangerous.

Note that ozone treatment is suitable for both lung cancer patients and emphysema patients.

Brain cancer

Brain cancer is one type of cancer for which conventional medicine has very little to offer, especially in children. Chemotherapy and radiotherapy cause horrific side-effects and permanent retardation often follow such treatment. Very few of these patients survive for 5 years following such treatment and the quality of life is ghastly: the patient is constantly sick from the treatment and the immune system is severely damaged, making ultimate recovery virtually impossible.

The prospects following surgery are not much better. It has been estimated that neurosurgeons do not do much better than one patient cured of every 1000 treated (24). Radiotherapy slows the growth of brain tumors in adult patients but usually does not gain more than one month of life whilst the cure rate is of the order of one in 500—1000 patients. Chemotherapy, after more than 30 years of development work and clinical trials, has not come up with a drug that specifically penetrates the brain to a significant extent.

This problem can be largely overcome by including DMSO in the treatment protocol. This is the only treatment available that will help target the cancer-killing drugs used to kill the cancer cells in the brain. IPT with DMSO included would be the therapy of choice (see DMSO Potentiation Therapy, DPT). DMSO has shown to effectively help transport drugs across the blood-brain barrier (Hauser).

Because of the danger of swelling of any kind (arising from dead and dying cancer cells), this type of cancer requires specialized treatment. Dangerous seizures may arise because of inflammation caused in this way. The CsCl/DMSO protocol is the preferred treatment, but the doses of CsCl are generally lower for brain cancer patients to prevent these complications. Immediately consult your oncologist/surgeon and do not start any treatment before your oncologist has identified the type and precise location of the cancer and whether there is any danger of lethal swelling and dangerous pressure build-up. If necessary, immediate surgical intervention should be considered. Do not depend on alternative cancer treatments to work fast enough to relieve such pressures in this situation, and let your oncologist decide whether surgery is indicated. Most alternative treatments will make swelling and inflammation worse before it gets better. These therefore require special care and surveillance in which your oncologist must play a major role.

Chemotherapy drugs generally do not penetrate the blood-brain barrier sufficiently and selectively and the other conventional treatments are equally of limited value. The brain cancer patient must therefore rely entirely on alternative cancer treatment methods. This is one of the reasons why you should work with an oncologist/surgeon who understands the value of the alternative methods.

Because of the dangers created by inflammation/swelling in the brain, it is essential that all brain cancer patients, either on alternative or conventional treatment, carry anti-seizure medication with them at all times. Such a patient should always be in the company of someone who knows how to use the anti-seizure medication. Note that DMSO greatly improves the penetration of the blood-brain barrier by CsCl, thus not only enhancing the anti-cancer effects but also increasing the chances of seizures.

When are you a Type IV brain cancer patient?

If you have one or more of the following types of brain cancer, you qualify as a Type IV brain cancer patient:

- Glioblastoma or any form of it
- Any fast-growing brain tumor
- A brain tumor in a dangerous anatomical location
- A high mortality rate brain tumor
- A dangerous swelling (see above)
- Any other cancer in addition to brain cancer.

In addition to the cancer treatment protocol chosen, the brain cancer patient, regardless of the Stage IV protocol he/she is on, must take the following supplements to combat inflammation/swelling:

- A powerful multi-enzyme formula such as Vitalzyme, but do not use enzymes if the patient is on blood thinners
- Barley powder (5g daily)
- MSM 5-15g/day. Must be a pure product with no additives
- Oxygen treatment (see below)
- Vitamin C high dose, buffered (7-10g /day)
- Alpalipoic acid (500mg).

Brain cancer is a very serious condition for which no effective conventional treatment exists. Alternative treatments are effective in most cases, but the treatment needs to be carefully fine-tuned to the patient's needs. The CsCl/DMSO protocol is effective, but dangerous if significant inflammation and swelling or seizures are already present. There are no professionals with sufficient experience available in South Africa whom you could approach for advice and guidance. In America, Larry of the company Essence of Life is a possibility (32).

The other alternative is to use the Bill Henderson protocol which we discuss elsewhere.

Multiple Myeloma (MM) and other bone marrow cancers

Multiple Myeloma is a Stage IV bone marrow cancer, but the high number of malignant plasma cells produced in the bone marrow carries with it the risk that these malignant cells may invade the surrounding bone. This may actually dissolve bone to create an osteoporosis-like bone structure, with all the accompanying dangers. These brittle bones may start to break, causing all the known complications of osteoporosis. The patient may also then suffer severe mental and emotional trauma.

> *For this reason, Multiple Myeloma needs to be treated as a bone cancer even though it is a bone marrow cancer.*

The CsCl/DMSO protocol is the recommended treatment for both, because the cesium chloride readily penetrates bones and enters the bone marrow where it can kill any cancer cells. IPT under professional guidance is an alternative possibility.

Bone cancer patients also need to take a full spectrum of mineral supplements including strontium chloride.

Note: Melatonin should not be used by patients with cancers directly involving the immune system such as leukemia, Hodgkin's disease, lymphoma or multiple myeloma. Melatonin's stimulating effect on the immune system might worsen these immune system cancers.

Leukemia and myelodysplastic syndrome (MDS)

Note: Leukemia patients should not be treated with melatonin, as the immune stimulating effect of melatonin may aggravate this condition.

These two conditions are similar and will therefore not be discussed separately.

Leukemia (excess white blood cells in the blood) is a cancer of the blood-forming organs, namely the bone marrow or soft inner part of bone and the lymph system. In this condition, abnormal and immature white blood cells (leukocytes) are produced in the bone marrow and lymph system. In some patients the leukocytes may be so numerous that the blood assumes a whitish tinge. With the increased production of abnormal leukocytes, production of normal leukocytes decreases and the ability to fight infections is accordingly decreased. The ability to fight infections decreases because, as the abnormal leukemic cells accumulate, the production of oxygen-carrying red blood cells and platelets (blood clotting cells) as well as the production of normal leukocytes decreases. If left untreated, the surplus abnormal leukocytes overwhelm the bone marrow and then enter the bloodstream. Eventually they will also invade other parts of the body, including the lymph nodes, spleen, liver, brain and spinal cord, with loss of function in these organs.

Typical symptoms

These include weakness and chronic fatigue, fever and weight loss of unknown origin. Frequent bacterial and viral infections, headaches, skin rashes, non-specific bone pain, easy bruising, bleeding from gums or nose, blood in the urine and stools, enlarged lymph nodes and/or spleen and abdominal fullness may all be present, although these symptoms do not occur in all patients. The diagnosis is made through blood tests and examination of the bone marrow.

Causes of leukemia

These are largely unknown to orthodox medicine, although we can now state with a reasonable degree of certainty that micro-organisms (fungi, yeasts) are involved (32). Exposure to chemicals (benzene) may be a secondary cause. It is quite possible that decreased intracellular oxygen levels are partly responsible for leukemia, as is the case in all other cancers, as previously discussed (Peskin, Warburg).

Types of leukemia
Different types are defined in terms of how quickly the disease develops and progresses, and secondly on the basis of the type of blood cells involved. On this basis, four different types may be distinguished:

- Acute, chronic, lymphocytic, and myelogenic. As their names indicate, acute leukemias (often seen in children) progress very rapidly, while chronic leukemias progress very slowly.

In acute leukemia, the abnormal cells are blasts (immature cells) that remain very immature and therefore cannot carry out their normal functions. The number of blasts increases rapidly, and the disease, with all accompanying symptoms, progresses rapidly.

In chronic leukemia, some blast cells are present, but in general these cells are more mature and can carry out some of their normal functions. In this condition the cells look mature, but they are nonetheless unable to fulfill all their normal functions because they are not completely normal. They also live too long, and therefore cause an accumulation of certain types of white blood cells. The number of blasts increases more slowly and the disease also worsens gradually.

Lymphocytic and myelogenous leukemia refer to the two different kinds of cells from which the malignancy develops. Lymphocytic leukemia develops from lymphocytes in the bone marrow. Myelocytic leukemia develops from either granulocyte white blood cells or monocyte white blood cells in the bone marrow. Acute lymphocytic leukemia is more common in children, while chronic lymphocytic leukemia is more common in adults.

Treatment of leukemia

Chemotherapy, radiation and bone marrow transplants are the methods of treatment used by orthodox medicine. In some patients this may cause remission, which may last for shorter or longer periods. Bone marrow transplants are the most successful, but permanent cures are very seldom achieved, because these methods do not address the original cause of the disease.

The treatment of choice is IPT under professional guidance, using the correct mix of 3 or 4 chemotherapeutic drugs and the CsCl/DMSO protocol. It should, however, be noted that these conditions are highly associated with microbial infections and that provision should be made in the treatment programme to treat these infections (11).

In this case microbes (fungi, etc.) in the bone marrow penetrate to the inside of immature cells (stem cells) and prevent them from becoming differentiated. It is very important for the leukemia patient to understand that in this condition fungi play an even more important role than in many other types of cancer. Every case of leukemia is associated with a type of fungus, to the extent that certain cases of fungal infection have been misdiagnosed as leukemia. In order to stop the spreading of the cancer, it is important to deal with all other kinds of microbes that may be present.

Chlorine dioxide (ClO_2) is a safe and stable substance that releases oxygen in the body. It is used in the form of a concentrated solution of sodium chlorite ($NaClO_2$) which is a precursor of chlorine dioxide (see later).

The chlorine dioxide liberates oxygen in the body, thereby both killing anaerobic microbes and inhibiting spore formation. At the same time, immune system response is enhanced.

The CsCl/DMSO protocol is also a strongly recommended treatment for leukemia, especially for those who wish to be treated at home. CsCl can attack the immature white cells (which accumulate in the blood in this disease) as well as any fungus without raising the pH of the cells. According to the *Cancer Tutor* (32), the usual microscopic methods used to study blood cells cannot distinguish between immature white blood cells that are alive and those that are dead. For this reason, the white blood cell count may be misleading after treatment that kills the cells.

Additional treatment

Apart from IPT, CsCl/DMSO and chlorine dioxide protocols, treatment should include antifungal medication as previously discussed (undecenylic acid, caprylic acid, olive leaf extract). Treatment should also include the powerful detoxification products MycoDetox I and MycoDetox II, available from InnerLight in America (see ref 32).

Because of the important role of micro-organisms in leukemia, it is also highly recommended for any leukemia patient to use the Bob Beck Electromedicine protocol in addition to the other treatments chosen. The Bob Beck protocol consists of four independent treatments (see the Bob Beck Protocol elsewhere in this book).

Note, however, that if a patient is on alternative cancer treatment, the other treatments cannot be used because of the dangers created by electroporation, which can be caused by both the blood electrification as well as the magnetic pulser. For several days prior to starting the Bob Beck programme, the patient must avoid any drugs and potentially toxic medication, nicotine, alcohol, laxatives, tonic, herbs and even potentially toxic nutrients which include certain vitamins. Because of electroporation, these substances may reach lethal concentrations inside cells (48). Because of this, patients who are using the Bob Beck protocol can only use colloidal silver, the water ozonator and supplemental unadulterated linoleic acid (to improve intracellular oxygenation) as additional treatments.

For additional information, please consult the *Cancer Tutor* (32).

Pancreas and gall-bladder cancer

Cancer of the pancreas is one of the most dangerous cancers, with most patients having less than 6-8 months to live. Treatment must therefore be both immediate and vigorous, using the most powerful treatment protocols available, such as IPT and CsCl/DMSO, preferably in combination with the Kelley enzyme protocol and unadulterated sunflower oil to improve intracellular oxygenation.

The common bile duct from the liver is attached to the head of the pancreas. Therefore, in pancreas cancer, the bile duct may become blocked and this may be manifested by yellow coloring on the skin (jaundice). This may, however, happen in any condition in which the bile duct is blocked. If the condition is due to cancer, you should see your oncologist/surgeon, who should decide whether surgical intervention is necessary. You should not rely on alternative treatments to shrink the tumor in this situation, since these treatments do no work fast enough.

Pancreas cancer is an extremely fast-growing and dangerous condition which requires the strongest possible Stage IV treatment as well as very strict attention to diet (the Robert O. Young diet with wheat grass is preferred).

In addition, it is vitally important to read the comments on pancreatic cancer under Dr. Kelley's enzyme treatment in this book.

My advice to patients with pancreatic cancer is to consult with their physicians, in case surgery is indicated and to immediately commence with IPT and/or CsCl/DMSO and the Kelley enzyme protocol, after consultation with their health adviser, and to work closely with their health professional. Under no circumstances should you attempt to treat this dangerous condition without professional guidance and assistance.

Breast cancer

Breast cancer is the second largest cause of cancer mortality in women, after lung cancer. In the USA, approximately 230 000 women are diagnosed with breast cancer each year, of whom 1 in 4 will die. Thus one in every 8 women will develop the disease which causes much morbidity and has staggering financial implications. Fifty years ago, 1 in 20 women suffered from the disease and now, in 2009, 1 in 8 women will develop it, with every indication of a sharp rise in the very near future. It strikes fear into the hearts of women because of its potential for disfiguring surgery and especially the possibility of metastatic spread with its high mortality and other associated consequences. Clearly the war on breast cancer is being lost, despite the large-scale use of the conventional methods of treatment which include surgery (ranging from the simple removal of a cancerous lump to radical removal of the breast), radiotherapy and chemotherapy or various combinations of these.

The incidence of the disease is now so high, and the rate at which it is increasing so alarming, that every woman must henceforth assume that unless she takes precautionary steps, she will sooner or later get the disease. This is particularly alarming when the low success rate of conventional treatments is taken into consideration. It also stresses the importance of understanding the message in this book and all the other good books on alternative treatment.

A particularly dangerous aspect of the disease is the fact that, by the time it is discovered, there is a strong likelihood that it has already spread to other tissues including the bones. The number of cancer cells present in the average tumor detected by mammography is 600 million, and by the time the patient can feel a lump, it has grown to 45 billion.

The first line of conventional treatment is usually surgery. Thereafter, oncologists usually recommend radiation therapy to reduce the risk of recurrence of the primary tumor in the breast. While this may be successful to some extent, it does nothing to prevent the spreading to the bones, brain and lungs, which is usually what kills the patient. Further follow-up treatment with combination chemotherapy may kill 98—99% of the metastasized cancer cells, but never 100 %. If only 1 % of the cancer cells escape destruction in this manner, it still means that 450 million are present and ready to multiply when conditions in the "inner terrain" are favorable. Moreover, growth of these cells is now greatly facilitated by the fact that the immune system has been significantly weakened by chemotherapy and other conventional treatments.

This is serious because the patient developed the cancer in the first place as a result of a relatively weak immune system and unfavorable "inner terrain" conditions (mostly due to lifestyle and diet). Our only hope to kill all the cancer cells lies in restoring the immune system and to correct all the unfavorable factors which determine the "inner terrain", including lowered intracellular oxygen levels.

As a result of all these considerations the long-term prognosis of the breast cancer patient using only conventional treatment methods is not good. The issue is sometimes confused by the fact that usually breast cancer is a slow-growing cancer. This often creates the false impression that the cancer has been permanently cured after initial conventional treatment, eg by means of surgery.

The most constructive approach to breast cancer can be summarized in the following steps:

- Immediately follow a cancer prevention lifestyle and dietary programme as detailed in this book
- Pay special attention to restoring your immune system, especially if you have received chemotherapy and/or other conventional methods (see the section "what is good for the immune system", in this book). Consider the most appropriate alternative methods, including as a first step IPT, in consultation with your doctor and after due consideration of what has been said in this book. Especially, try to prevent conventional chemotherapy in isolation and any kind of treatment without dietary support and due consideration of what has been said in this book.
- At an early stage and especially if the tumor is in a clearly defined area, surgery may be an option to be considered by you and your doctor
- Pay careful attention to the steps you can take to restore immunity, and remember that Beta-1.3DGlucan is one of the strongest immune stimulants known
- Reduce the saturated fat content of your diet. Swedish workers have found that by raising the fat content of the diet by as little as 10 %, the rate of breast cancer recurrence increases 4 to 8 times (49).

Timing of surgery in relation to the menstrual cycle

If surgery for breast cancer is indicated, choosing the correct time for the operation within a woman's menstrual cycle may make a significant difference in survival chances. One study on 289 premenopausal women destined for mastectomy or lumpectomy showed that those who had the surgery between days 18-20 of their cycle fared best in terms of survival (76 % better survival rate over a follow-up period of 18 years) compared to women who had surgery during days 3-12 of their cycle. This is due to progesterone levels which increase as the menstrual cycle progresses, but especially after ovulation until about day 23. In this study the desirable level of progesterone was found to be 4µg/ml.

In general, matching surgery to menstrual cycle in this manner doubles the survival rate for patients with cancers involving the lymph nodes (50).

How to prevent breast cancer

Conventional medicine has a number of approaches to prevention, which look impressive on paper but which are not entirely safe because they may aggravate the problem. Moreover, they are hugely profitable to the industry. Most of these practitioners honestly believe that what they are doing is beneficial for the patient, which ultimately it is not. As we have often stressed before, the corruption does not lie with the ordinary well-meaning clinician who truly has his patients' interests at heart; it lies with the system as it has developed over the years and within which he is forced to operate.

First of all, they have a Breast Cancer Awareness Programme, with the motto "Early detection is YOUR best PREVENTION". While the message as such is true, the way they propose to achieve the early diagnosis and early treatment are not.

Breast cancers may be either oestrogen receptor positive or negative, which can be clinically assessed either by means of biopsies or on tumor tissue after surgery. Oestrogen receptor positive tumors respond to oestrogen in the blood, which then stimulate the tumor to grow and proliferate. Oestrogen suppression therapy is widely applied as adjuvant therapy in the treatment of breast cancer.

Many doctors use the drug Tamoxifen to suppress oestrogen activity. It is supposed to block the entry of the strong oestrogen Estradiol into the tumor cells which, initially at least, are dependent on this hormone for growth.

However, this effect wanes with time, and after two years Tamoxifen no longer blocks oestrogen absorption by the cancer cells. Moreover, when entry into the cancer cells is blocked, the Tamoxifen may go elsewhere and stimulate growth in the lining of the uterus, causing endometrial cancer (1). An even greater problem with Tamoxifen is its relationship with insulin-like growth factor (IGF), a hormone produced in the liver after stimulation by growth hormone. As is generally known, the main function of IGF is to stimulate growth in young animals. The problem is that it also accelerates cancer in women sensitized by Tamoxifen, according to Drs. Wiseman and Martini of the Royal Victoria Infirmary. Thus cows treated with growth hormone have increased levels of IGF in their milk, which is linked to breast cancer in women.

In 1996 the WHO declared Tamoxifen to be a carcinogen, but drug companies continue to market Tamoxifen for the limited advantages that it offers. These advantages last for less than two years, after which it may actually cause breast cancer (1).

Therefore do not take Tamoxifen in order to prevent breast cancer (1).

There are other important causes of breast cancer that can be easily avoided by women, thereby considerably reducing their chances of ever getting the disease. Here are a few:

Mammograms. Dr. C. Simone, a well-known expert on breast cancer, says bluntly:

> "Mammograms increase the risk for developing breast cancer and raise the risk of spreading . . . an existing growth."

It has been said repeatedly in the medical literature that all the applications of X-rays in medicine increase the risk of cancer. A mammogram is an X-ray image of the breast that can reveal cancerous growths before they are detectable by other methods such as a physical exam. The use of mammograms can not only be hazardous, but does not always yield reliable results. One study on 60 000 women revealed that 70 % of tumors detected in this manner turned out to be false positives, which amongst other things were responsible for treatments that are unnecessary and distinctly hazardous (1). There are many other similar studies which confirm the risks associated with mammograms and their doubtful advantages.

The only reason why this practice is still continued and much promoted by the medical profession appears to be, according to Dr. Bollinger, the fact that it is such a lucrative source of income (1).

So, in order to prevent breast cancer, do not let doctors do regular mammograms on you. Consider other diagnostic procedures such as thermography.

Exposure to environmental chemicals. Although on first impression it may not sound all that important, this is in reality very important, albeit not readily visible. Many of these chemicals are oestrogen "mimickers", meaning that they can partly take over the role of oestrogen in the body, substantially increasing the patient's oestrogen load, which results in increased pressure on cells to proliferate and to become cancerous. Even more significantly, it has been shown that some of these carcinogenic pesticides ultimately find their way into breast tissue, where they are lodged and are concentrated, probably as a result of the high fat content of the tissues in that area.

Topical application of chemicals such as in shaving creams and antiperspirants appear to be another major cause of breast cancer ([1](#)). Toxins in the body accumulate mainly in certain areas, eg under arms, behind knees and ears and in the groin area where the toxins are eliminated in the form of perspiration. Antiperspirants prevent you from sweating, thus preventing the body from eliminating accumulated toxins in these areas. The body then finds somewhere else to deposit these toxins, and one such area appears to be the lymph nodes under the arms. The toxins accumulating there then create conditions favorable for the development of cancer. Numerous studies over many years have shown that all breast cancers develop in the upper outer quadrant of the breast precisely in proximity to the lymph nodes in that area.

At least one clinical study has demonstrated a connection between antiperspirants, underarm shaving and cancer. Women who regularly use these products develop breast cancer 22 years earlier than those who do not use them. Aluminium chlorohydrate is an important ingredient in these products.

A group of preservatives known as the parabens is also implicated as a cause of breast cancer These compounds, used as preservatives in underarm cosmetics and deodorants are derivatives of para-hydroxybenzoic acid, which is structurally similar to oestrogen. One study found traces of parabens in every sample of tissue taken from 20 different breast tumors.

An Israeli study found that the concentration of toxic environmental chemicals such as DDT and PCB was much increased in cancerous breast tissue compared to non-cancerous tissue from elsewhere in the same woman's body (51). The message is clear: there is some factor or factors present in breast tissue that attracts these toxins and concentrates them. This means that everybody, but especially women, should make a special attempt to avoid exposure to such environmental toxic organochlorine compounds.

Wearing a bra. Medical scientists Singer and Grismaijer, in a study involving 4700 women, found that women who wear a bra 24 hours a day are 125 times more likely to get breast cancer than those who do not (52).

- Further important conclusions from this study were: women wearing bras more than 12 hours a day but not in bed had a 1 in 7 chance of developing breast cancer women wearing bras less than 12 hours a day had a 1 in 152 chance of developing breast cancer women who rarely or never wore bras had a 1 in 168 chance of developing breast cancer

It is possible that the wearing of a bra restricts blood and lymph flow in the breast tissue, thus suppressing tissue oxygenation and toxin elimination, which are conducive to the growth of cancer cells, as we have seen.

Although these figures as they stand have staggering implications, it is still probably too early to take them at face value until the study has been repeated. But then, preventing disease has never been a popular subject, so that it is unlikely that we will soon see further studies in this regard. However, we can-not just totally disregard these findings, and in the meantime it seems that not wearing a bra is one of the options to prevent breast cancer. Taken together with all the other known risk factors such as exposure to chemicals, correction of nutritional deficiencies, etc., it seems that there is a real possibility of largely preventing breast cancer, which is much better than treating it.

Hormone Replacement Therapy (HRT). This is often recommended for postmenopausal women to reduce the risk of osteoporosis and prevent some of the unpleasant effects of the menopause. For this purpose, oestrogens are usually given in the form of Estradiol. Until recently, pregnant mare urine (Premarin) was used by doctors as a source of oestrogen, until it was shown to be ineffective and not without side-effects. Premarin contains conjugated horse oestrogens, some of which do not occur in humans.

It has also been shown that the side-effects are partly due to the fact that oestrogens were given without progesterone. The correct way to give hormones to postmenopausal women to replace hormone production lost during the menopause is to give bio-identical hormones, which means to give oestrogens as well as progesterone, and in quantities that are comparable to those produced in healthy premenopausal women and not more. It is also wrong to give progestogens (synthetic analogues of progesterone) instead of natural progesterone, as these are known to have serious side-effects of their own since they are not natural compounds.

Using the older type of Hormone Replacement Therapy formulations has shown that Hormone Replacement Therapy significantly increases the risk of breast cancer (53).

How one woman doctor treated her own breast cancer

This is reported in greater detail in Bollinger's book (1). Briefly the facts are: Dr. L. Day was diagnosed with invasive breast cancer which she had surgically removed. However, the tumor soon returned, in a more aggressive form which grew rapidly. As a doctor, she was aware of the fact that chemotherapy is seldom successful. She chose to treat herself and was cured with the Gerson protocol as detailed elsewhere in this book.

Preventing breast cancer metastasis

In all cancers, spreading of the cancer to other anatomical sites is a dangerous complication which is often the real cause of cancer deaths. Bone metastasis, with its accompanying severe loss of bone, is a particular problem associated with breast cancer.

Cancer cells that attach to bone cause its breakdown by promoting the activity of osteoclasts, a population of bone cells that break down bone as a normal part of a cycle in which bone is broken down and then rebuilt by another class of bone cells called osteoblasts. The balance of these two processes ensures maintenance of a healthy bone structure.

Metastatic cancer cells lodging in bone presumably break down bone by stimulating osteoclasts in order to obtain the minerals which they themselves require for growth.

> *By preventing orthoclastic activity, the biphosphonate drugs such as clodronate have been found to prevent metastatic tumor growth.*

Clodronate is a biphosphonate drug that has been used for nearly 20 years for the treatment of malignant bone diseases, and its clinical uses are well documented. It inhibits bone destruction, prevents bone fractures, relieves bone pain and prevents new bone lesions. It has been shown to be particularly valuable for the bone metastasis associated with breast cancer (54). It reduces the number of bone metastases in breast cancer patients by at least 50 %, which was associated with a simultaneous reduction in metastasis in other organs as well as leading to an overall reduction in mortality. Tumor-induced hypercalcemia (too much calcium in the blood) resulting from osteoclast-induced bone destruction is another common problem associated with breast cancer metastasis which responds well to clodronate. The biphosphonates also have analgesic (pain killing) activity. This is important in the treatment of bone metastatic growths, since these are often accompanied by intense pain.

An interesting property of the biphosphonates is their capacity to limit adhesion of cancer cells to bone.

There are obviously many advantages attached to the use of biphosphonates in breast cancer patients.

Because clodronate is relatively non-toxic and well tolerated, at least one source suggests that it is justified to start taking the drug as soon as a diagnosis of breast cancer has been made, especially in view of the fact that it has been shown to improve survival in these patients (55).

There is no reason why clodronate should not be used in conjunction with any of the treatment protocols discussed in this book. There is no reason to hesitate in suggesting such a step since in a way biphosphonates, being derivatives of phosphoric acid, can be considered to be natural compounds.

Breast cancer: what to do
M: medical supervision essential
S: medical supervision not essential

- *Conventional therapies* (M). Study the track record of these therapies together with your oncologist in an open-minded fashion. Whatever you do, do not rush into conventional chemotherapy. It has a dismal long-term success record. Depending on the location of the cancer and whether it is clearly localized, surgery may be useful to reduce the burden of cancer cells that the immune system has to fight.
- If the cancer has already metastasized to the bones or lungs, conventional treatments hold very little chance of long-term success. In that case, your best option is one of the stronger alternative therapies such as IPT and/or the CsCl/DMSO protocol or Gerson therapy as discussed in this book. Consider IPT and supplementation with unadulterated sunflower seed oil as the treatments of choice
- *Melatonin* (S): 3-30mg sublingually in slow release form at bed time
- *Indole-3-carbinol* (M): Two to three 200mg tablets daily as a substitute for Tamoxifen
- *Vitamin D3* (M): 75-100mcg daily on an empty stomach with monthly blood testing for toxicity and blood calcium levels
- *Multinutrient* (S): 4-6 tabs daily in divided doses
- *Omega-3 fatty acids* (S): 2 one gram fish oil capsules daily
- *Omega-6 fatty acids* (S): 2-4g daily of first virgin cold pressed sunflower seed oil

- *Dostinex* (M): 0.25-0.5mg twice weekly to suppress prolactin blood levels to below 3μg/ml.
- *Coenzyme Q10* (S): 200mg in an oily base taken in divided doses, preferably with oil or an oily meal)
- *Topical progesterone* (S): Apply daily as directed but do not exceed recommended dosage levels
- *Clodronate:* Use as directed.

Breast self-examination

While early detection and prevention is the best way of not getting breast cancer, the heavy emphasis placed on mammography by the medical profession is not the best way of achieving this. As previously pointed out, mammography in itself significantly increases the risk of breast cancer. Regular breast self-examination is a simple, effective and much safer means of achieving the same objective. To do this, firmly press the breast tissue against the chest with the fingers moving in a circular pattern from the outer edges of the breast toward the nipple. Palpate first lightly then deeper and be sure to examine the entire breast, covering the area up to the collarbone and over the shoulder to the armpit where numerous lymph nodes lie. Do the examination while standing and again while lying, preferably with the arm on the side being examined above the head. Look for any unusual features, including swelling, breast enlargement, dimpling and skin or nipple changes.

- Premenopausal women should examine their breasts 6-8 days after onset of menstruation, or shortly after their period ends. At these times the breasts are least likely to be tender.
- Postmenopausal women should examine their breasts monthly on a fixed date—perhaps the first day of the month to ensure constant checking.
- Women who have had a mastectomy should inspect the incision to feel for any nodules or skin changes.
- Any abnormalities detected should be immediately reported to your doctor or gynecologist.

Prostate cancer

Breast and prostate cancer are not only major health hazards in the Western World, but also appear to respond particularly favorably to treatment with natural products. They are also cancers that can be most easily prevented if one understands the underlying nutritional causes. It is extremely important to understand when to treat and how. In America, 244 000 cases of prostate cancer were diagnosed in 1995 and the incidence is increasing at an accelerated rate of approximately 20 % per year. The number of new cases almost doubled between 1990 (106 000) and 1994 (200 000) in that country.

Prostate cancer is generally classified as latent or benign, moderately progressive or rapidly progressive and extremely malignant. Screening by means of the prostate specific antigen test appears to be only of value in the case of moderately progressive prostate cancer, because in the case of tumors of the first type, there is no need to detect the tumor, whereas the extremely malignant tumors progress so rapidly that timely screening detection becomes nearly impossible and when accomplished may serve no useful purpose.

The latent harmless form of prostate cancer is the most prevalent. One study found that 15 % of autopsies of thousands of men in their 50s who had died suddenly from other causes had evidence of prostate cancer. This increases to 40 % for men in their 70s and to 80 % in the case of octogenarians. This means that in South Africa, approximately more than 1 million men have microscopic signs of prostate cancer that are relatively harmless. In such men, prostate specific antigen tests may cause unnecessary worry and premature, possibly harmful treatment. In such cases, prevention is much better than treatment. Prevention should include lifestyle and dietary changes as discussed in this book.

The prostate gland

Prostate cancer develops in the prostate gland, which is situated at the neck of the bladder. During the initial stages, the cancerous growth is physically isolated by a capsule surrounding the gland. As long as the cancer remains encapsulated (early stage prostate cancer), it responds well to treatment, including testosterone-blocking therapy as discussed later. At this stage, the condition is also known as testosterone (male hormone) dependent prostate cancer. This means that the cancer cells cannot grow without testosterone.

Hormone dependent prostate cancer

Gaining time—testosterone blockage therapy

Several drugs are used as testosterone blockers (eg Flutamide and Lupron). These drugs may be used to block testosterone activity at more than one metabolic point, including blocking testosterone production at both the hypothalamic level or at the testosterone receptor sites. In both cases, the cancer cells are deprived of testosterone which they require to grow.

It is critical to use these drugs at the right time and in the right manner, which only an experienced oncologist who specializes in the treatment of prostate cancer can do correctly. Early stage prostate cancer treatment with testosterone blockers usually causes the cancer to go into temporary remission, which may last for up to 3 years. Increased long-term benefit may be derived if the drugs are used intermittently to prevent the development of resistant cancer cells (non-androgen-dependent forms). This gives the patient time to make the necessary lifestyle and dietary changes and to follow other treatments that may bring about a permanent cure as discussed in this book.

Intermittent androgen therapy is monitored by means of blood PSA (prostate specific antigen) determinations. The drugs are given until the prostate specific antigen value drops below 0,5 µg/ml, when treatment is interrupted. This usually occurs after a few months. Thereafter the prostate specific antigen values will start to increase again (monthly monitoring of prostate specific antigen values). As soon as values have risen to 5.0µg/ml or 40-60 % of its initial value, another cycle of testosterone suppression is started in the same manner.

Other strategies to produce such temporary remission include inhibition of Prolactin (by means of Dostinex) and of the enzyme 5-alpha reductase. If these are used in combination with testosterone blockage, significant temporary remissions may be obtained which may even be permanent in some cases.

Prolactin suppression therapy

The female hormone prolactin, which induces lactation in pregnancy, also occurs in men. Rising prolactin levels in the cancer patient indicate progression of the disease.

It is assumed that prolactin facilitates entry of testosterone into the prostate cells, thus promoting progression of the cancer. Drugs such as Bromocriptin and Dostinex, which suppress prolactin secretion, are relatively safe and have been used for this purpose for a long time. This can be advantageously combined with intermittent anti-testosterone therapy (3 to 8 month cycles depending on prostate specific antigen levels). During the course of such therapy, the prolactin therapy can be continued for longer periods; up to 15 months.

It is interesting to note that high doses of Vitamin B6 (25-100mg of pyridoxine) also have a suppressing effect on prolactin secretion.

In the meantime, antioxidants and especially Lycopene (10-20mg per day) and other therapies discussed elsewhere in this book can be instigated. It is quite likely that during the periods of hormone deprivation, when the cancer cells are still dependent on testosterone for growth, the effects of these natural therapies will be more effective against the "weakened" hormone-deprived cancer cells.

Intermittent vs. continuous hormone blockage

Unless the testosterone blockage is continued indefinitely, it is unlikely that the tumor will end its testosterone dependence since, during periods when the blockage is interrupted, testosterone will once again be available to the cells.

However, during the periods of interruption, the cancer cells will now have another battle to fight—that of the patient's altered lifestyle, antioxidant and other supplements as well as the natural compounds used to treat the disease, a stronger immune system and the removal of the carcinogenic compounds in the patient's environment. This, in many cases, is sufficient to ensure a permanent cure.

The relative advantages of intermittent hormone blockage, compared to continuous testosterone blockage, have been studied in animals (56). The results showed that it was possible to maintain prostate specific antigen levels for 5-6 cycles of intermittent blockade in mice, which resulted in a 66 % increased time of cancer control in the intermittent group compared to the continuous group. During the final stages of the study, the intermittent group had prostate specific antigen levels 3.78 times lower than the continuous group.

Some oncologists report that clinical experience shows that in humans the situation is much the same, and that the time gained in this manner, is significant to remove the causes of the cancer and to institute nutritional therapy.

The significance of prostate specific antigen monitoring

In recent years, clinicians have looked at prostate specific antigen monitoring as a way of catching prostate cancer early, when treatment could be more effective. The disease can develop and spread with few or no warning signs. Especially in young patients, many cases are discovered too late, when the disease has spread beyond the prostate itself. Such cases are, from the conventional point of view, very difficult to reverse. Traditionally, conventional medicine believes that prostate cancer cannot be cured once it has spread beyond the prostate gland (57). With the aid of the various multimodal alternative therapies discussed in this book, such a view is no longer accepted by alternative therapists.

Clinical studies have shown that regular prostate specific antigen measurements and prostate specific antigen doubling times, together with recent refinements of analytical methodology (determination of "total" as well as "free" prostate specific antigen which allows determination of the malignancy-associated portion of the total PSA reading), will indeed facilitate early diagnosis, which will result in a better cure rate, even when only conventional treatments are used (58).

It is important to understand what a particular prostate specific antigen value means in terms of patient risk. In one study, 22 % of men with PSA values between 2.6 and 4.0µg/ml had prostate cancer, which was localized in the prostate gland in all cases. In another study on 559 men with initial prostate specific antigen values of 2 or less, only 3 (0.5%) had persistently raised PSA values above 4.0µg/ml for the following period of 3 years. In only one (0.2%) cancer was detected. In yet another study, the cancer incidence was 4.5 % in men with initial prostate specific antigen values of 2.1—4.0, which was 15 times higher than that of a second group with initial prostate specific antigen values of 2 or less (59). These figures give some idea of the risk in terms of PSA values at the lower end of the range. From these studies it may be concluded that men over the age of 40 should have regular prostate specific antigen determinations (at least once every 6-12 months) and if values are above 4.0, there is some reason for concern. If this happens to you, discuss the situation with your doctor in the light of the abovementioned and further information given below. You should avoid rushing into a biopsy at this early stage and especially avoid surgery and other conventional treatments at this early stage. Rather examine your lifestyle, diet and other risk factors critically, including exposure to carcinogenic factors such as smoking, and make amendments where necessary. In addition, your follow-up medical surveillance should include monthly prostate specific antigen determinations which will allow you and your doctor to discern the direction and rate of change of the readings. The doubling time of your prostate specific antigen readings is of particular significance.

On the other hand, one should clearly understand that there are strict limitations to the significance of a single prostate specific antigen reading. A reading above 4.0µg/ml is by no means proof that cancer is present, since other conditions may also cause a high reading, eg benign prostate hyperplasia, inflammation of the prostate (prostatitis), as well as mechanical pressure on the prostate. False positive tests based on a single prostate specific antigen reading are extremely common (50 % of tests). Such tests have more significance if they are considered together with other findings, eg a digital investigation of the prostate.

Hormone independent prostate cancer

In this condition, the disease progresses—as shown *inter alia* by rising prostate specific antigen values and other parameters—despite castrate levels of testosterone below 200μg of testosterone per liter. The condition is further confirmed by a lack of response to androgen suppression therapy.

The drug Nizoral is widely used in the treatment of this condition. It rapidly reduces testosterone levels and is often combined with hydrocortisone to correct for the simultaneous suppression of cortisone production. Its many advantages in the treatment of both androgen-independent as well as androgen-sensitive prostate cancer have been stressed (60). It lowers testosterone to castrate levels within 48 hours by mechanisms that differ from those of the anti-testosterone drugs. Nizoral blocks the production of testosterone by the testes and also suppresses the production of testosterone precursors (eg DHEA) which are converted in the testes into testosterone.

One of the main advantages of Nizoral—as in the case of hormone suppression of prostate cancer—is that it allows the patient to gain time for the nutritional and lifestyle factors and other natural treatments to take effect.

A complicating factor in the case of prostate cancer is the fact that cancer cells inside the prostate capsule are not homogenous—they occur in the form of clones or families. Some of these clones may be hormone dependent while others are testosterone independent. This obviously creates the possibility that treatment with hormone blockers may ultimately create a tumor mass that consists only or predominantly of hormone-independent cells, which is in fact what one sees in practice. In this manner heterogeneity is related to tumor size or burden. With increasing tumor burden, gene mutations also occur which may stimulate the multi-drug resistance gene, adding to the problems that may occur in the treatment of prostate cancer with drugs. This also leads to resistance to chemotherapy drugs. Therefore, tumor burden, testosterone resistance and resistance to chemotherapy drugs appear to go hand in hand.

All of this stresses the importance of other natural products that can be used in such cases. Of these, Lycopene (15-30mg/day) and, depending on the severity of the condition, the CsCl/DMSO protocol and/or IPT are of particular importance. In the light of what was previously said regarding oxygenation and its effects on cancer, all prostate cancer patients—regardless of stage of cancer and age—should be given a daily supplement containing the unadulterated w-6 and w-3 fatty acids as detailed in this book.

Some nutritional therapies in the treatment of prostate cancer

1. Lycopene

Lycopene is one of 500 carotenoids that occur as colored pigments in plants. Lycopene is the pigment that gives the red color to tomatoes and watermelons. It is the strongest antioxidant of all carotenoid and, perhaps because of this, it affords 10 times more cancer protection than beta-carotene, being particularly effective against breast, lung, endometrium and prostate cancer cells (61).

In one particular study, some 500 carotenoids were evaluated as protectors against prostate cancer in 47894 men. Only Lycopene, the most abundant carotenoid in the prostate gland, was found to have a protective effect against cancer (62). In men who ate at least two daily servings of tomato containing foods, the prostate cancer risk was reduced by 35 %. Fresh tomatoes did not have a similar effect and the reason for this is the extremely low solubility of Lycopene in water. Fats and oils (eg prepared foods) are necessary for the absorption of the fat soluble Lycopene.

Lycopene is the predominant carotenoid in serum and in a number of tissues including the prostate gland.

In 1990, Kucek reported one of the first controlled studies on the preventive effect of Lycopene on human prostate cancer. In this study, Lycopene supplementation was compared to placebo with regard to various cancer indicators (63). The study involved 30 men with localized prostate cancer destined to undergo radical prostatectomy. They were divided into two groups, a placebo group and an experimental group that received 15mg of Lycopene orally twice daily for 21 days before surgery. During surgery, prostate specimens were collected for evaluation of cancer status which included cancer volume, Gleason score, pathological stage and biomarkers for cell proliferation, apoptosis and differentiation. Serum Lycopene determinations showed that serum Lycopene levels had increased by 22 % in the experimental group.

The following results were found (experimental vs placebo groups): percentage of patients with organ confined prostate cancer (67 % vs 44

%); tumors smaller than 4ml volume (84 % vs 55 %). In addition, the serum prostate specific antigen levels and biomarkers for proliferation decreased, whereas the biomarkers for differentiation and apoptosis increased significantly in the experimental group.

The effect of Lycopene supplementation was unexpectedly large in view of the short time of supplementation and the fact that no provision for optimal absorption of the water insoluble Lycopene was made.

These results suggest a significant role of Lycopene in both the prevention and treatment of prostate cancer.

In order to improve absorption of supplemental Lycopene, I suggest that a concentrated tomato extract be used in conjunction with the Lycopene supplement.

Concentrated tomato extract in an oil base
500g of fresh, washed, ripe, organically grown tomatoes, cut into small pieces
100ml olive oil
100ml of first virgin, cold-pressed sunflower oil
900mg of Lycopene

Blend in a liquidizer or an electric mixer for 5 minutes. Then heat the mixture for another 5 minutes until warm (60 ºC). Allow to cool, and then seal properly in an opaque glass bottle.

Use 10—20ml (2—4 teaspoonfuls) daily over food.

The use of the abovementioned oily Lycopene rich extract is to be strongly recommended.

Alternatively, Lycopene capsules should be used but in combination with oil such as cold pressed sunflower or olive oil. Take 15—30mg of Lycopene in capsule form together with one tablespoon of the oil daily.

2. *Multinutrient supplement*
A good multinutrient supplement supplies other micronutrients that are important for the prostate cancer patient. These include Vitamin E (400-600 iµ) and selenium (200mcg).

3. *Green tea extract*
The polyphenols in green tea inhibit vascularisation (new blood vessel formation) in cancer tissues, which is one mechanism that can be used to limit the growth of cancer. Take 2 capsules daily.

4. *Zinc supplements*

Zinc plays an important role in the prostate. The prostate patient should ensure a daily intake of 30mg of zinc in the form of supplements.

Lifestyle factors in the treatment and prevention of prostate cancer

Smoking

If you smoke and persist with that evil habit, there is nothing I can do to help you. It is not only important to stop smoking, but also to avoid passive smoking at home and at work.

Exposure to industrial and toxic chemicals

The average person in the UK ingests more than 4kg of foreign chemicals a year from a multitude of sources: fried foods, soft plastics, pesticides, agricultural chemicals, air pollutants, industrial wastes, food additives and colorants, hormone residues in foods such as meat, milk and many other foods.

In the context of prostate cancer, it is important to note that many of these chemicals are "hormone mimickers". This means that they have some (but not all) of the properties of natural hormones. At the molecular level they send the wrong signals to cells when they occupy hormone receptors at the cell surfaces, which in turn mean that processes that culminate in cancer may be "switched on".

Heavy metals like mercury and lead in drinking water are another source of contamination. Avoid this by using only suitably purified (reverse osmosis) drinking water. Mercury in dental fillings is another serious source of contamination. Otherwise reliable treatments often fail as a result of a high level of toxic contamination. Teeth with mercury fillings should be removed by an expert dentist who knows how to accomplish this without spilling mercury. In addition, the patient should take oral chelating agents beforehand as a protective mechanism.

The prostate cancer patient should make every attempt to clean up his environment.

Alcohol consumption

The prostate cancer patient should avoid alcohol completely, especially during the initial phases of treatment, until such time as the disease is well under control. Even then, alcohol intake should be limited to one drink a day.

Diet

This is of the utmost importance. No cancer treatment can succeed without due and strict attention to diet. Follow the cancer diet given in this book. Foods containing tomatoes reduce prostate cancer risk by 45 %. You should have at least 10 servings of these per week. Lycopene supplements (15—30mg per day) have much the same effect, especially when taken in combination with a fatty meal or fish oil supplements as indicated above

- Fish oil supplements (1—2g/day) will also reduce risk
- Sunflower seed oil: use 2—4g of first virgin, cold pressed oil
- Selenium (400—600mcg/day) as part of a multinutrient supplement suppresses the growth of prostate cancer cells (64)
- Exercise: physically active men have a much lower risk of prostate cancer
- Overweight increases the risk.

Prostate cancer: what to do
M: Medical supervision essential
S: Medical supervision not essential but desirable

Early stage prostate cancer

- IPT (M)
- Intermittent hormone blockage (M) if cancer is still hormone sensitive
- For hormone insensitive cancer (M): Nizoral
- Lycopene (S): 30mg daily in an oily base, preferably with a fatty meal or with other oils (eg flaxseed oil; see concentrated tomato extract above)
- Omega—3 fatty acids (S): 1—2g of fish oil (*Fortifood*) or 1 tablespoon of flaxseed oil
- Sunflower seed oil (S): 2—4g of first virgin, cold-pressed sunflower seed oil
- Vitamin D (M): 75—100mcg daily on an empty stomach with monthly blood testing to control toxicity and possibly rising blood calcium levels
- Lifestyle factors: as discussed
- Multinutrient (S): 4—6 tabs daily
- Regular prostate specific antigen monitoring (M).

Advanced prostate cancer with metastases
Follow the abovementioned protocol where appropriate (M)

- Insulin Potentiation Therapy (M)
- CsCl/DMSO or Henderson protocol (M)

Skin cancers (squamous cell carcinoma and melanoma)

Skin cancer is the most common of all cancers, one out of every 3 new cancers being skin cancer. Fortunately not all skin cancers are dangerous. Chronic over-exposure to sunlight and a deficiency of unadulterated fatty acids is the cause of most skin cancers, which occur most frequently on exposed areas of the body such as the face, ears, neck, scalp, shoulders and back.

The following are the main types of skin cancer:

- Melanoma, a malignant and dangerous tumor that originates from the melanocyte cells in the skin
- Basal cell carcinoma, originating in the basal cells of the skin
- Squamous cell carcinoma, originating in the squamous cells in the skin.

Of these cancers, melanoma is by far the most dangerous and notorious for rapid spreading to distant sites. In this case spreading does not occur in the usual way where cancerous cells are detached and move to different parts to start new growths. It seems possible that a deficiency of w-6 fatty acids originally caused the cancer, or perhaps that certain micro-organisms come out of the cancerous tissue and move in the bloodstream to burrow into the normal tissues elsewhere to start new growths ([1](#)). For this reason the spread is extremely rapid and treatment should in the first place be aimed at removing the causes. For this purpose there are antifungal and other drugs as well as high-quality w-6 supplements available which may be used topically.

Melanoma is a very dangerous cancer and must be correctly handled from the onset. Once metastasis (spreading) has occurred, it is extremely dangerous, with a very low success rate, at least with conventional treatment. It calls for a strong Stage IV treatment such as IPT and/or CsCl/DMSO with strict attention to diet. Dr. Max Gerson and the Gerson Institute in

Mexico have listed an impressive number of melanoma patients successfully treated by means of the Gerson protocol as outlined in this book.

Basal cell carcinoma begins in the deep basal cell layer of the outer layer of the skin (epidermis). It occurs 6-8 times more frequently than melanoma but is much less dangerous, being a slow growing cancer that does not spread to other tissues.

Squamous cell carcinoma begins in the squamous cells of the epidermis. It is less common than basal cell carcinoma but grows faster than basal cell cancers, especially when located near the eyes, ears, mouth or pubic area.

Ty Bollinger describes the successful use of escharotics pastes in the treatment of skin cancer (1).

Bone cancer

Bone cancer is difficult to treat, both by means of orthodox and alternative methods. The treatments of choice are the CsCl/DMSO protocol and IPT in combination with a bone mineral supplement containing strontium chloride.

Quite often cancer in other areas tends to spread to the bones, which means that treatment for the original cancer should include pre-emptive steps to treat bone cancer. Regardless of what treatment protocol for the primary cancer is followed (eg the CsCl/DMSO protocol) it must also include a supplement to rebuild bone. Such a supplement should include a strontium salt such as strontium chloride or carbonate as well as other bone-building minerals (details available on the Internet). The correct balance of these minerals, which may require some experimentation to determine, will reduce and even prevent pain in the bones. The bones of bone cancer patients often become so brittle that they might easily break, even during normal activities. This has an adverse effect on the patient's morale and his/her will to fight the disease. It is therefore critical to strengthen the bones as indicated above, even if bone metastases are only in the initial stages.

Note that not only calcium is required to build bones, but there are several other minerals that are required:

- Strontium (the natural mineral in the form of chloride or carbonate) (1)
- Magnesium
- Various micro minerals (34)
- Silicon (34).

Note: Never supplement with phosphates as a bone supplement or for any other purpose as is often recommended by dietitians. The reason is that calcium and phosphate have to be present in balanced quantities of roughly 1:1. The Western diet provides 2-4 times more phosphate than calcium. Typical Western foods such as meat and poultry contain 10-20 times as much phosphate as calcium, and most soda pops and cola drinks, apart from being acidifying, contain large excesses of phosphate. In the presence of excess phosphates, the body withdraws calcium from bones, thus weakening the bone. This can lead to osteoporosis and osteopenia that make bones brittle and fragile. Too many phosphates may not be the only reason for bone brittleness in bone cancer patients, because the cancer itself contributes to this. Phosphates should be avoided by people with bone cancer. As long as a patient does not have a cancer that is more dangerous than bone cancer (eg cancer of the pancreas), it is best to design the treatment around the requirements for bone cancer, including steps to strengthen the bone structures

Liver cancer

Because the liver is such a vital organ, the body does everything in its power to maintain liver function, even when it is seriously diseased as in the case of liver cancer.

Two vital steps are necessary in any treatment programme of liver cancer. Firstly, toxic chemicals may have accumulated in the liver; these have to be removed before healing can begin. Secondly, the healing process which entails the killing of the cancer cells and restoration of the patient's inner terrain can then begin.

Because of its capacity to detoxify, the Brandt Grape Cure is one of the first protocols to be considered for treatment. The variation of the Brandt protocol, in which vegetable juices are substituted for grape mush, is also acceptable. One study done at NHS looked at the effect of various carotenoids on the invasion of liver cells by tumor cells. All the carotenoids investigated inhibited the invasion in a dose-dependent manner. The results suggest that the anti-invasive action towards the tumor is the result of the antioxidant properties of the carotenoids.

Essiac tea is also strongly recommended, on the strength of numerous personal reports of the successful treatment of liver cancer. This product can be combined with the Grape juice protocol. One problem is that good quality Essiac tea may not be easy to obtain in South Africa. Consult the

Internet to find overseas vendors, but make very sure of the quality of the product that you buy.

These treatments can be combined with IPT under medical guidance.

The Bill Henderson protocol, which has the Budwig diet as the core of its procedure, is another treatment for liver cancer recommended by the *Cancer Tutor* and which can be combined with Essiac tea.

Other natural compounds that have been used in the treatment of liver cancer include: Vitamin D3 (4000-6000IU daily on an empty stomach), copious quantities (2-3 liters a day) of clean, chlorine free water, curcumin (used with black pepper to improve absorption) and Inositol hexaphosphate (IP6).

The latter is of particular interest in that it was demonstrated reverting human cancer cells back to normal cells (1). Moreover, IP6 has been studied in the treatment of a variety of other tumors in cell culture and experimental animals.

The lymphomas

These are a group of diseases of the lymph system, affecting mostly the lymph glands. The treatment of choice is IPT and the CsCl/DMSO protocol, but in certain cases (mantle cell lymphoma) and depending on the severity of the condition and where the tumor is situated, the CsCl/DMSO protocol may be contra-indicated, especially where there is evidence of a lymph node pressing on a critical anatomical site (trachea, esophagus). The cesium treatment does not cause sufficient decrease of the tumor size (and might even increase it). In such cases immediate medical attention may be required, and often chemotherapy or, better still, IPT is indicated as a temporary measure. Conventional chemotherapy will not cure the condition but will resolve the lymph node size more than the temporary swelling caused by cesium therapy. At a later stage, when the tumor size has decreased sufficiently, cesium therapy may be used to kill the cancer cells.

Lymphomas may be difficult to treat, and in problem cases it is best to seek advice from experts who have specific experience in handling any particular problem. The *Cancer Tutor* recommends Larry from Essence of Life for this purpose, who can provide advice on the telephone. Alternatively, the Wolfe Clinic in Canada can be approached for assistance (32).

The Bob Beck protocol (discussed elsewhere in this book) is another option strongly recommended by the *Cancer Tutor*. In this case electro medicine is used to treat the lymph fluids. The Magnetic Pulse Generator is used specifically to clean the lymph system of parasites. The complete cure lasts only 4-8 weeks, so that it is necessary to follow this with some other suitable remission treatment which may even be the CsCl/DMSO protocol or IPT.

As previously pointed out, both the Magnetic Pulse Generator and the Electromedicine treatment cause electroporation, which means that absolutely no drugs or other chemicals must be present when the protocol is used. This is critical. The only other products that are allowed during this treatment are Colloidal Silver and Ozonated water. It is strongly recommended that before using the technique, the patient and his doctor should read the article by J.C. Weaver (70).

Colorectal cancer

Colon cancer is the second most common cause of cancer deaths. Many studies have linked it firmly to lack of fiber in the diet. Insoluble fibers (eg wheat bran, brown rice, pulses, lentils, Brussels sprouts) reduce the incidence of colorectal cancers by binding bile acids, increasing stool bulk and decreasing transit time. Soluble fibers (oat bran, apples, citrus fruits, carrots and psyllium husks) lower cholesterol levels, nourish friendly bacteria, slow the rate of entry of sugars into the blood and bind heavy metals.

Before treatment of this condition is commenced, it is vital to know exactly where the cancer is situated and whether any danger of critical occlusions may occur. The treatment selected must take this possibility into consideration.

This is another situation where dead cancer cells may cause swelling and obstruction. Where possible, such cancers should be surgically removed, followed by IPT, CsCl/DMSO or Bill Henderson protocols. If the intestinal tract is already blocked, no alternative treatment should be given until such blockages have been removed surgically.

Colorectal cancer is the second most prevalent cancer in the world and at the same time one of the deadliest. It is responsible for one out of five cancer deaths, and more than 50 % of colorectal patients will die. One reason for the high death rate is the fact that it is usually detected at a late stage. Detected early, progression of the disease is entirely preventable using the methods discussed in this book.

Early detection of colorectal cancer
Visible blood on the surface or mixed in the faeces is a reliable early indicator of the disease. Blood in the faeces can also be detected by means of

a chemical test ("occult blood test"). In rare cases, pain and tenderness may be present in the lower abdominal area, but in general no symptoms appear until the tumor has grown so big that it causes functional disturbances such as obstruction or rupture of the intestine. This is an emergency situation which calls for immediate surgery and the strongest possible form of treatment. Under no circumstances should the patient try to treat this dangerous condition without expert medical guidance.

The Guiac test or Haemocult test is a simple test that reveals the presence of colorectal cancer. In this test, a sample of faeces is applied to a card impregnated with a plant gum called guiac. This gum turns blue when it comes into contact with the red pigment (hemoglobin) in blood. The test is carried out by applying a liquid haemocult developer to the faeces on the card. The test may yield a false positive result if the patient has recently consumed certain foods such as red meat (which also contains hemoglobin) iron tablets, anti-inflammatory drugs, aspirin, certain fresh foods and vegetables, which should all be avoided for a 24 hour period before the test.

A positive result should be followed up by sigmoidoscopy, which is a more reliable method of revealing polyps and tumors. The presence of polyps may serve as a warning that colorectal cancer may develop in the near future

To lower the risk of colorectal cancer, many clinicians recommend a vegetarian high fiber diet in which meat and fat are restricted. Other authorities like Dr. Hauser prefer the anti-cancer diet previously discussed. In persons older than 50 years, regular sigmoidoscopy every 2-3 years is advisable. It has been claimed that the consumption of red meat (but not poultry, fish or other white meat) is the most important risk factor for colorectal cancer. Refined sugar, wheat flour products, diet low in fruits and vegetables and low in fiber are other important risk factors (65). Dairy products, with the exception of yoghurt, should also be limited. In general, a diet rich in cereal grains, fresh vegetables and low GI fruits should be followed. Legumes, fish, and pulses are the healthiest sources of protein for everyone at risk of colorectal cancer or already with the disease. Other protective dietary factors are garlic, onions, cruciferous vegetables and chives (66). Alcohol, processed meats and smoking are also risk factors, initiating and promoting colorectal cancer or recurrence of the disease (67).

In addition, people who drink chlorinated water have a 20-40 % higher risk of developing the disease (67).

If colorectal cancer has been detected, the dietary steps indicated above and one of the alternative treatments described in this book, including IPT, should be considered in consultation with your oncologist.

It should be noted that the CsCl/DMSO protocol is a highly effective therapy for the treatment of many cancers including colorectal cancer. It should only be used if the danger of occlusion has been assessed or removed by means of surgery as advised by your oncologist. Thus the time to implement alternative treatments would be immediately after surgery.

Antioxidants, especially Vitamins C and E, and calcium, Vitamin D and folic acid supplements may also reduce the risk and even aid in reversing cancer in its early stages.

There are a number of alternative cancer treatment methods that are suitable for colorectal cancer:

- The Brandt Grape Cure protocol. There are several reports of successful treatments of advanced/terminal cancer patients by this method.
- Johanna Brandt suggested that in these patients a grape juice enema using 30 % grape juice should be added to her normal protocol.
- The Budwig Protocol. There are many testimonials on the Internet which report on the successful use of the Budwig diet in the treatment of this condition. The main ingredients in this diet are flaxseed oil and cottage cheese. Lignans are constituents of flax seeds, but mostly not of flaxseed oil. They are powerful cancer-fighting ingredients and are especially effective against breast, colon, uterus and prostate cancers by their effects on hormones in the body. They *inter alia* flush excess oestrogen from the body. It therefore seems advisable to include flaxseeds as part of the Budwig protocol.
- Essiac tea. There are many convincing testimonials of the successful use of Essiac tea in the treatment of terminal colorectal cancer patients, even after unsuccessful medical treatment with chemotherapy and radiation. Native Essence is a reputable brand of Essiac Tea in the USA. More info is available on the Internet.
- Raw food. As with many cancers and many cancer diets, raw food is a major item in the fight against colorectal cancer. I have described the essentials of the raw food diet in the cancer diet. Basically it consists of only raw fruits (low GI) and vegetables as solid dietary items combined with 1-3 liters of freshly extracted carrot juice daily.
- Coenzyme Q10. One of the principal characteristics of cancer cells is the anaerobic metabolic pattern and the breakdown of the energy producing electron transport system in the mitochondria. Q10 is a vital coenzyme in this system. Beneficial effects of restoring Q10

levels in cancer patients with different types of cancer, including rectal cancer, have been reported. The usual dose is 400mg per day.
- Diet. Cruciferous vegetables (Brussels sprouts, cabbage, cauliflower, broccoli, etc.) contain a variety of anticancer compounds such as glucinolates, sulphoraphane, lutein, zeaxanthin and other cancer-killing nutrients. Even conventional medicine knows that a diet rich in broccoli and cauliflower is an important step in preventing colorectal cancer. These patients should consume the vegetables on a daily basis. This relationship appears to be most consistent for colorectal, stomach and lung cancers and least consistent for ovarian, prostatic and endometrial cancers.

While these foods are beneficial, there are others that should be strictly avoided. Most important amongst these are meat, processed foods, sugar, preserved foods, etc. Especially meat is thought to increase the risk of cancer and also specifically of colon cancer.

Cervical cancer

It is vital to detect and treat cervical cancer at the earliest possible stage. If untreated, cervical cancer cells tend to move into the deeper layers of the cervix and glands of the uterus and then spread into nearby organs like the bladder, vagina and rectum, and eventually into other organs. Usually such cancers will metastasize after 10-12 years if left untreated, but in rare cases the period may be as short as 1-2 years. Cervical cancer develops through a series of changes including dysplasia to a precancerous state (carcinoma *in situ*). In the early stages of this process, the chances of successful treatment are excellent. Abnormal changes in the cervix are usually detected by means of a Pap smear, which is strictly a screening test and not a diagnostic test. Other tests are used for a definite diagnosis.

Treatment, according to one expert, consists of three phases:

- Local treatment with enzymes performed by a doctor
- Systemic treatment to improve immune function with oral supplements of Vitamin C, selenium, folic acid
- Improvement of overall health by means of diet and lifestyle changes.

This is essentially a preventative treatment for cases where the cancer has been detected early.

Once the disease has spread to neighboring organs, more drastic measures may be required, such as the CsCl/DMSO protocol and IPT as described later.

Cachexia and loss of appetite in the cancer patient

This is a term used to describe the considerable loss of weight and often near-complete loss of appetite seen in advanced cancer patients. This loss of weight is not only due to a change of diet from a typical Western diet of refined foods and fats to a cancer diet as described in this book, but often the weight loss is also caused by aggressive cancer cells which are "hungry" for the nutrients (especially glucose) in the patient's body. This may be so strong that the patient may start to lose his/her muscles, food reserves and even bone, to ultimately present in the emaciated appearance of the advanced cancer patient.

> *As many as 40% of cancer patients die as a result of this problem, which in practical terms means the patient dies of starvation and not in the first place of the cancer.*

The "cachexia cycle" depends on the conversion of glucose into lactic acid in the cancer cell. The lactic acid then goes to the liver where it is reconverted into glucose. Both of these processes require much energy, which is obtained from the body's energy reserves. This cycle consumes an enormous amount of energy (15 times more than the aerobic metabolism of glucose which occurs in normal cells). The result is that the body starts to consume its own tissues (eg muscles and bones) in order to feed the cancer cells (wasting syndrome).

Fortunately there is a product (hydrazine sulphate) available now, which effectively addresses this problem when used in combination with CsCl. In this cycle, the CsCl blocks the glucose from entering the cells while hydrazine sulphate blocks the cycle in the liver by preventing the formation of glucose from lactic acid. The use of hydrazine sulphate for this purpose is described under the CsCl/ DMSO protocol.

In addition to its effects on the lactic acid cycle, hydrazine has also been shown to have a direct anti-tumor activity of its own.

All cachexia patients have some degree of bone loss. Therefore it is advisable to include a bone mineral supplement in the treatment.

The cardinal rules of alternative cancer treatment

The following rules (summarized from the *Cancer Tutor* and other sources) apply in the case of seriously ill patients.

RULE 1: Always have at least one true Stage IV alternative cancer treatment in your protocol as listed above

Your first choice should be IPT with CsCl/DMSO as a possible alternative.

This is the very first requisite for successful treatment. However, it is equally important not to have two or more Stage IV treatments at the same time, except perhaps in a clinic setting. This is because each of these treatments has been designed to kill the maximum number of cancer cells and the combined load of dead cells may be more than the body can handle.

In alternative cancer methodology, killing cancer cells is not the problem. There are several methods in alternative medicine that will do that. The problem is safely killing the cancer cells and avoiding an overload of debris.

The exception to this rule is hydrazine sulphate, which can be combined with any other treatment (with the exception of high doses of Vitamin C) because it does not kill cancer cells. It is used to treat cachectic patients as detailed above.

RULE 2: The cancer diet is as important as the treatment protocol selected

No cancer treatment can be successful unless the patient also meticulously adheres to the cancer diet given here. There are several powerful alternative cancer treatments available, but none of them can successfully fight some of the more dangerous and fast-growing cancers without significant outside help in the form of a highly alkaline diet. The major cancers cannot survive and spread in an alkaline environment in which the pH is higher than 7.8. The diet determines the inner milieu or terrain of the body and in this manner determines the amount of resistance that the body will put up in a fight with invading cancer cells. A bad cancer diet (eg the typical Western diet high in refined products) will feed the cancer cells. A mediocre cancer diet will not only feed the cancer cells but it will not assist the body in its fight against the cancer cells.

A good cancer diet (see later) will assist the body in its fight against the invading cancer cells by creating an inner terrain or environment (eg an alkaline pH) in which cancer cells cannot survive.

The diet plays an especially important role in the treatment of fast-spreading cancers such as pancreatic cancer, and it can stop the growth and spreading of the cancer better than any treatment. I have seen many cancer patients on good treatment lose their battle because the cancer was spreading faster than it could be contained by the treatment alone, although this may have been the best available treatment. The only means of winning the battle in this situation is to have both an optimum anti-cancer diet (as described later) and a superb cancer treatment such as IPT or the CsCl/DMSO protocol described in this book.

For an optimum anti-cancer diet, you have at least four options to choose from:

- The cancer diet previously described
- The Robert O. Young alkaline diet as described in his book (13). Be careful not to include any food item that contains a significant amount of glucose. If you are serious about overcoming your cancer, it will be necessary for you to buy this book. It is the key to surviving fast spreading cancers
- The Brandt Grape Diet. Grapes are very alkaline and detoxifying at the same time. Although this is also a Stage IV cancer treatment in its own right, it is permissible to use it in combination with any other Stage IV cancer protocol although it is generally not allowed to use more than one of these treatments at the same time. This diet can be used as the "cancer diet" item, for example in combination with the very powerful CsCl/DMSO protocol.
- The Hauser diet (see later).

RULE 3: Work under the guidance of an experienced professional

This is automatically ensured if you work with a clinic. It is not always easy to find a suitable clinic in South Africa. Consult the Internet for advice and guidance. The other alternative is for the patient to depend on active telephone or e-mail support. Here again, the Internet may be able to provide advice. Whatever you do, do not treat yourself or design your own treatment programme.

RULE 4: Buying time

The critically ill cancer patient needs time to implement the various treatments suggested in this book and elsewhere (32). This can be achieved by using a product (or products) that acts quickly, does not necessarily cure the cancer but retards it sufficiently for the patient to implement other more powerful protocols that do not act fast enough.

An example is the use of high-dose Vitamin C in terminal cancer patients. Many years ago the two-time Nobel Prize winner Linus Pauling and a well-known oncologist and surgeon, Dr. E. Cameron, did a series of clinical studies in cancer patients in Scotland (7) that proved beyond doubt that daily Vitamin C doses of 10g extended the life expectancy of the patients 6 times or more compared to controls. Patients with a variety of cancers were included in the study and in addition to the significantly extended life expectancy, other benefits of the Vitamin C treatment were noted which included a meaningful improvement of quality of life (7). A similar study was later completed in Japan with even more impressive results. Typically, the average life expectancy of untreated control patients was 6 months, compared to 36 months in the treated patients. This shows that the treated patients had an additional 30 months to live during which time they could implement different other treatments that could be life-saving. Although the Vitamin C treatment was found to cure only 5 % of the patients, it did gain valuable time. It should be noted here that high doses of Vitamin C should not be given together with hydrazine in the treatment of cachexia in cancer patients.

There are other treatments that can be used to buy time in a similar manner for terminally ill cancer patients (32).

Cancer cells "steal" nutrients from normal cells, thus depriving the patient of valuable nutritional support. This may be one of the reasons why these patients develop severe cachexia which may be responsible for their death. It is therefore essential to supply vital nutrients in the form of concentrated nutritional and mineral supplements, of which several are available in this country. In this manner time can be bought for the patient. In addition, it is also necessary to include antifungal agents in the treatment. Almost all cancer patients have severe microbe infections which may include fungi and various other pleomorphic micro-organisms (32). Removal of these by means of appropriate products which may contain more than one active ingredient is therefore necessary and is another means of buying time for the patient. MycoDetox I and MycoDetox II are examples of such products which are available in America (see (32) for more details).

RULE 5: Using several Stage IV protocols in sequence

As a general rule, more than one Stage IV treatment should not be used at the same time because of the increased load of dead cancer cells that the body has to dispose of. However, sometimes the patient is in such a critical condition that it becomes necessary to use several Stage IV treatments in sequence. This may also happen for example when a particular patient has reached his or her "cesium limit" as discussed later in the section on the CsCl/DMSO protocol. This may happen before the cancer has been totally removed by the cesium treatment. In such a case it becomes necessary to use one or more other Stage IV treatments such as IPT, ozone therapy, the Budwig diet and others as suggested by your consultant.

Another typical example is the following: In the case of a patient with a fast-growing pancreatic cancer which has already spread to the bones, treatment might be initiated by going to a suitable clinic for a course of ozone therapy combined with IPT. Following that or in conjunction with the IPT treatment, the CsCl/DMSO protocol may be used, preferably together with a bone mineral supplement until the patient reaches the cesium limit, which should then be followed by the remission treatment described in this book

RULE 6: Treat the patient's mental state

Under no circumstances must the patient be allowed to lose hope. It is crucial to remove from his mind all thoughts of fear and hopelessness. This is where family and friends can play a major role. There are now so many potent cancer treatments available, especially alternative cancer treatments, that one can genuinely be optimistic of the prospects no matter how critically ill the patient is. The patient should be told success stories of cancer treatment and a general optimistic atmosphere should be created by those in contact with the patient. Frequently cancer follows some traumatic event to which the patient had been exposed. It is absolutely necessary to break this mental barrier. To achieve this, major changes must be made in the patient's mental attitude towards the negative factors and especially the enemies in his life. The worst possible thing that could happen is for someone close to the patient to express doubts about the chosen course of treatment. There is absolutely no room for negativity around a cancer patient

RULE 7: Determine your degree of success

Start by making an assessment of how much cancer there is in your body and repeat this test or tests from time to time to make sure you are making progress. One method is to do PET scans, about which your doctor will be able to advise you. The number of PET scans must be reduced to a bare minimum as the X-rays used in the scan may themselves cause cancer.

A number of other "cancer markers" such CA-125 is available, but these are not very reliable except in the case of certain cancers. The Navarro Test is more reliable, but may be more expensive since urine samples have to be sent to the Philippines. Alternatively, the AMAS test may be used.

RULE 8: Attending to the patient's liver function is a required part of any cancer treatment programme

Ideally, it should be done (together with a colon cleanse) before the cancer treatment programme is started. A coffee enema is frequently used for this purpose (see Gerson therapy). Coffee enemas open the bile duct, thus allowing the liver to flush out the toxins. This greatly enhances the success of the treatment—it is absolutely critical to saving a cancer patient. Even the best treatment protocol may not succeed if the patient's liver is not attended to. There are also other methods of supporting the liver which you could consider—details in (1) and on the Internet).

RULE 9: Treat the fungi which every cancer patient has

There are many different secondary causes of cancer, but one important cause is pleomorphic yeasts/fungi that thrive in a highly acidic diet or a wrong diet. It is therefore vital to remove these as a first step in the treatment. The most important antifungal products are caprylic acid, undecylenic acid, olive leaf extract, garlic, bromelain, Aloe Vera extract and Grapefruit Seed extract (not grape seed extract). Details are available in Dr. Young's book (13). Much of the danger posed by cancer is caused by these microbes. One reason is that they feed on the same things as the cancer cells, because of their similar anaerobic metabolic patterns. This means that some of the anticancer compounds used in the treatment may be diverted away from the cancer cells towards the yeast/fungus invaders. Many of the cancer-killing foods also have antifungal properties. If you have leukemia, you should pay special attention to controlling fungal infections; you may need several antifungal preparations (1). Also bear in mind that the Bob Beck Electro Medicine treatment previously discussed is one of the most effective treatments for microbes.

RULE 10: Enzymes and Barley powder

These may play an important role in removing the proteins from the exterior of the cancer cells so that they become accessible to the immune cells which kill them. Two key enzyme preparations are used for this purpose: Wobenzyme and Vitalzyme (consult the Internet).

Note that patients on anti-coagulant therapy should not take the enzymes, but they may take Barley powder.

Buying time for the seriously ill cancer patient

First and foremost, we should look at the work of Cameron and Pauling at the Vale of Leven Hospital in Scotland many years ago (already referred to in a different context). Now I would like to concentrate on the fact that they found that by giving 10g of Vitamin C daily to terminal cancer patients who were beyond medical treatment, they could extend the lives of these patients 6 times over that of the controls (7). Typically, the controls lived 6 months as against 36 months in the case of the Vitamin C patients. Although only 5 % of the treated patients ultimately survived, the significance of this work lies in the fact that for these patients a 30 month period was "bought" by the Vitamin C treatment, during which time all kinds of life-saving alternative treatments could be instigated. Thus, this treatment allowed the patients sufficient time for more powerful treatments to work. In addition, the quality of life of the patients was significantly improved during these terminal 30 months of their lives (7). For weak, terminally ill cancer patients with little energy and generally feeling miserable, this tactic brings very significant advantages. These weak cancer patients need treatments that will "buy time" for more powerful treatments to work and, above all, that will give them hope and restore their will to live. This aspect of the Vitamin C treatment is extremely important. Unfortunately, it has been completely overlooked by the medical profession.

Some general remarks on cancer and carcinogenesis

The process of carcinogenesis is intimately connected to the concept of energy production in cells, aerobic (with oxygen) and anaerobic (without oxygen) mechanisms of energy production and also with the process of angiogenesis (formation of new blood vessels). Aerobic energy production takes place in the mitochondria (subcellular structures) in cells where fuel molecules (glucose) are broken down stepwise in a process called the Krebs Cycle. Electrons generated in this process are then passed down stepwise in the electron transport chain and finally to oxygen, with the creation of large amounts of ATP energy. If for some reason not enough oxygen is available for this process, the Krebs Cycle is disrupted and the cell now has to look at another way of extracting energy from glucose. This it does by metabolizing glucose anaerobically, which is also called fermentation. Anaerobic fermentation is an inefficient way of producing energy from glucose (only $1/18$ of the energy available in glucose is liberated in this way) so that a lack of energy develops. Hence the severe weight loss seen in cancer patients. All this critical information was published 70 years ago by Otto Warburg in a series of brilliant publications which earned him two Nobel prizes.

Angiogenesis is the process by which new blood vessels are formed to supply growing cells with nutrients. This also happens in growing cancer cells. It is by means of this mechanism that cancer cells attempt to compensate for lack of oxygen: cells deprived of oxygen emit antigenic emergency signals. An important discovery was that if they can somehow succeed in restoring oxygen supply to the cancer cells, cellular respiration can be restored, thus transforming the cancer cells back into normal cells.

In other words, cancer is reversible

As previously explained, anaerobic microbes inside cancer cells are assumed to play a major role in establishing the anaerobic conditions inside cancer cells. It is not clear at this stage whether this can also happen without the participation of such microbes.

In evaluating success of treatment, it is important to note the difference between "survival time" and "five year survival time"

- *"Survival time"* is the time interval between the time when the diagnosis of cancer was first made in a patient and when that patient dies from the diagnosed cancer.
- *"Five year survival time"* is a survival interval of five years from the time when the diagnosis of cancer was first made. If the patient is then still alive, he is considered cured. If, however, the patient dies after five years and one day, he will be counted as cured for purposes of statistical analysis.
- Although these two concepts may sound similar, they are in fact vastly different. Much false information is published on the basis of the five year survival rates, which is the norm used in the evaluation of most of the conventional methods. Many cancers such as breast and prostate cancers are slow-growing and may in fact be present for many years before the patient dies. Dr. P. Binzel summarizes the situation rather well in his book (71):

In the past fifty years, tremendous progress has been made in the early diagnosis of cancer. In that period of time, tremendous progress has been made in the surgical ability to remove tumors; tremendous progress has been made in the use of radiation and chemotherapy in their ability to shrink or destroy tumors. But the survival time of the cancer patient today is no greater than it was fifty years ago. What does this mean? It obviously means that we are treating the wrong thing.

What kills the cancer patient, is the lack of nutrients and the spreading of the tumor. The tumor itself presents no danger to the patient, certainly not in the case of solid tumors unless they block vital fluids in critical areas such as the brain or the common bile duct.

It is necessary to understand the precise structure of a solid tumor as presented by Webster Kehr in the *Cancer Tutor*. The majority of cells in such tumors are healthy cells and there are therefore not enough cancer cells in such a tumor to kill the patient. Cancer cells on their own cannot form tissue since they are autonomous and do not respond to growth-regulatory mechanisms in the body. Typically, in prostate cancer, and if the cancer is contained inside the prostate, there is no danger to the patient's life. This sometimes happens in elderly patients. Even if the cancer cells in such a tumor were killed or if the tumor was cut out, it would not save the patient's life if the cancer has already spread, as shown by the breast cancer example previously discussed. Quite clearly, then, it is the spreading of the cancer that kills the patient, not the cancer cells inside the primary tumor.

Ironically, orthodox medicine focuses on the shrinking of tumors (killing of cancer cells inside the tumor) and often uses this as evidence of successful treatment. This creates false expectations by the patient, who inevitably has to face the consequences of metastases later on, which is the real reason why the patient may die.

A further complicating factor arises in the case of chemotherapy because the drug itself is so toxic (due to insufficient selectivity) that if enough of the drug were given to kill the cancer cells, the patient would also be killed. The doctor is therefore forced to limit dosage levels so as not to kill the patient, but at these low doses the cancer is not prevented from spreading. We will show how this problem may be addressed, at least partially, by means of IPT later in this book.

That is why chemotherapy may put a patient in remission, which is then claimed as successful treatment. However, virtually every cancer patient who goes into remission eventually comes out of remission and then dies as a result of the now more widely disseminated cancer.

This scenario is replayed every day in many cancer wards the world over. Frequently, solid cancers may either be surgically removed or treated with radiotherapy even after the cancer has already spread, because the doctors are interested in shrinking the tumor as mentioned above. But the tumor is not the problem—it is the spreading of the tumor that kills the patient.

As a method of saving the patient's life by ensuring long-term survival, conventional medical treatments are practically worthless, as shown by the recorded survival rates of 2 % previously discussed. However, many alternative treatment protocols are no better, because many alternative practitioners do not use the best treatments for financial reasons, or they do not have sufficient knowledge. In addition, different vendors promote their own product lines for selfish reasons, which are not necessarily the best.

On the other hand, there are some good alternative doctors and there are some good products, but these have to be identified and found.

Clearly then, the cancer patient and his/her doctor are in a very difficult situation. They have to wade through a maze of uncertainty and deception, which is further complicated by the fact that drug authorities strictly prohibit doctors from using or even investigating alternative treatment methods. This means that there is no or very little reliable information available on which to base decisions. So what must the cancer patient do? Although it may not sound like a million-dollar solution to the problem, the only way forward for the cancer patient is the old-fashioned way of finding people with integrity to work with who are interested in curing your cancer and not in their own bank account in the first place. In addition, the patient and doctor must be prepared to study and gather the necessary knowledge in order for them to make the right decisions. Much information is available on the Internet, where very good websites such as the *Cancer Tutor* are to be found (32).

Evaluation of some cancer protocols

Only a few of the more than 300 different published alternative cancer treatments are strong enough and act fast enough to treat a cancer patient who has been given up on by conventional medicine and sent home to die.

You should not feel that you are entering uncharted territory if you select an alternative cancer protocol. More patients visit alternative medicine practitioners than conventional doctors for treatment of a wide variety of diseases—and this number is rapidly increasing. A survey by the Life Extension Foundation in America found that 80 % of cancer patients take one or more alternative treatments, and that half of these do not tell their doctors, from which one gathers that these patients were also getting some form of conventional treatment. There are literally thousands of personal reports of the successful treatment by means of alternative methods of most types of cancer. Many of these can be viewed on the Internet.

In the following pages I list 17 of the most preferred treatments according to my judgment from reading the literature.

Out of these, I have selected the following six most preferred treatments which could be used in the emergency situation of a Stage IV cancer patient who has been given up on by the medical profession and has only weeks to live. Provided it is not contra-indicated (build-up of pressure in critical anatomical areas such as the brain), I judge the overall two best single protocols in general to be the CsCl/DMSO protocol and IPT. Please note that all cancer patients should receive a daily supplement of the correct mix of unadulterated w-3 and w-6 essential fatty acids in addition to whatever other treatment protocol(s) may have been selected.

Also please note that all cancer patients should be treated under the supervision of medical doctors who also have experience and knowledge of natural methods of treatment, regardless of the type of cancer or treatment the patient is receiving.

Preferred list of treatments

1. IPT (possibly combined with DMSO)
2. CsCl/DMSO
3. Supplementation with the correct fatty acid mix
4. Ozone therapy
5. Brandt Grape Therapy (possibly substituting vegetable juices for grape mush)
6. The Bill Henderson protocol which includes the Budwig Diet (flaxseed oil + cottage cheese)
7. The sodium chlorite method.

This does not mean that the other protocols are less effective. For particular cancers they may even be better, eg Gerson therapy for the treatment of melanoma and laetrile therapy for long-term follow-up treatment.

These treatments are best used in conjunction with an immune system building protocol such as Beta-1.3DGlucan (see "Building the Immune System").

These 7 protocols can be used to treat any type of cancer with the provisos mentioned in each protocol.

Please note that they are my own personal assessments based on information in the literature.

Not I, nor anyone else, can in any way guarantee success or safety. The patient and his/her doctor must study the evidence and reach their own conclusions.

It is not wise to treat yourself with one of these protocols without telling your doctor. Ideally, your doctor should be involved in your treatment programme; if he objects to alternative treatments, you should find another doctor.

1. The CsCl/DMSO protocol

The theory behind the use of cesium salts for the treatment of cancer was developed by Dr. K. Brewer, an American physicist. He showed that for reasons that are well understood, cesium and rubidium ions enter cancer cells when other minerals cannot.

Once inside the cancer cell, the cesium ion does several things:

- The inside of the cancer cell is made alkaline (pH 8.0 or more). It is important to realize that only the intracellular pH is made alkaline by cesium—not the blood.
- Intake of glucose into the cell is limited, thus starving the cancer cell.
- Lactic acid inside the cells (which causes the cells to multiply uncontrollably) is suppressed.
- Fermentation in the cells is stopped, thus limiting lactic acid production. Fermentation is also suppressed as a result of the limited supply of glucose.
- CsCl stops the spreading of cancer to distant sites (metastasis).
- It also stops cancer-associated pain within 24—48 hours, depending on the location.
- Cesium absorption by the cancer cells is supported by Vitamins A and C and also by the minerals zinc and selenium. Hence the necessity that the patient should take a good multinutrient supplement.

The CsCl/DMSO protocol targets the cancer cells directly, because normal cells do not readily ingest CsCl. The presence of DMSO increases the selectivity of CsCl for cancer cells even more (13). DMSO is a natural product which is *inter alia* obtained as a byproduct of the wood industry. It is closely related to and often used together with MSM (which is DMSO with an extra oxygen atom)—therefore $DMSO_2$. MSM or $DMSO_2$ also occurs in fruit and vegetables. DMSO and $DMSO_2$ are interconvertible in the body and as such act as an oxygen transport pair which enhances aerobic metabolism:

$$DMSO_2 = DMSO + O$$

Trials with CsCl on humans have been carried out by several researchers, including Dr. Nieper in Germany and Dr. Sartori in Washington. On the whole the results have been very satisfactory given the variables associated with such trials. Many more clinical studies would have been published, but the FDA and other authorities in America have forbidden doctors to publish such studies. The original Sartori studies have, however, been published. Other studies on the mechanism of action of CsCl are available and have been published by Dr. D.W. Gregg and others (see Internet). The ground-breaking work of Dr. K. Brewer has also been published (32).

The CsCl/DMSO protocol and IPT are perhaps overall the best of all secondary alternative cancer treatments. CsCl can (and must) be administered through the skin, and it can be taken by those still on chemotherapy or even on IPT treatment, which may even be a preferred combination. It is an absolutely obligatory treatment for bone cancer unless contra-indicated by the presence of another type of cancer. It works fast, shrinks tumors and also rapidly reduces pain (11).

Another advantage is that a less stringent cancer diet than usual is permitted because the CsCl and potassium used in the treatment prevent glucose from entering the cancer cells. This means that more foods with higher glucose content are permissible. This less restricted and more nutritious diet benefits the cancer patient, whose normal cells already have a deficiency of vital nutrients.

In the past, the use of CsCl/DMSO was limited in the case of tumors where restricted blood flow in critical anatomical areas could be caused by the treatment. There are now substances available (including chemotherapy and IPT) that will counter this problem. These new technologies allow CsCl to be used in situations where it was previously not possible. There are also a limited number of other alternative cancer protocols that can be used where swelling may be a problem (see later).

For brain cancer patients, the CsCl/DMSO protocol is especially valuable, provided that steps are taken to deal with the swelling problem.

The CsCl/DMSO protocol is one of the major alternative cancer treatments, with many advantages. It can be done at home and is suitable for those who cannot take oral supplements. It can be combined with chemotherapy and IPT. In fact, it seems to act synergistically with chemo, and when using this combination, swelling is far less of a problem because fewer cancer cells are killed. There are, however, natural products that can replace chemotherapy for this purpose and these are to be preferred (see later). A contact for more info in difficult situations is Larry at Essence of Life in the USA (details on the Internet).

It is absolutely essential to use the remission treatment as detailed in this book when you have reached your cesium limit (see later) and you can therefore no longer continue with the CsCl/DMSO protocol.

The other advantage attached to the CsCl/DMSO treatment is that it works fast. Different vendors in America are available with much information and a long record of successful use. The only disadvantage is that it creates an unpleasant odor, not detected by the patient, which is a small price to pay for such a good treatment. For details of usage, see "Protocols" later.

Although this is a very safe and harmless treatment, it is nonetheless necessary to adhere strictly to the application rules, and above all to arrange for active telephone support if the services of a clinic are not available.

If you are a Stage IV patient with advanced cancer and with a history of previous medical treatment, your chances of survival on further conventional treatment are less than 5 %. Also, with advanced cancer there are very few alternative treatment protocols that will give you a fighting chance. The CsCl/ DMSO protocol and IPT are probably the best ones, and the more strictly you follow the rules, the better your chances are. Even with a history of unsuccessful medical treatment, you may still have a 50 % chance of success if you go about it in the correct way (32).

CsCl and its effects on potassium levels

Blood potassium levels are affected by CsCl treatment, so that correction of these by means of supplementation is urgently required. Some patients on cesium develop potassium depletion. This also results from the alkalosis caused by the treatment. Alkalosis drives potassium into the cells, thus lowering serum levels (hypokalemia). In addition, the cesium as such also drives potassium into the cells, with the same result. Most potassium in the body (98 %) is present within the cells, with only a small amount circulating in the bloodstream. The balance between potassium in the intracellular (inside cells) and extracellular (outside cells, eg in blood) compartments is critical in many ways, however, and affects many vital systems including heart rhythm. It affects the functionality of cell membranes and governs the action of the heart and pathways between the brain and muscles. Excess potassium is usually eliminated via the kidneys, but if these are not functioning optimally, blood potassium levels may increase excessively. Another cause of rising blood potassium values during cesium therapy is the potassium released into the circulation by the dead cancer cells.

However, the most common effect on blood potassium levels during cesium treatment is declining blood potassium levels leading to too low levels (hypokalemia) for reasons mentioned above. Alkalosis (increased blood alkalinity) causes the movement of potassium into the cells, which may then also result in too low blood levels. This movement of potassium into the cells which depletes serum (blood) levels may result in critically low blood levels which require immediate correction by means of supplementation. In addition to the alkalosis effect, potassium is also driven into cells (especially cancer cells) by the cesium ions. It is therefore critically important for patients on the CsCl/DMSO protocol to have their serum potassium levels monitored regularly, initially every few days, and later, when the condition has stabilized, once every 1-2 weeks. Kidney damage may result if serum levels rise too high, and effects on heart rhythm may develop when levels decline too much. In addition to monitoring serum potassium levels as explained above, the patient should be alerted to the clinical symptoms of hypo and hyperkalaemia.

- *Symptoms of hypokalemia (too little serum potassium)* fatigue, muscle weakness and cramps intestinal paralysis accompanied by constipation and bloating abdominal pain abnormal heart rhythms may develop that can be fatal.
- *Symptoms of hyperkalaemia (too much serum potassium)* tingling of hands and feet muscular weakness and temporary paralysis abnormal heart rhythms that can be fatal.

If these symptoms occur, you should immediately consult your doctor.

Note that both conditions can lead to muscular weakness and abnormal heart rhythm. Supplementation levels should therefore be adjusted to keep serum potassium levels within the normal range (3.5—5.5mmol/L). The trend that may become evident in successive serum potassium values gives an early warning of possible future problems. For example, if successive serum values taken at weekly intervals are 4.7, 4.1 and 3.9, this indicates that the patient may soon become hypokalaemic and early adjustment of supplementation levels may forestall future problems.

In addition to regular checking of blood potassium values, blood uric acid, magnesium, calcium and sodium serum levels should be checked at least once every 3-4 weeks. Magnesium and calcium values may become too low, which can be corrected by taking appropriate quantities of coral calcium or some other suitable supplement.

Uric acid levels may become too high as a result of the DNA released by the dead cancer cells. At the normal dosage levels of 3g CsCl per day, this is unlikely to occur, but if it does, the attending physician who will most likely prescribe Xyloprim, should be alerted.

Although it is a very safe treatment, it is best not to take CsCl on your own without at least active telephone support. The names and addresses of doctors who have some experience of the use of CsCl, whom you may want to contact, are available on *www.fortifood.co.za*. Like all other treatments, there is really no such thing as "one size fits all". The treatment should be adapted to the patient's weight, type of cancer, stage of cancer and many other variables in order to attain the best results. Cancer patients also need to know what to expect during the treatment, and especially to be alerted to the symptoms of the so-called "cesium limit" (see later). The patient needs to be advised on the best high-density nutritional supplements, enzymes, bone-building supplements, etc. In addition, it is necessary to know whether there is any evidence of bone loss, with possibly brittle bones and bone cancer, and what the most appropriate steps are in any particular situation. This has been discussed previously (see bone cancer).

There is an address in America where you can buy products and also get advice on the various problems mentioned (72). This company will mail products and return phone calls to anywhere in the world. Unfortunately, it is a bit expensive for South African buyers.

The CsCl/DMSO protocol requires precise information on diet, the correct supplements, the correct combination of minerals including strontium chloride, and the correct amounts of each.

Dosage levels of CsCl and potassium

Although there are exceptions, as a rule CsCl and DMSO should not be taken orally. There are no significant advantages attached to taking both orally, and in any case, there is no necessity to do so, since the DMSO promotes rapid absorption of CsCl through the skin when they are applied together, and the DMSO itself is also absorbed in a similar manner.

The CsCl/DMSO protocol is provided in a ready-to-use standard kit which can be used as a nutritional supplement in most cancer treatment programs.

The following is an example of how the ingredients in the kit are used. The procedure involves mixing a solution of CsCl and a DMSO solution (both supplied in the CsCl/DMSO kit) and applying the mixture to the skin on a suitable area of the body. Do not apply directly above a cancerous growth or touching any surface cancer cells or any area where there is a dense concentration of cancer cells. The normal dosage levels are such that 1500mg of CsCl is mixed with DMSO and the mixture applied twice daily (a total of 3.0g daily of CsCl). In addition, the patient has to take 3 capsules, 500mg each, of the special potassium complex provided twice daily one hour after the CsCl application. In addition the patient has to take 6-8 capsules of the alkalinizing formula. Note that the potassium supplement and the alkalinizing formula should be taken one hour *after* each CsCl/DMSO application and not simultaneously with it.

The procedure and effects may be summarized as follows:

- Three grams of CsCl are daily taken in 2 divided doses of 1.5g each with DMSO (applied topically).

- The mixture may be applied by means of a spray or dropper bottle. Alternatively, it may be applied to the skin using your finger (wash your hands immediately afterwards—do not use gloves). The mixture should be applied over a relatively large skin area (approximately 100-200mm^2).
- 5-6 capsules daily of the potassium complex (depending on blood potassium levels) in 2 divided doses taken orally, each dose at least 1 hour after the last CsCl application. Under no circumstances should the potassium supplement be taken at the same time as the CsCl, since the potassium can block (compete with) cesium from entering the cancer cells, thereby nullifying the treatment.
- It is advisable to include several potassium-rich foods in your daily diet. Examples of potassium-rich foods are: green vegetables, potatoes, apples, prunes. You should get at least as much potassium from food as from the supplement. Potassium from food is better utilized by the body, since foods also contain other nutrients which are required for the optimal use of potassium.
- Drink lots of purified (reverse osmosis) water during this treatment. Try to drink at least 2 liters per day.
- Pay careful attention to when and which doses are to be taken. Although these are arranged in the kit in such a manner that errors can be easily avoided, it is nonetheless advisable to have someone else check the whole procedure.
- A rash may sometimes develop at the application site of the DMSO/CsCl mix. This is due to the dehydrating effect of the DMSO. Spray the area with clean water and wash.

Note that even though DMSO is considered a non-toxic substance, certain precautions are necessary. For example, it should never be used by pregnant women (or women who may be pregnant); it should not touch cloth, gloves or anything else before application, because everything it comes into contact with will be carried into the body when it is subsequently applied to the skin.

Note that DMSO, used as described above, may impart a significant body odor (garlic or oyster-like smell) which you will not notice personally. This may cause social problems, but is a small price to pay to rid you of cancer. For example, you may have to make appropriate arrangements in your work situation.

Continue to take CsCl every day until you reach your cesium limit (see later).

Note that certain tumors may even increase in size during treatment before they start to shrink. This is because of the inflammation caused as a result of the treatment as discussed above. Also note that shrinkage of tumors is not necessarily a reliable indicator of successful treatment (11).

Once you have reached your cesium limit as discussed later, you should stop taking cesium, but it is vitally important to continue monitoring your blood potassium levels regularly (and to correct these by a suitable supplementation programme) for at least another 3 months.

If you have cancer anywhere in your digestive tract, do not use the CsCl/DMSO protocol except under professional guidance, especially if there are signs of obstruction and inflammation.

Cramps may occur if the patient has a deficiency of potassium, but magnesium and/or calcium deficiencies are also frequently the cause of cramps. A potassium deficiency is further recognized by the fact that if you curl your toes they do not immediately return to their normal position. If that occurs, the patient should be checked for deficiencies of all the abovementioned minerals and appropriately treated by means of supplements. Increasing the amount of potassium-rich foods is another good method of correcting a potassium deficiency. If cesium and potassium administration are not separated in time, cramping may be promoted. If cramping persists after you have been separating them for one hour as indicated above, then you should increase the time between the two doses by more than 1 hour (2 hours or more).

The cesium limit occurs when a patient has been on cesium therapy for some time (1-3 months). In some patients it occurs sooner than in others. While it is not a dangerous situation, cesium therapy should be stopped but, if this becomes necessary, monitoring blood potassium, magnesium and calcium should be continued for at least another 3 months under medical surveillance.

- The cesium limit can be detected when one or more of the following symptoms occur: your feet turn purple, they feel cold and/or they feel as if you have frostbite your finger tips feel like needles and pins; they hurt if you bump them against something, especially something cold.

Some patients on the CsCl/DMSO protocol may reach their cesium limit before their cancer is completely cured. If they then stop the treatment, there is a strong possibility that the cancer may return with its full fury. This situation usually develops when the cesium treatment has reduced the initial Stage IV cancer to perhaps a Stage I or II cancer without completely curing the patient.

As a general rule, the patient has the option to go on another round of cesium treatment as soon as the evidence of the cesium limit has disappeared. But, whatever decision is made, every person who has been on cesium treatment needs to play safe and go on a different but less potent alternative cancer treatment such as the Bill Henderson Protocol which includes the Budwig diet or, in serious cases, on IPT. Another good option would be to follow up with the Protocel protocol as suggested by the *Cancer Tutor* (32). Protocel is simple to use, easy to go on and costs less than R20 per day.

It has the disadvantage that it has to be imported and the patient needs to take the product every 6 hours, 24 hours per day. The Protocel treatment should be followed for at least a year after finishing one or two cesium treatments. More details are available in the book by Tanya Pierce, *Protocel and Cancer* (available from *Amazon.com*).

Instead of the Protocel protocol, any one of the strong Stage III treatments could be considered as a follow-up treatment after one or two courses of the CsCl/DMSO protocol (see later). After all signs of cancer have disappeared following cesium treatment, a small number of cancer cells may still remain which are impossible to detect. It is for this reason (and just to make sure) that the patient should consider a final round of treatment as suggested above. Another possibility: if the patient prefers to have yet another course of cesium treatment, he/she may opt for another round of the CsCl/DMSO protocol, this time, however, reducing dosage levels by 50 %. You should wait a month before going on this last round of cesium treatment, and you also need to be constantly on the lookout for signs of the cesium limit. You will obviously have to continue monitoring your potassium levels and treat these if necessary. Cesium takes about 3 months to leave the body completely and there may be some cesium build-up in some of the healthy cells.

The following symptoms may occur *during* cesium therapy:

- *Prickly and tingly feelings*, particularly in your fingers but sometimes also in lips and face. This is a common side-effect of cesium therapy and does not indicate that the cesium limit has been reached. It is generally seen during the first 3 weeks, and has no particular significance other than the fact that it indicates that cesium is being absorbed. It is no reason for alarm, since it usually goes away after a few weeks. It is interesting to note that this side-effect is also seen in some patients on conventional chemotherapy.

- *Dry, scaly skin which may be accompanied by itching.* This happens when the patient does not drink enough water, especially on hot days, and indicates systemic dehydration. As indicated above, the patient should drink at least 2 liters of purified water per day and more on hot days.
- *Frequent urination, especially at night, and sleeplessness.* The kidneys do most of their work of eliminating toxins from the body while you are sleeping. This also happens with the debris caused by dead cancer cells. This fills up the bladder quickly, which compels you to get up frequently at night. Sleeplessness may also be a problem, which is aggravated by frequent trips to the bathroom. Applying both your CsCl/DMSO doses before lunchtime may help. In addition, the CsCl may cause mild hypertension which contributes to insomnia and is another reason to take both your CsCl/DMSO doses earlier in the day. Eating fruit also helps in this situation, although it runs against the rules of the cancer diet. Eating low glucose (low GI fruits) will help.
- *Blood (dark, dried) in the urine.* This is usually no reason to be alarmed if your kidney function is normal, because it indicates that the kidneys are performing their task of getting rid of the dead cancer cells. It is generally seen in the morning following the night-time cleansing action of the kidneys while you sleep. However, fresh, bright red blood is never a good sign and may indicate internal bleeding and possibly kidney damage. The situation therefore requires immediate medical attention.

Monitoring your progress

After some time, all cancer patients want to know if they are winning the battle. It is important to understand, as explained above, that the shrinking of solid tumors is not a reliable indicator of treatment success or otherwise. The size of solid tumors may even temporarily increase in the beginning of cesium therapy. As previously explained, this is due to inflammation. However, generally the size of the tumor should start to decrease after 1-3 months or sooner.

The tumor markers sometimes used by oncologists to monitor treatment progress or otherwise are not of much real significance. They are generally specific types of proteins which occur in the blood of patients with particular types of tumors. They are often used to indicate the presence or absence of cancer, for which purpose they are not particularly reliable. Changes in the level in the blood over time may have greater significance on whether a particular tumor is increasing or decreasing. They are, however, not of absolute value for this purpose because of the large number of false negatives and false positives that have been recorded (see further comments on cancer markers).

You may use the AMAS and Navarro tests to assess your cancer status as discussed elsewhere in this book.

Measuring Acidity

Since the principles of the CsCl/DMSO treatment are based on altering the intracellular pH in the cancer cells, the patient might wonder whether this can be measured during treatment as an indicator of successful treatment. It was previously mentioned that cancer cells die at an intracellular pH of 8.0 or higher. pH measurements can be made on various body fluids such as blood, urine, saliva, mucous, etc. Such measurements indicate systemic or extracellular acidity. In addition, these measurements do not indicate a static value, since the fluids analyzed are constantly running through the tissues, attempting to remove acid wastes. They do not indicate the pH value inside the cancer cells. And this is what we want to know. The bad news is that we have no useful means of measuring the pH value inside the cancer cells. The only practical way to ensure that your tissues are alkaline is to follow a highly alkaline diet (see "Cancer Diet") and to make sure that you limit acidifying foods as much as possible in your diet.

Warnings: what not to take with the CsCl/DMSO protocol

Do not take any other Type IV cancer treatments or any other treatment that kills large numbers of cancer cells together with this protocol. Most treatments have been designed (by varying concentrations, etc.) to kill the maximum number of cancer cells that the body can safely handle. Additional cancer-killing treatments may cause excessive accumulation of cancer cells which the body cannot safely dispose of. However, IPT is the preferred therapy, and it can be combined with most other treatments under medical supervision.

However, other treatments for example those that build the immune system, improve the patient's nutritional status, protect the kidneys or the liver, etc. can be taken together with the CsCl/DMSO protocol. It is interesting to note that IPT or chemotherapy is one of the other treatments that can be advantageously combined with the CsCl/DMSO protocol.

Although CsCl is available in tablet form for oral consumption, I do not recommend taking it orally. It may cause stomach bleeding and irritation, especially if it is not taken with food.

Protocol

The CsCl/DMSO with potassium and alkalinizing calcium supplement treatment (suppresses lactic acid production in cancer cells and blocks cachexia cycle)

NOTE:
CsCl = cesium chloride
Potassium supplement = corrects potassium lost during CsCl treatment
DMSO = dimethylsulfoxide
K= potassium
Cs = cesium
Ca = calcium

This, and IPT, are the treatments of choice for the advanced cancer patient. There are, however, some important points to note:

- CsCl treatment (application to the skin) must include DMSO and preferably also a calcium supplement—all this can be provided in one convenient pack (available from *www.fortifood.co.za*). Note that the CsCl-DMSO mix must be applied to the skin.

    NB Cesium should never be taken orally!

- The calcium and potassium supplements are taken orally.
- It is highly preferred that patients should not self-medicate; at the very least they should have active telephone support or, even better, be treated at a clinic or by a doctor who has experience in the use of CsCl. The Internet is able to supply patients with a list of competent health professionals who may undertake that function. CsCl is actually a very safe procedure when carried out correctly, which means that due attention should be given to the following points: dosage and timing must be precise potassium must be supplemented as detailed below in order to facilitate the use of the different products required in the protocol, a complete supplement protocol pack is now available on the Internet.

Cancer cells develop when there is a deficiency of oxygen. The cells then revert to a primitive mechanism to extract energy from glucose, by converting glucose into lactic acid through a process of fermentation for which oxygen is not required. The lactic acid produced lowers the cell pH and the resulting acidity suppresses the ability of DNA and RNA to control cell division. The acidity may increase from a normal pH 7.4 to as low as 5.8 in cancer cells. The increased acidity also suppresses numerous other critical cellular reactions and the cancer cells begin to multiply in an uncontrolled manner. The lactic acid simultaneously causes intense local pain and destroys other cellular enzymes. The developing cancer then appears as a rapidly growing outer cell mass with a core of dead cells (in the case of solid tumors).

- The very cause and nature of cancer (oxygen deficiency followed by acidity) is the thing that CsCl and DMSO address. Cesium has been shown to enter cancer cells when other nutrients cannot, and the main effects that result are: the inside of the cancer cells is alkalinized—not the blood glucose absorption in the cancer cells is limited, thus starving the cell it neutralizes lactic acid (which is the real cause of the unlimited growth and pain) it stops the fermentation process which produces lactic acid
- CsCl solution makes cancer cells highly alkaline (pH 8 or higher) making them weak so that the immune system can destroy them normal cells do not ingest CsCl.

Dosages
Note: CsCl and DMSO should never be taken orally.
Mix the CsCl (solution) with the liquid DMSO (70 %solution) as indicated in the protocol and apply to the skin, NOT ABOVE any area with a dense concentration of cancer cells and not touching any surface cancer cells.

- For days 1-10: Use bottles marked "Day 1-10"(A1) supplied in the pack
- This CsCl solution contains 1.5g of CsCl per teaspoon (5ml). Mix 5ml of this solution with one tablespoon (10ml) of 70 % DMSO solution (A2). These products are conveniently supplied, ready for use in the Protocol Pack.
- Wait several minutes before applying the mixture to the skin. (*Do not mix the potassium supplement into this solution*). Apply liberally

to a conveniently large area of skin (eg 10-20cm²) using a different area each day. Use your finger tip or a sprayer to apply the solution, but wash your hands thoroughly immediately afterwards without touching anything else. Alternatively use a dropper.
- This mixture is applied twice daily (total daily dose of 3.0g = 10ml of CsCl + 20ml 70 % DMSO) to the skin, not near or above the cancer, meaning that the cancer must be nearer to the heart than the application site. Alternate application sites so that the mixture is not applied to the same site on consecutive days. Use your finger to apply the mixture over a conveniently sized portion of the skin, eg on the upper arm or leg. Do not use plastic or any other type of glove to apply the mixture. Wash your hands thoroughly after applying the mixture and do not touch anything while your finger is still wet with the mixture.
- In addition, take 1.2g (2 tabs) (depending on your blood potassium level) of potassium supplement (KCl) (A3) orally daily, also divided into 2 equal doses of 1 tablet each. Note that the daily dose (g) of potassium supplement is less than half that of the CsCl.
- Do not take the potassium supplement within 1-2 hours after the cesium application.
- One bottle containing 100 tabs of potassium supplement (A3) is supplied for the whole 40-day course. Two tabs are equal to one daily dose of potassium supplement (1.2g).

This is taken in two equal doses of one tablet daily at least 1 hour after each CsCl dose.

Important: take the potassium supplement one hour or more after applying each dose of CsCl. The reason for this is that if they are taken at the same time, the potassium ions may block (compete with) the cesium for entry into the cells.

- Include several high potassium foods in your diet (eg green leafy vegetables, avocados, plums, prunes, almonds, beets, spinach, tomatoes)
- During this treatment, drink lots of water—at least 4 glasses of purified, toxin free water daily.
- For days 11-20, 21-30 and 31-40 proceed in a similar manner using the bottles supplied in the pack and marked accordingly to complete the course.

- One course of treatment is 40 days
- Immediately after completing course 1 (40 days) continue with course 2 (also 40 days) if no signs of the cesium limit have appeared (see later).

Warnings

To a certain extent, cesium accumulates in the body until mildly toxic levels are achieved. This is called the cesium limit. The cesium limit in a person is recognized by the symptoms listed below.

- A rash may develop at the application site before the cesium limit is reached. This is not the same as the cesium limit. It is caused by dehydration of the skin by DMSO and is completely harmless. Spraying water on the site and rubbing it will help.
- Some cancers may actually temporarily increase in size before they shrink during treatment. This is due to inflammation. For certain types of cancer, this may create a dangerous situation because of the additional regional pressure exerted. It is particularly dangerous in patients with brain cancer, cancer of the pancreas or cancer of the gastrointestinal system. Therefore seek medical advice if such a possibility exists.
- Muscle cramps are one of the symptoms of a potassium deficiency. Another sign of a potassium deficiency is that if you curl your toes, they do not go right back into the normal position. In both cases, a deficiency of magnesium and/or calcium may also be involved. One reason for separating the CsCl from the potassium is specifically to avoid cramping. If you still get cramps and you have been separating the potassium and cesium doses by at least an hour, it indicates that you should separate them by more than one hour or that you should take a calcium-magnesium supplement.
- Some cancer patients reach their cesium limit before their cancer has been completely cured. In this case the cancer has probably been reduced from a Stage IV to a Stage I or II cancer. These patients have two options. One is to resume the cesium treatment after a while (20-30 days after completing two courses as directed above). Alternatively, the patient can go on to another alternative cancer treatment. In the meantime, the patient should continue with the basic diet.

Additional compounds to be used in conjunction with the CsCl/ DMSO protocol

1. **DMSO and MSM** *(promote absorption of CsCl by the cancer cells)*

   - Apart from their use in combination with CsCl, additional DMSO and MSM have many other advantages for the cancer patient.
   - Prepare a 70 % DMSO solution by mixing 70ml of pure DMSO with 30ml of purified water and use this solution topically if more DMSO is required.
   - While DMSO is very non-toxic systemically, it can be mildly dangerous if handled incorrectly. It should not be given to pregnant women and should not come into contact with any other material than glass or the site of application on your skin. Remember that DMSO will carry anything that it comes into contact with into your body. For example, if it first comes into contact with plastic material, the plastic may dissolve in the DMSO and be subsequently carried into your body.
   - One mild disadvantage of DMSO is the breath and body odor that it imparts to the user. This has been described as an oyster or garlic-like smell. Although it can be quite unpleasant or even embarrassing, the cancer patient has little choice in the matter and it is up to him/her how best to deal with the situation. It is in any case harmless.
   - Because of the danger of overloading the body with the debris from dead cancer cells, the CsCl/DMSO protocol should not be combined with any other treatment that kills cancer cells quickly. It may be combined, however, with treatments that build the immune system, improve the nutritional status, protect the liver and kidneys, and with IPT or chemotherapy. The Kelley enzyme therapy described later is another example of a protocol that can be combined with CsCl/DMSO.

2. **Hydrazine sulphate** (For cancer patients with cachexia and severe weight loss)

   Hydrazine blocks cachexia in the liver. Cancer cells burn glucose to produce energy by means of a very inefficient mechanism (fermentation). The cancer cells therefore only partially metabolize glucose to produce lactic acid. The lactic acid produced is expelled by the cancer cells and then goes to the liver, where it is converted back into glucose by means of a process requiring a huge amount of energy (gluconeogenesis). The glucose produced in this manner then goes back to the cancer cells and the cycle starts again. In this manner, the patient's healthy cells are starved while the cancer cells grow vigorously.

The conversion of lactic acid into glucose in the liver and the conversion of glucose into lactic acid in the cancer cells both consume much energy, which is effectively taken from the normal cells that burn glucose for energy production (aerobically, using oxygen) much more efficiently. This drains energy from the cancer patient, leaving him extremely tired and emaciated (cachexia). The lactic acid cycle is present in virtually every cancer patient and increases sharply as the cancer grows.

- With cachexia, healthy cells have a deficiency of both energy and vital nutrients. This is what is responsible for severe fatigue and approximately 40 % of all cancer deaths.
- Hydrazine blocks the cachexia cycle in the liver while CsCl blocks the cycle in the cancer cells as a result of the increased pH in these cells induced by the CsCl. Combining these two is therefore a very effective means of combating cachexia.

Further benefits associated with hydrazine are:

- Hydrazine has been shown to stop growth of both animal and human cancers.
- Hydrazine works by stopping gluconeogenesis by the cancer cells because these cells *are starved of glucose. Normal cells do not suffer in this way, because, unlike the cancer cells, they can also derive energy from burning fats.*
- Hydrazine is relatively non-toxic at normal dosage levels, but higher doses may be toxic. Therefore do not overdose.
- Hydrazine may produce a significant reduction in pain levels accompanied by a feeling of euphoria, increased appetite and a sense of improved well-being This usually happens within 1-2 days.
- Hydrazine does not destroy white blood cells (immune cells) or bone marrow cells as standard chemotherapy does.
- Hydrazine can be combined with other therapies, eg CsCl/DMSO.
- Cachexia patients should be treated with a flood of highly nutritious foods and supplements such as the vegetable juice and carrot juice

previously mentioned. They should also be given easily digestible fats such as olive oil or the correct mix of w-3 and w-6 fatty acids to nourish the normal cells.
- Hydrazine's main benefit is that it prevents loss of protein and body mass caused by cancer while at the same time exerting indirect anti-tumor effects. Experience with hydrazine shows that it leads to significant subjective improvements (notably in controlling pain and nausea) as well as improving the outcome in the treatment of many types of cancer (73).
- Studies conducted at the Petrov Oncology Research Institute at St. Petersburg, Russia, produced research results supporting the use of hydrazine on six important aspects, including the fact that it was selectively non-toxic and that it could control cancer growth in humans. It produced objective, measurable improvements in 33 % of cancer patients and subjective improvements in 58 %. This amounts to a positive response in 91 % of patients.
- Dr. R. Chlebowski, a former director of the NCI, conducted 4 double blind placebo controlled studies with hydrazine sulphate in the treatment of cancer patients (see (11) and *J Clin Oncol*, 1990) which convincingly demonstrated the efficacy of the drug in the treatment of lung cancer patients.

In June 1989, FDA agents raided the offices of 2 USA distributors of hydrazine sulphate, seizing supplies and documents.

Hydrazine: dosage

The following is an example of a hydrazine treatment protocol for a 55kg patient:

- One 60mg capsule of hydrazine sulphate every day (before breakfast) for the first 3 days.
- Then, for the next 3 days, one capsule each with breakfast and dinner.
- Then, one capsule in a similar manner three times a day beginning with breakfast and then one capsule every 8 hours.
- For patients weighing less than 50kg, these doses are halved. Under no circumstances must hydrazine be overdosed.

Hydrazine is most effective when given alone (no other medications given ½ hour before or after the hydrazine). If an adequate response is obtained on 2 capsules a day, the patient should continue with this dose level, since patients have been maintained successfully on this dosage level.

The greatest success has been achieved by maintaining daily treatment as above for 40 days, followed by an interruption of 14 days before recommencing treatment. It has been reported that this schedule prevented the development of peripheral neurotic symptoms.

Warning

- Patients on hydrazine treatment should avoid alcohol, tranquilizers and barbiturates. They must also not take more than 250g of Vitamin C daily.
- It is also important to avoid MAO inhibitor drugs and high tyramine foods to prevent dangerous rises in blood pressure. Typical examples of such foods: most cheeses, lunch meats, cottage cheese, hot dogs, yoghurt and many other similar foods (2) and drugs. Most of these foods should in any case be avoided by the cancer patient.
- It is important to interrupt treatment for a 14 day period after 40 days.

About half of all patients who take hydrazine sulphate experience weight gain, improved appetite, extended survival time and a significant reduction in pain. Many also report feelings of well-being and optimism.

Clinical trials have shown that hydrazine affects every type of tumor at every stage. It can be administered alone or in combination with other treatments including chemotherapy, IPT and radiation.

Cachexia is an important cause of death in cancer patients, which suggests that cancer patients die as a result of the associated complications. Dr. H. Dvorak, chief of pathology at Beth Israel Hospital in Boston, comments as follows:

> *In a sense, nobody dies of cancer . . . they die of something else—pneumonia, failure of one or other organs.*

Cachexia accelerates infections and the building up of metabolic poisons.

Cachexia treatment plan summarized

1. Use hydrazine to stop the cachexia in the liver.

2. If a temporary increase in tumor size (due to inflammation) will not cause any danger, then use the CsCl/DMSO protocol for treatment and to stop the cachexia in the cancer cells by blocking glucose.
3. Do not use more than 250mg supplementary Vitamin C together with hydrazine.
4. Use a highly concentrated and easily absorbable amino acid mix (SON) or other similar product (e.g. whey powder) to provide large amounts of energy to the patient.
5. Use other concentrated sources of nutrients in the form of juices to provide a concentrated source of vitamins and minerals (eg carrot juice, youngberry juice) to nourish the nutrient-deprived normal cells in the patient.
6. Use a concentrated source of enzymes (barley powder).
7. Use MSM (3-5g) to block formation of lactic acid (optional).
8. Use ribose (3-5g) to get glucose into the cells (optional).
9. Follow the cancer diet (mandatory).

3. More on potassium supplementation (with the CsCl treatment plan)

Most (98 %) of the potassium in the body is within the cells, but the remaining 2 % outside the cells is very important for a number of critical functions, including the heart and blood pressure. The balance of intra and extra cellular potassium is critical to the body and many of its functions, including cardiac action. It affects the ways the membranes work, apart from controlling heart function including the pathways between the brain and the heart. Normally, potassium levels in the body are controlled by the kidneys and hyperkalaemia (excess potassium in the blood) may develop in certain kidney and other conditions. Hyperkalaemia is a serious condition which must be treated promptly. Some patients on CsCl may develop evidence of potassium depletion, which necessitates monitoring blood potassium and uric acid levels. Any alkali therapy, including CsCl therapy, causes movement of extracellular potassium to the intracellular compartment, thus lowering serum potassium levels which may become critically low. CsCl therefore lowers blood potassium levels by driving potassium into cancer cells. Patients on CsCl therapy must be constantly monitored (preferably weekly) for either hyper or hypokalemia in order to maintain blood potassium values within normal limits. Kidney damage may result if potassium levels rise too high, but this may be corrected by drinking copious quantities of purified water.

Typical symptoms of hypokalemia

- Fatigue, muscle weakness and cramps, intestinal paralysis with constipation, bloating and abdominal pain. Severe hypokalemia may also result in muscular paralysis and abnormal heart rhythm (arrhythmia) that can be fatal.

Typical symptoms of Hyperkalemia

- Tingling in hands and feet, muscular weakness and temporary paralysis.
- The development of arrhythmia which can lead to cardiac arrest is one of the most important and dangerous symptoms.

Conclusion: Blood potassium levels should be regularly checked in patients on CsCl—at least every few days in the beginning and later at least once every 2-3 weeks. In addition, patients should be closely monitored clinically with special attention to the signs of blood potassium deviations (muscle weakness, abnormal heart rhythms)

> *Other blood abnormalities that may develop if you take the recommended doses of supplemental potassium and the alkalinizing calcium supplement in the CsCl/ DMSO protocol*

Regularly (at least once a month) do blood determinations of uric acid, electrolytes, potassium, magnesium, calcium and sodium (under medical supervision).

- Potassium levels may become too high or too low as explained above. Generally, however, potassium levels tend to be too low, meaning that supplementation (by means of diet or otherwise) is indicated.
- Calcium and magnesium levels may be too low (correct with coral calcium).
- Uric acid, when too high, may cause kidney damage. (Large masses of DNA-containing dying cancer cells may cause blood uric acid levels to rise). If levels are too high, use Xyloprim to normalize (under medical supervision). At a level of 3g of CsCl daily, it is unlikely that uric acid levels will rise to dangerous levels, but the potassium status of the patient must nonetheless be checked regularly (every week)

during treatment. Early signs of possible developing problems may be picked up by watching initial trends in the values of succeeding analyses, even though the values may still be in the accepted normal ranges.
- Individualizing dosage levels: although standard dosage levels are given below which work best for the average patient, there is no such thing as "one size fits all". Based on patient response and experience, dosage levels have to be adapted to best fit the patient. This is why it is advisable to work with an experienced health professional or clinic or even over the telephone if medical supervision is not possible. For those who can afford it, there is a specialized service in America at *life.com/info/cesium.htm* which offers this type of service. Fortifood can provide the names of doctors who may be willing to perform this function in South Africa.

Additional supplements

- *Wobenzyme (or Vitalzyme) and bromelain.* Strips protective enzyme coating from cancer cells, thus exposing them to attack by the immune system. Also liquefies mucus.
- *High-dose Vitamin C.* Improves immunity and prolongs life of cancer patients. Note that patients treated with hydrazine should not take more than 250mg of supplemental Vitamin C.
- *Concentrated vegetable juices* (carrots, beetroot, etc.). Strengthens normal cells.

4. **The calcium protocol (alkalinizing calcium supplement)**

An alkalinizing calcium supplement has been developed which not only alkalinizes the extracellular fluid but also corrects for the increased intracellular potassium concentration accompanied by declining extracellular potassium levels, which is the hallmark of many cancers.

The calcium supplement alkalinizes and normalizes DNA replication. It combines very well with the CsCl treatment.

- The alkalinizing calcium supplement provides calcium (Ca), magnesium (Mg), potassium and trace elements
- Dissolved in water, it has a pH of 10-12 (very alkaline) and therefore it helps to make the cells alkaline.

- As a *treatment,* use 4.5-5.0g of calcium supplement daily in divided doses (one teaspoon of the supplement = 4.5g).

It is almost a waste of time to take calcium products without also making sure that you are getting enough Vitamin D. You can ensure this by taking Vitamin D supplements (eg one tablespoon of codliver oil or 5000IU of Vitamin D) and also ensuring adequate (eg 1hour) daily exposure to direct sunlight.

- The strongly alkaline supplement induces a condition of alkalosis, which causes a shift of potassium ions from the extracellular fluid (circulation) into the cells accompanied by an increased urinary loss of potassium. To compensate for this loss of potassium from the circulation, the calcium supplement contains a source of potassium.
- Although using both the Calsiumsupplement and the CsCl/DMSO protocol in cancer patients has many advantages for the patient, these two treatments should not be administered at the same time. It is best to stagger the doses over a 24 hour period. Since both products have to be administered twice daily, one way of achieving this is as follows:

Time	Product
06h00	CsCl/DMSO
08h00	One potassium supplement tablet
12h00	CsCl/DMSO
18h00	Calsium supplement
19h00	One potassium supplement tablet
21h00	Calsium supplement

NOTE: In the case of cachexic patients, hydrazine doses have to be taken between, but not at the same time as, the other products. For example, the hydrazine may be taken at any time but not within 1 hour of any of the other products. Typically, the first hydrazine tablet of the day can be taken at 07h00 in the abovementioned programme.

- You should also ensure that your daily magnesium intake is adequate (300-400mg daily of elemental magnesium) and in an absorbable form. Check regularly by means of blood analysis. Several good magnesium products are available.)

Summarizing: the cancer protocol pack

In order to facilitate dispensing of the various products in the cancer protocol, all components of the cancer protocol are conveniently supplied together in the form of a Cancer Protocol Pack which contains the following:

1. CsCl powder. 100ml bottles containing 30g of CsCl per bottle for the first 10-day period. Add purified water to dissolve and make up to 100ml. Mix with 70 % DMSO as described above and apply twice daily.

   NOTE that for the other periods of treatment (day11-20, day 21-30, day 31-40) there are increasing quantities of CsCl per bottle (3.3g for day 11-20; 3.6g for day 21-30 and 3.9g for day 31-40).

2. 70 % DMSO. 200ml bottles containing 200ml of 70 % pure DMSO is supplied.
3. Potassium-supplement tablets. One bottle containing 100 potassium-supplement tablets is supplied in the pack. The usual dose is 2 tablets daily, but should be adapted to the prevailing blood potassium values.
4. Calcium supplement. This is supplied as a powder or capsules. Use 1 teaspoonful mixed with water as directed above, or 9-10 capsules daily.

How to judge your progress

The size of your tumor may increase in the beginning of the CsCl treatment. This is because of inflammation, which will disappear after a few weeks. In general, the size of your tumor should start to decrease permanently after 1-2 months or less. Note that shrinking of tumors is not necessarily an indicator of successful treatment. Tumor markers are also not a good indicator of success or otherwise. The best analytical method to monitor treatment is the Navarro method. The AMAS test may also be used.

NOTE: Dr. H. Nieper was a famous but controversial oncologist in Hanover, Germany, before his death a few years ago. He was one of the foremost proponents of alternative medicine in Europe and has made many valuable contributions, including the use of CsCl. As might be expected, he was strongly criticized and opposed by Big Pharma, especially in America where he was prohibited from practicing by the FDA. In spite of this, many famous personalities from all over the world came to consult him, including leading personalities in the Medical Establishment and even ones from the institutions that violently opposed Dr. Nieper. In this regard, he commented as follows:

> *You would not believe how many FDA officials or relatives of FDA officials come to see me as patients in Hanover. You would not believe this, or directors of the American Medical Association, or American Cancer Association, or the presidents of orthodox cancer institutes. That is the fact (74). As stated elsewhere, these even included one American president and other famous personalities such as John Wayne, Yul Brynner and Princess Caroline of Monaco.*

5. **The Bill Henderson protocol**

- This is a modified form of the Budwig diet based on cottage cheese and flaxseed oil which must be taken orally. It does not cause nearly as much inflammation and swelling as most other treatments and is therefore the treatment of choice if swelling is a major problem, for example in patients with brain cancer. In some patients it does not create swelling at all. One problem is that many weak cancer patients cannot take food. However, there are ways of overcoming this problem (discussed elsewhere).
- Diet is extremely important for every cancer patient and its purpose is *inter alia* to create an alkaline inner terrain in which cancer microbes and cancer cells cannot exist.
- The Bill Henderson protocol provides the patient with much needed essential nutrients such as certain fatty acids to build essential new cells. It should not be combined with other Stage IV treatments because of the resulting excessive load of dead cancer cells possibly created in this manner, even though the Henderson treatment normally does not create much inflammation and swelling. It should

- for the same reason preferably also not be combined with the CsCl/DMSO protocol.
- The Bill Henderson/Budwig protocol should not be stopped for at least one year after starting, until the patient is in full remission. Sometimes it may be necessary to stop the treatment in favor of a more suitable treatment for a particular situation. This is permissible as long as all treatment is not stopped altogether.
- When the patient is in full remission on the Bill Henderson protocol, the full remission treatment should be instituted as discussed in this book.
- The Henderson protocol includes the requirement of a very strict cancer diet which the patient must follow meticulously. The treatment actually consists of the strict diet plus the Budwig cottage-cheese-flaxseed-oil protocol. See the Budwig Protocol for details. The cancer diet plus the supplements buy time for the rest of the treatment.
- The Bill Henderson/Budwig protocol is a "gentler" treatment, meaning that cancer cells are killed at a slower pace, thereby producing less congestion and swelling. This is of particular importance for lung and brain cancer patients. This protocol is therefore particularly suitable to buy time for patients who may need other treatments, for example patients who have had prolonged conventional chemotherapy treatment and therefore suffered much damage to the immune system.

The Bill Henderson protocol: modified

The entire Henderson protocol rests on 5 legs, each of which is important:

1. *The diet.* Follow the cancer diet outlined in this book. Pay special attention to the forbidden items (processed food, sugar, dairy products and gluten-containing foods such as bread). Maximize raw and lightly cooked whole vegetables and sprouted seeds. You may include cereals such as millet and quinoa, steamed potatoes and almond milk.
2. *Cottage cheese/flaxseed oil as in the Budwig diet.* Five to six tablespoons of flaxseed oil mixed by hand with $2/3$ cup of organic, low fat cottage cheese. To improve the taste you may blend this mixture with nuts,

berries and/or apple juice and a little Stevia to taste. Eat as soon as finished and do not leave the rest for later consumption.
3. *Barley powder.* Five to six tablets 15 minutes before each meal (20 tablets or capsules per day).
4. *Green tea extract.* Three to four capsules daily in divided doses before meals.
5. *Immune system stimulation.* Use the Transfer Point Beta-1.3DGlucan. Source: Internet or directly from *http://www.AboutBetaGlucan.com/bspecial.asp (username: save; password: save).* You may also call the following number in the USA: (800) 746-7640

- If the Beta Lucan product cannot be obtained, you may use Aloe Vera extract.

A rather difficult problem in connection with the Henderson protocol is the requirement that the cottage cheese used must contain a certain amount of essential sulphur proteins. For this purpose, Henderson specifies the use of certain brands of cottage cheese in the USA. This information may not be available in all countries. In South Africa, the Simonsberg brand of cottage cheese may be used.

Summarizing: This is a good treatment that works gently but reasonably fast in the presence of a previously damaged immune system. It alters the inner terrain in such a way that cancer-causing microbes cannot survive. The cancer cells are killed slowly over a period of 3 weeks, which allows the body the opportunity of disposing of the dead cells. Some detoxifying effects may, however, be noticed, such as mild pain in the kidney/liver area, increased bowel movements and urine production, mild nausea and rashes. These are quite normal and are no cause for concern. During this period the cancer markers used to detect cancer may increase temporarily due to increased antigens liberated by the dying cancer cells. Your oncologist may view this as a cause for concern, thus causing unnecessary panic. In particular, do not allow your oncologist to start immediate chemotherapy treatment. This would be very wrong since the symptoms will disappear after a few days.

- More information and further details are available in Bill Henderson's book *Cancer-free—Your Guide to Gentle, non-toxic Healing*, available as an e-book or from the publishers Amazon.com.
- For more info on the Budwig Protocol, see the "Budwig Protocol" in this book.

Additional supplements

- Vitamin D (at least 10000IU = 250mcg of Vitamin D) or codliver oil, 1 tablespoonful daily.
- Multivitamins (eg multinutrient, 6 caps daily).

Remarks about the special features of the Bill Henderson Protocol

- It addresses the four characteristics of cancer (lack of oxygen, excess acidity, excess toxins, and a weak immune system) and not just the symptoms (the cancerous growth).
- The cancer cells are slowly killed over a 2-3 week period.
- Detoxification symptoms may appear (pain in the liver/kidney area, unusual bowel and urine movements, rashes, mild nausea, etc.) This is quite normal.
- During this treatment, some of the cancer markers usually used to assess patient status may temporarily increase (spike). This is normal and is caused by the increase in antigens from the dying cancer cells. This may cause panic and your oncologist may suggest immediate chemotherapy treatment. We all know what the result of that treatment will be. Relax and wait a few days.

All products indicated above can be shipped to any address in the world by the vendors cited.

- There are 3 other major causes of cancer which, unless removed, will prevent success with this regimen. These are: heavy metal toxicity due to heavy metals in root canals severe emotional trauma and stress wrong diet and lifestyle deficiency of unadulterated w-6 fatty acid.

You can expect to see positive results after 6-8 weeks on this regimen. If not, then you are doing something wrong. Maybe you are not being strict enough with your diet? Reassess the position and continue treatment.

6. The Brandt Grape Cure

This is the oldest cancer cure still in use. It was introduced to the USA in 1920 by a South African born woman, Johanna Brandt. There are 2 different variations of this treatment. The first and preferred one uses black, red or purple grapes crushed to a mush. Since grapes are not always available, they can be replaced by vegetable juices (carrots, beets, etc.) in the second variation. The grape-based variation is preferred and considered a full Stage IV treatment, whereas the vegetable juice variant is rated Stage III. The grape cure is considered a "juice fast" in which no other foods (but purified water) are permitted. The reason for this is that if no other food is taken, the cancer cells have no other food than the grape mush, which is the intended effect, since black and purple grapes contain a variety of cancer-killing compounds like resveratrol, anthocyanidins, bioflavonoids and others. In other words, the cancer cells are forced to consume only what is to them toxins and which are harmless to normal cells. In this manner, the cancer cells are selectively killed. Resveratrol is of special importance. It is a polyphenol which inhibits the growth of cancer cells at several stages. It also activates the p53 gene which controls the process of apoptosis (normal cell death which is the mechanism by means of which the body disposes of unwanted, old cells). In addition grapes, especially colored grapes, contain a variety of other cancer-killing compounds and polyphenols.

A complicating factor is the fact that grapes are notorious for the load of pesticides on them. It is therefore vitally important to use only organic products and to wash the grapes well before use. Grape juice alone—especially the commercial variety which is prepared by means of chlorine-containing tap water, is not suitable. In addition, whole grapes are required because they contain enzymes necessary for digestion of the other components.

> *An extremely important aspect of the treatment is the fact that the patient is required (every day) to fast for 12 hours followed by nothing but the grape mush for the next 12 hours.*

In this manner the cancer cells are first starved for 12 hours and thereafter they get nothing but the grape mush with its cancer-killing ingredients, which the cancer cells consume voraciously *inter alia* because of its glucose content.

During this period, 2-4 liters of the grape mush should be consumed slowly in small portions over the entire 12 hour period (and not only during meal times). The grape mush is prepared by means of a food processor. To avoid nausea and to maximize the effectiveness of the treatment, the daily portion of the mush is divided into 8 equal portions, one portion being taken every 1½ hours.

- The treatment usually lasts 6 weeks, after which the patient can stop for 14 days and then go on the treatment for another 6 weeks, or the patient can go directly on to the remission protocol.
- This is not an easy protocol to follow; many patients find it very hard to eat nothing but grape mush for 6 weeks. It is, however, a proven treatment that has been around for a very long time and should be seriously considered in certain situations as an alternative Stage IV treatment if the problems surrounding it can be overcome.

Other supplements that go with the grape cure
These should be taken between 8 am to 8 pm to ensure that there is always a period of at least 12 hours during which only grape mush/grapes is given:

- Grape seed extract (proanthocyanidins), 500mg
- Grape skin extract (resveratrol), 10mg
- Vitamin c, 10g a day in divided doses)
- Cayenne pepper and niacin (1g). Both of these increase blood flow, which helps to improve delivery of glucose and oxygen to the cells. Take as much pepper as is convenient.
- A good multinutrient supplement which provides alpha-lipoic acid (300mg), vitamin e (400iu), Vitamin A (4000IU), Selenium (200mcg) and zinc (30mg).

The Brandt grape protocol is very effective but difficult to comply with and must be very strictly adhered to. In practice it can be very demanding on the patient to exist for weeks on nothing but grape mush. Also, there are the distressing symptoms that result from the elimination of large amounts of toxins. Together these can be just too much for the patient who, after a few weeks, may be tempted to give up. The patient should be highly motivated (eg by reading about the many success stories of others) and especially by active support of friends and family. During critical periods, it may be necessary for someone to phone the patient a few times during the day. More sources of information are available on the Internet and in the *Cancer Tutor* (32).

7. **Ozone treatment**

There are different variations of this procedure available. Since the equipment is rather expensive and possibly too complicated to handle at home, I suggest that it is best to have this treatment in a clinic setting. It is, however, a very effective way of treating cancer (see later).

8. The Robert Barefoot calcium treatment

This protocol is based on the use of coral calcium to increase systemic alkalinity. Since the extracellular fluids are alkalinized in the first place, this method will not have a major direct effect on intracellular alkalinity, including cancer cells. It does, however, have some effect on intracellular alkalinity to the extent that the extracellular fluids are in equilibrium with the intracellular compartment. But this effect is not a major one. It is therefore not considered to be strong enough to be rated a Stage IV cancer treatment. It is, however, considered a strong Stage III treatment (32). The information presented here was mainly obtained from the book by Robert Barefoot and Carl R. Reich (75) in addition to that summarized in the *Cancer Tutor* (32).

In this protocol, coral calcium is used as the alkalinizing agent. The usual dosage levels are 3.0-4.5g of pure coral calcium per day, which equals 6-9 capsules, each containing 500mg of coral calcium.

- This daily dose should be spread over your *3 daily meals and taken during the meals.*
- To improve mineral absorption, your meals should consist largely of fresh and lightly cooked vegetables.

In addition, I suggest that you include apple cider (or apple juice) with the meal to supply the organic acids which improve mineral absorption.

- Since the dosage level of coral calcium is not critical, you can also buy coral calcium powder and use the powder instead of the capsules. This is not only more economical, but in this form the minerals may be slightly better absorbed. One level teaspoonful of coral calcium powder is approximately 4g. Half a teaspoonful with each meal will ensure that you get enough coral calcium.
- It is important to make sure that you buy the best quality coral calcium (32) such as the product that comes directly from the coral reefs in Okinawa. Some vendors market a cheap product as "coral calcium" which consists of a mixture of calcium carbonate and coral calcium. This is not acceptable, because coral calcium contains 20

% of calcium and 10 % of magnesium, and if calcium carbonate is added, the patient gets too little magnesium, which is an important ingredient of coral calcium. The Okinawan coral calcium is also an important source of micro minerals which are important for the cancer patient.
- As rain falls on the earth, water runs down mountains and rocks, extracting many different minerals from the soil. Micro-organisms in the sea take up these minerals, which are eventually precipitated in the ocean bed as islands or coral reefs. Over thousands of years this process can build entire islands like Okinawa. It is important to realize that the mineral deposits in such coral islands do not only contain calcium carbonate but, in addition to the carbonates of calcium and magnesium, it is also a rich source of natural marine nutrients, which has become known as coral calcium. Mixtures of calsium and magnesium carbonates (often sold as "coral calcium") therefore can in no way replace the real coral calcium. In addition, when you buy coral calcium, make sure that the product comes directly from the coral reefs and that it does not consist of coral deposits collected on beaches in Okinawa.
- It is vitally important that the patient also gets enough Vitamin D, which is necessary for mineral absorption. I therefore suggest that the following supplements be included in the protocol:

  > Vitamin D2 (at least 12000IU or 300mcg) (32) or 1 tablespoon of codliver oil daily with meals
  > Multinutrient (4-6 tabs) (32)
  > CellFood (20 drops daily on an empty stomach—optional)
  > A balanced source of w-6 and w-3 unadulterated fatty acids in the correct proportion
  > Vitamin C powder, 3 heaped teaspoonfuls daily, in divided doses away from meals (1 heaped teaspoonful = 4.0g) (32)

- MicroRuboCes 10 (1 capsule providing 10mg of CsCl and 10mg of rubidium chloride) (32). This is optional.
- Vitamin E (at least 1000IU = 1000 TE) (32)
- Magnesium (6 caps of Biomag daily = 435mg of magnesium) (32).

Vitamin D is particularly important. The Vitamin D status of the patient can be further improved by daily exposure to sunshine (1-2 hours a day exposing your skin and face, including indirect sunlight to your eyes). Do not use any type of sun blocker or sun glasses. Sunlight exposure also prevents excessive increases in blood calcium levels, according to Robert Barefoot's book.

I suggest a blood mineral analysis at the beginning of the treatment and thereafter at monthly intervals to monitor calcium and magnesium status. It is impossible for coral calcium alone to lead to excessively raised Calsium levels (hypercalcaemia) (75).

Note that this protocol is not for Stage IV cancer patients. It is, on the other hand, a strong treatment for Stages III, II and I. Stage IV patients require the strongest possible treatment, which are IPT and/or CsCl/DMSO protocol in combination with a strict cancer diet. However, as previously pointed out, the CsCl/ DMSO protocol can be combined with the Barefoot calcium protocol.

> *It is essential that the patient should follow the cancer diet given in this book. Although fruits are generally forbidden in the cancer patient's diet because of their glucose content, those on the Barefoot protocol are allowed apple juice and some whole, low GI fruits (eg apples, pineapples, avocados) with meals.*

Possible "side-effects" of the Robert Barefoot protocol

The alkalinisation of the body fluids that takes place on the Barefoot protocol releases toxins attached to the outside of the cell membranes into the blood. The body recognizes these as foreign invaders and responds by attacking them with a powerful immune response which may cause flu-like symptoms (diarrhea, stomach aches, headaches and fever). This merely indicates that the body is ridding itself of these toxins which may be cancer-inducing.

9. The Laetrile protocol

Laetrile is a cyanogenic glycoside (a sugar derivative which contains complexed hydrogen cyanide) which occurs in many edible plant species. It also occurs in many foods, such as lentils, beans, etc. For the treatment of cancer, it is usually obtained from apricot kernels, which are an especially rich source of the active glycoside. Cyanogenic cyanohydrins are formed when certain aldehydes react with hydrogen cyanide (HCN). When that aldehyde is part of a sugar molecule, a cyanogenic glycoside is formed. The cyanogenic glycoside that occurs in apricot kernels is called laetrile or Vitamin B17 (amygdaline). Cancer cells contain certain enzymes which hydrolyze the cyanogenic glycosides to liberate free hydrogen cyanide and benzaldehyde, both of which are highly toxic and kill the cancer cells. The active form of the compound as it occurs in plants is in a laevorotatory form, but other, less active forms also occur, especially in the plant glycoside amygdaline. I therefore prefer the natural form as it occurs in apricot kernels for the treatment of cancer.

Laetrile is one of the most widely used alternative cancer treatments. It is very safe and simple to use and highly effective if high enough doses of a high-quality product are used for a long enough period of time. It needs to be combined with a strict anti-cancer diet (as with all other cancer treatments) and certain supplements have to be used with it (see later). As in the case of all other cancer treatments, the cancer patient using laetrile as well as his/her doctor must be prepared to study widely and gain a working knowledge of the product. They must also ensure that the patient receives an adequate amount of a balanced w-6:w-3 fatty acid supplement as in all other cancer treatments.

- The history of how laetrile was developed by a few doctors and scientists, and the long personal histories of successful treatments as well as the violent opposition by conventional medical establishments to the product, form one of the darker chapters of medical history (1). In America, the FDA has made the availability and distribution of laetrile effectively impossible although it is a perfectly safe and natural compound. In 1975, a comment by the FDA stated:

Laetrile has been sold for treating cancer for around 25 years, yet there is still no sound, scientific evidence that it either effective or safe.

The FDA, however, fails to add that doctors are not allowed to use laetrile in the treatment of cancer patients, and that this is the main reason why no proper clinical studies have been conducted. One consequence of the official campaign against laetrile is that only illegal sources are now available, and that the quality of such products is often dubious. It is, therefore, better to use unrefined apricot kernels.

In the meantime, the FDA is continuing its strong-arm tactics and raids against distributors (1). For example, in 1977 the FDA took the unusual step of posting large "Laetrile Warning" posters in 10 000 post offices in the USA and sending an FDA "Drug Bulletin" on the subject to hundreds of thousands of health workers. All of this happened in spite of the fact that laetrile is a common food component which occurs in hundreds of foodstuffs and that it is used in large amounts by certain communities in the world. In this manner the authorities succeeded in implanting the idea of laetrile toxicity in the minds of many uninformed people.

Clinical studies with laetrile

Fortunately, it has been possible to conduct some clinical studies, mostly in countries outside the USA. One study, by Ellison, found an 82 % response rate (various degrees of response) in cancer patients (1).

One of the main proponents of laetrile therapy has been Dr. Contreras in Mexico (1). At his institute in Tijuana, he has been treating terminally ill cancer patients with laetrile since 1960. Dr. Contreras claims that 65 % of a large number of terminally ill patients that he has treated derived some benefit as a result of the treatment, but that half of these had recurrences after the treatment was terminated.

Dr. J.A. Richardson published detailed case histories of 4 000 patients he claims to have treated with success (1).

Dr. H. Nieper is a well-known German oncologist who practiced in Hanover for many years. He used laetrile widely in his medical practice. He is the author of several papers on laetrile, including one on the results of 60 patients treated with laetrile (1).

Dr. M.D. Navarro is another prolific author in this field. He has published almost 20 articles in various journals on laetrile since 1954. He has called laetrile "the ideal drug for the treatment of cancer".

Numerous other authors have commented on their experience with laetrile as an anti-cancer drug. These reports indicate that most of the patients treated with laetrile were preterminal—many after immune system-destroying chemotherapy. Most of these patients responded in some way to laetrile therapy, but only a small percentage (approx 5 %) was actually cured. Many others went into remission. One possible reason for the low cure rate in these chemotherapy-pretreated patients may be that the patients were preterminal, which did not allow enough time for the laetrile therapy to work.

In summary, laetrile appears to be particularly suitable as a "second treatment" after or during treatment with a strong Stage IV treatment such as the IPT or CsCl/DMSO protocols.

Laetrile works by killing cancer cells and building the immune system, *but it works slowly.*

In spite of the violent opposition by some authorities, laetrile continues to be widely used for the treatment of cancer. It has been used for centuries as a cancer remedy and it is interesting to note that in Nepal, where apricot kernels form part of the national diet, the incidence of cancer is very low or completely absent.

In view of what was said before, my advice would be to use apricot kernels (24-40 per day) instead of capsules or pills. The apricot kernels can be made more palatable by grinding the kernels and mixing the powder with an equal quantity of ground nuts (eg almonds, walnuts). The taste can be further improved by mixing the resulting powder with apple juice.

The reaction of orthodox medicine

After years of refusing to do so, the National Cancer Institute in the USA finally agreed to test laetrile in 178 patients with advanced cancer. The tests were conducted at four major medical centers, including the Mayo Clinic where the abortive Vitamin C trial was conducted. Dr. C. Moertel, who also conducted the controversial Vitamin C trial, played a major role in the overall study design and was in charge of the trial at the Mayo Clinic. Dr. Moertel, as previously pointed out, was outspoken in his sentiments against the use of natural products in the treatment of cancer. The study was intended in its design and conduct, to close the book on laetrile (76). For various reasons, 22 patients were excluded from the final analysis, leaving 156 evaluable patients. According to Moertel, 50 % of the patients showed evidence of cancer progression within one month of starting laetrile therapy. Ninety did so after 3 months and 50 % had died before 5 months. This led Moertel to conclude that "laetrile is ineffective as a treatment of cancer."

The laetrile lobby reacted bitterly, because there was a suggestion that the material tested in the study was not laetrile. The Committee for Freedom of Choice in Cancer Therapy and American Biologics Inc. had offered to provide free laetrile for the trial, but this was refused by the investigators. When the offer was refused, these bodies unsuccessfully tried to have the trial stopped.

"Real laetrile is not the material being tested," said one Pro-Choice publication flatly. In addition, they pointed out that 66 % of the trial patients had already received immune system-destroying chemotherapy, a fact which was not mentioned by Moertel in his presentation of the trial results.

In their comments the Committee for Freedom of Choice in Cancer Therapy and the publication *Choice* stated that genuine laetrile was never tested (77). But to the general public, laetrile was a dead duck, partly because of the status of the Mayo Clinic.

Thus the same scenario as in the case of the Vitamin C studies was being replayed: the trial was conducted under conditions which ensured a negative outcome and nobody was conspicuously guilty. In this case, the uncertainties that were identified were introduced by patient selection (pre-treatment with chemotherapy) and by uncertainty of the quality of the product used. This ensured the negative outcome.

This conclusion is supported by the fact that, 10 years after the trial, more laetrile was being used than ever before by over a dozen centers to treat cancer patients (1). In addition, laetrile was forcibly defended by Dr. K. Sigiura, one of the most senior and most respected cancer scientists at the Memorial Sloan Kettering Cancer Center in New York. A lengthy report on the role played by this esteemed scientist in connection with the laetrile saga is available in (1).

Mechanism of action of laetrile

In cancer cells, the laetrile molecule is broken down by the action of the enzyme beta-glycosidase into 2 molecules of glucose, 1 molecule of hydrogen cyanide and one molecule of benzaldehyde. Apart from hydrogen cyanide, benzaldehyde also appears to play an important role in killing cancer cells.

> *The selective action of laetrile against cancer cells is based on the fact that beta-glycosidase enzyme occurs in minute quantities in many cells but it occurs in huge quantities in cancer cells.*

Thus the two toxins hydrogen cyanide and benzaldehyde are unlocked selectively in cancer cells, providing the highly selective action against cancer cells in the presence of normal cells. It has further been shown that, although both these toxins are highly toxic when they are combined, the result is 100 times more toxic than either on its own.

The selective anti-cancer action further depends on the presence of another enzyme, rhodanese, which is present in far greater concentrations in normal cells than in cancer cells. This enzyme breaks down the two toxins in laetrile (HCN and benzaldehyde) into derivatives of salicylic acid, which aids in pain control. Interestingly, cancer cells were found to contain no rhodanese, so that cancer cells do not have the same protective mechanisms as normal cells. Normal cells contain a high level of the enzyme rhodanese, which converts cyanide into isocyanate (CNS), thus effectively detoxifying cyanide.

The action of laetrile as a coenzyme is based on the trophoblast theory of cancer (see Dr. Kelley's metabolic protocol for the treatment of cancer). This theory is based on the role of the pancreatic enzymes trypsin, chymotrypsin and amylase to digest the protein coating covering cancer cells. These enzymes are inhibited by certain inhibitors in the blood, but they can be reactivated by cyanide to become active again.

> *By supplying cyanide, laetrile acts as a coenzyme to trypsin and the other enzymes.*

Thus, in the absence of *cyanide*, these pancreatic enzymes will not be able to remove the protective protein coating on the cancer cells as effectively as in the presence of cyanide. Cyanide (from laetrile) therefore reactivates the pancreatic enzymes necessary to digest the protein coating on the cancer cells, thus rendering them susceptible to destruction by the immune system.

In normal cells, the laetrile molecule is altered in such a way that it loses its cancer-killing capacity. Thus it is important to take enough laetrile to ensure that enough cancer-killing capacity remains after contact with normal cells. The optimum daily dose appears to be 24-40 apricot kernels per day in divided doses, each preferably opened immediately before use.

A second important component of laetrile therapy is the laetrile diet. This differs somewhat from the normal cancer diet. It is also important to provide enough of the proteolytic enzymes trypsin and chemotrypsin. These enzymes break down the enzymes that surround the cancer cell, thus providing access to the cancer cells by the immune cells (see discussion of the Kelley Metabolic treatment).

> *Note that patients on anti-coagulant therapy should take these enzymes only under medical supervision.*

The laetrile diet

The cancer diet is always a very important part of the overall treatment plan, no matter what treatment protocol has been selected. This is also the case with the laetrile diet, which is not much different from other cancer diets. A good summary of the laetrile diet is given in Dr. Binzel's book

(71). However, the diet given there is less than ideal, because it does not include fruits and vegetables with cancer-killing components, and other fruits and vegetables. The base diet should therefore be the raw food diet with modifications (see the cancer diet).

The most important modifications are the inclusion of laetrile-rich fruits and vegetables, and secondly the inclusion of "laetrile friendly" supplements. You should give preference to laetrile-rich foods such as almonds and macadamia nuts.

Supplements for the laetrile diet

These supplements contain nutrients that are required for the optimum action of laetrile in the body. Many of these nutrients (eg manganese, magnesium, selenium, iodide and Vitamins A, E and B6) are present in a good multinutrient supplement (32). Therefore, there is no need for extra supplementation.

It is, however, necessary to take extra zinc (50mg) and Vitamin C (build up to at least 5g a day in divided doses).

Zinc is one of the most critical supplements. It is essential for the transportation of laetrile in the body to the active sites.

> *Laetrile will not perform its anti-cancer action without adequate amounts of bioavailable zinc.*

The enzymes mentioned above can be taken as extra supplements (trypsin, chemotrypsin, bromelain) or they can be obtained in the form of commercially available multi-enzyme preparations (eg Wobenzyme and Vitalzyme). More information is available in reference (32).

It is vitally important to take these enzymes during laetrile therapy using the particular vendor's maximum dosages.

Cancer is best treated with a total nutritional programme which includes the abovementioned supplements as well as a good multinutrient and the correct diet based largely on fruits and vegetables indicated in the cancer diet, with protein largely in the form of vegetable proteins (grains, nuts, beans, etc.). Cottage cheese (eg in the form of the Budwig diet) is permissible. This, however, increases the importance of proteolytic enzymes.

Do not rely on laetrile treatment as the only treatment in seriously ill patients. Its action is too slow. It does, however, make an ideal second treatment in combination with another strong Stage IV treatment. Thus it combines very well with the IPT and CsCl/DMSO protocols because of its immunity-stimulating effect, which the cesium and IPT do not do. Laetrile should be used as a supplemental treatment or as a remission treatment.

Laetrile warnings

Proteolytic enzymes increase the effect of anti-coagulants. This is ordinarily not important, but patients already on blood thinners should take notice of this. Blood coagulation monitoring should be done regularly and, if necessary, the proteolytic enzymes should be discontinued. Extremely high doses of proteolytic enzymes should in any case be avoided (see Dr. Kelley's protocol).

For maximum effect, laetrile treatment should preferably be part of a comprehensive protocol of diet, enzymes and supplements, and should be supervised by a medical professional. For example, laetrile only works in the presence of adequate quantities of zinc and Vitamin C. High level Vitamin A supplements should not be taken.

- Do not take laetrile on a full stomach.
- Intravenous laetrile should be given only under medical supervision. The patient's reaction must be monitored closely and the dose adjusted over a period of 3 weeks.
- On the other hand, there is no reason not to use laetrile as secondary treatment in combination with other treatments.
- Laetrile is also an excellent preventative treatment for cancer.
- Laetrile may occasionally cause a decline in blood pressure due to the conversion of cyanide into thiocyanate. This may be of importance only for those who are on blood pressure medication.
- Laetrile should only be combined with other alternative treatments with due attention to possible contra-indications. Thus Vitamin C should be used with laetrile, but is contra-indicated in patients on hydrazine therapy.
- Do not take laetrile with probiotics.
- The conventional medical establishment has tried to scare patients away from laetrile by claiming that it contains toxic cyanides. This is just a scare tactic, since the actual quantities of cyanide present in laetrile are minute in comparison with the toxic dose of cyanide (calcium 200mg in the form of sodium cyanide).
- For more information consult the website of Dr. Contreras in Mexico (*www.oasisofhope.com*).

Summary: what the patient must do

In collaboration with his/her health professional, the patient must:

- Take 24-40 fresh apricot kernels daily in divided doses
- Strictly adhere to the laetrile diet
- Take the supplements indicated above, especially zinc and Vitamin C.

Do not use this as the principal treatment protocol in severely ill patients, but rather use it as a second or auxiliary treatment protocol.

10. Dr. Max Gerson therapy

This is essentially a dietary protocol developed by Dr. Gerson (a specialist in internal medicine) in Germany in the early 20th Century. He noticed that, while working in a sanatorium, patients, after spending the weekends at home, had gross exacerbation of their symptoms on Mondays. He concluded that diet is an important factor in the cancer patient. The foods that the patients ate at home were—compared to the hospital diet—high in saturated fats, salt, preservatives, pickled goods and alcohol, and relatively low in fresh fruits and vegetables. This contrasts sharply with the bland hospital diet. He subsequently found that he could reverse the symptoms of many diseases such as lupus, tuberculosis and cancer by putting these patients on a diet of grasses and vegetables, which he would juice. He became famous in Europe for his dietary treatment of disease, and later went to the USA, where he continued to treat cancer patients with a diet consisting of 13 glasses of fresh vegetable juice a day. He also eliminated from the patient's diet extra sodium (eg in the form of salt) and all animal proteins except yoghurt and cultured buttermilk. He also gave extra potassium and iodide by means of supplements.

One unusual aspect of his protocol included daily coffee enemas to promote elimination of toxins from the liver and cleanse the body.

In this manner he succeeded in providing a treatment schedule that no one could match. In fact, his work was so impressive that early in his career in the USA the prestigious *JAMA* published one of his articles.

In 1945 Gerson was called to testify before a US Senate Committee investigating cancer. He brought with him five patients who had had some of the most common forms of cancer. In addition he submitted X-ray photos, pathology reports (including some from the prestigious Memorial Hospital in New York) as well as testimonials from many other patients and relatives of cancer patients.

Gerson's credentials were impressive. He had graduated from a leading German medical school and had studied with noted medical experts. At the time when he appeared before the committee, Gerson was affiliated with the Gotham Hospital in New York and he also had a private practice in that city. In addition, he was the author of fifty articles in medical journals.

Gerson's methods were gaining popularity just at a time when the newly introduced chemotherapy was seeking public acceptance. This prompted a rapid response from the orthodox forces that were not slow in responding to the challenge.

Possibly also because of the public attention that his methods were attracting in the newspapers and on the radio, the orthodox medical establishment decided that he had to be silenced, and the same *JAMA* which had earlier published one of his articles, later attacked him and called him a quack. He was also subsequently reviewed in the *JAMA* and it was concluded that his methods were of "no value". This was followed by other drastic and orchestrated steps to discredit and harass him.

The official position of the medical establishment on the role of nutrition in the treatment of cancer is reflected by the following official statement by the American Medical Association:

> *There is no scientific evidence whatsoever to indicate that modification in the dietary intake of food, or other nutritional essentials are of any specific value in the control of cancer (78).*

I predict that this is one of the official statements made by the American Medical Association which they will regret in times to come.

At the height of his career in the USA, a special Senate committee headed by Senator Claude Pepper of Florida was appointed to investigate his work. Sen Pepper then invited Dr. Gerson to bring forward medical documentation and patients in support of his work. Gerson brought forward 50 terminally ill cancer patients who were alive and well 5 years after treatment with the Gerson therapy.

> *His results were especially impressive in the treatment of the much dreaded malignant melanoma.*

Pepper and his committee were so impressed that not only did they not condemn him (which apparently was the objective of the exercise) but they actually commended him. Not only did this not change the official medical assessment of Gerson's methods, but in fact he was forbidden to continue his practice in the USA and had to continue his work elsewhere.

In spite of being unmercifully vilified, harassed and even persecuted by the American Medical Association in a manner that is difficult to understand, Dr. Gerson continued his work as best he could. Fortunately, there were also others who did understand the importance of his work—amongst them the famous missionary doctor and Nobel Prize winner, Dr. Albert Schweitzer, who declared: *I see in Gerson one of the most eminent geniuses in medical history."* Today, his work is continued in Mexico by his daughter Charlotte Gerson Strauss.

The essence of the Gerson diet

The Gerson programme consists of three components:

- an intensive nutritional programme high in raw, unprocessed food and raw vegetable juices, supplying healing nutrients naturally present in the best organically grown foods accelerated detoxification and elimination of waste products and accumulated metabolic poisons that interfere with normal healing processes in the body, *inter alia* by means of coffee enemas raw liver injections, thyroid extract, digestive enzymes and supplements of important minerals and vitamins, including a relatively high intake of Vitamin C.

The juices are prepared from organically grown vegetables (eg carrots) and permitted vegetables. The preferred fruits are low GI fruits such as apples and pineapples, although Gerson permitted grapes, cherries, mangos, oranges, grapefruit, and papayas.

The protocol specifies 13 glasses of freshly prepared juices (carrots, beetroot) taken hourly during the day. In this manner the patient receives high concentrations of antioxidants, vitamins and minerals that will actively support the immune system. In addition, the patient also receives large quantities of phytochemicals (known and unknown) that kill cancer cells. Among these are also chemicals with pronounced anti-cancer properties such as isothyanates and glucosinolates now known to occur in members of the Brassica family (broccoli, Brussels sprouts, cabbage, etc.). These are examples of known anti-cancer compounds. They have such powerful anti-cancer properties that regular consumption has been shown to reduce the risk of cancer by 50 % (79). All these details were of course not known to Dr. Gerson when he did his pioneering work in the 1930s.

In his protocol, Gerson strictly forbade animal proteins, smoking, alcohol, salt, sodium bicarbonate, all smoked foods, sharp condiments (pepper, ginger), all cooking equipment made of aluminum, microwave ovens, pressure and steam cookers. Interestingly, he did not advise his patients to drink large amounts of water as the full capacity of the stomach was required for the large volumes of juices and soups.

The potassium-sodium ratio

Dr. Gerson placed great emphasis on potassium (high potassium plant foods, partly in the form of juices) and on the potassium-sodium ratio in the diet. He realized that our ancestors ate a high potassium plant-based diet in which the potassium-sodium ratio was 4:1, which is very different from today's Western high sodium (salt) diet in which this ratio is reversed to 1:4. (80).

In this respect, as in many others, Dr. Gerson was way ahead of his time. Nearly 50 years later convincing evidence was published by Dr. M.M. Jacobs which supports Gerson's thinking on the significance of this ratio in relation to cancer (80, 81). An important finding in these studies was that a decreased potassium-sodium ratio is associated with accelerated metastatic spreading of colon cancer.

Today it is also known that an elevated potassium level together with a strongly reduced sodium level in the tissues suppresses tumor formation (82).

- Much of what Dr. Gerson said about diet and cancer 50 years ago is now accepted by many, in the light of newer knowledge. In his publication *Cancer therapy: Results of 50 cases,* Gerson details his therapeutic programme, and documents his clinical experience over a period of 30 years. He also includes a clinical summary of 50 patients who had recovered completely from end-stage cancer.
- The National Cancer Institute and the American Cancer Society heavily criticized Gerson's work for several decades—until 1980. Then the American Cancer Society published its official anti-cancer diet (after a previous strong statement that diet has nothing to do with cancer, as pointed out above) which in many ways resembles the Gerson diet.

The Gerson programme also included supplements such as potassium, iodide, vitamins, thyroid extract, minerals and digestive enzymes. All animal proteins were excluded for a period of 6-12 weeks and then kept to a minimum. The diet is further largely fat free, but does allow non-fat and unflavored yoghurt, cheese varieties, and cottage cheese, buttermilk and flaxseed oil. The latter is remarkable, since at that stage the important cancer-preventing effects of prostaglandin E3 (derived from alpha-linolenic acid in flaxseed oil) had not yet been described (83).

For detoxification and toxin elimination, Dr. Gerson used self-administered coffee enemas several times a day. He believed that cancer patients do not die of the cancer itself, but rather of the mass of toxins liberated during the break-down of cancer cells, which the liver cannot handle. (In this he was well ahead of his times; the reader may recall that when we discussed the CsCl protocol, the accumulated toxins resulting from the massive killing of cancer cells by the cesium were one of the problems encountered.) In addition, the numerous environmental toxins to which we are exposed contribute to our systemic toxin load and also raise the sodium content of the soil whilst at the same time lowering potassium levels.

Caffeine, taken rectally, stimulates and supports liver function by increasing bile flow and by opening the bile ducts so that the liver can excrete tumor breakdown products more easily.

Gerson claimed an overall cure rate of 30 % in his terminally ill cancer patients, although others who have used the procedure subsequently have claimed a much higher success rate. The Gerson Institute claims that it is particularly effective for melanoma (84) and other skin cancers as well as for ovarian and colorectal tumors.

Gerson: cancer prevention vs treatment

Two variants of the procedure were developed by Gerson: one for treatment and one for prevention.

For prevention of cancer, the patient was allowed to select 25 % of all food eaten according to his/her own preferences. The other 75 % had to be strictly according to the principles of the protocol, with the main aim being to protect the patient's vital organs and to strengthen the surveillance capacity of the immune system to guard against cancer cells that may have developed.

For treatment, the usual more stringent protocol was prescribed as detailed above. For detoxification purposes, castor oil every second day was used in addition to the coffee enemas.

Clinical efficacy

There are hundreds of personal reports of near miraculous recoveries of terminally ill cancer patients who had resorted to the Gerson therapy in an attempt to save their lives. These do not strictly count as scientific evidence of efficacy. Large scale double blind clinical studies at official institutions are, however, very difficult to get off the ground because of official prejudice, that makes it nearly impossible to get the necessary funding and permission for such studies. The large number of extremely positive anecdotal reports of advanced malignant melanoma and other cancers has inspired a group of scientists at the University of California to conduct a broad-based retrospective study on similar patients. In this study, advanced melanoma patients who had followed the Gerson Protocol were compared on a five-year survival rate basis with a similar control group who had followed other courses of treatment (84). Over a period of 15 years, 153 adult melanoma patients entered the study and were treated according to the Gerson method. The results showed that 100 % of the 14 Stage I and II Gerson melanoma patients survived for at least 5 years, compared to 79 % of 15 798 similar patients treated by other methods (85). Of the 33 Stage III Gerson patients, 70 % survived after 5 years compared to 41 % of 134 of the control patients. Of the 18 Gerson patients with Stage IV, 39 % survived after 5 years, compared to 6 % of the 194 other patients reported in the literature (84).

Although this is a retrospective trial, conducted on different populations of patients, the differences are so large and consistent with other similar studies that they may be considered strongly supportive of the Gerson method, especially considering the fact that most of the patients were end-stage. They also emphasize the overall importance of diet in the management of the cancer patient.

A remarkable case history of a melanoma patient

This is the case history of patient (J) with melanoma treated successfully with the Gerson protocol. I repeat this study here because it is so typical of what happens to many patients in practice. In March 1982, J found a mole on the right side of his forehead, which did not concern him much because it was not big: about half the size of his finger nail. However, J's doctor suggested taking it off and doing a biopsy. The result was shocking: the growth was malignant, Clark level 4. Surgery was immediately performed, but within 10 days the cancer was back at the primary site and thereafter several tumors appeared, within days, all over his upper body, chest and arm. Different doctors gave different advice, but they all agreed that there was very little they could do to stop the cancer. Different alternative doctors were also not very optimistic, but the Gerson Institute pointed out that Gerson therapy is known to be effective against melanoma. The fact that J had not had any previous immune-destroying conventional treatment (eg chemotherapy) was considered a positive point in his favor. The Gerson Institute thought that J's chances were good, but warned that he would suffer a great deal from nausea in the beginning due to the detoxifying effect of the Gerson therapy. J did get quite sick in the beginning, the type of symptoms one would expect in the case of stomach flu. The situation became so bad that J nearly lost faith after a week, but nonetheless continued after the amount of juices and tablets were cut back somewhat. Thereafter, he felt better again. The heart of the therapy consisted of an 8 ounce (250ml) glass of half carrot and half apple juice every hour starting at 8 in the morning and continuing until 7 o'clock at night. Actually, the juices were varied somewhat: basically, J had at one hour a juice that consisted of half carrot juice mixed with half apple juice and the next hour there was a green juice (mixture of lettuce, green pepper, red cabbage and apple). The juices were laced with a supplement consisting of potassium salts and the other supplements prescribed by the protocol. In addition, the patient was allowed 3 meals which conform to the requirements of the protocol (see above).

In the beginning, one starts to kill and digest the cancer cells, which are then eliminated from the body by the liver in the form of metabolic toxins which are also responsible for the influenza-like symptoms. To help this process, J was given a coffee enema every 4 hours (6 am, 10 am, 2 pm, 6 pm and 10 pm). The coffee enemas put the drug caffeine directly into the portal vein. This allows the liver to detoxify much more efficiently than it could otherwise do. J found the coffee enemas to be of great help: they relieve pain, relieve digestive discomfort and therefore form a crucial part of the therapy. This was more or less the daily routine for 2 months. By that time, every visible tumor in J's body had started to regress, and then the tumors started to shrink, dry off and then to fall off. In May 1982 J's body had several tumors and he was told by 4 medical doctors that he had very little chance of survival. In July he had been on Gerson therapy for 3 months and all visible cancers had regressed and disappeared.

The Institute advised that although the visible cancers had disappeared, J had to stay on the therapy for another 18-24 months. Now, after 13 years, J is still cancer free.

J's subsequent experience in trying to help others is as illuminating. He states that he could easily identify those that would succeed and those who would not. People used to the passive mode, where they just sit and the professionals are the ones who do things for them, are the ones that fail. These people are often horrified when they find out the extent to which they have to cooperate and do things on their own.

Note: The supplements referred to in the abovementioned report consist of potassium (500mg), niacin (100mg), thyroid extract, Lugol's solution, pancreatin, pepsin, Vitamin B12 and liver injections. These are required to be taken on a daily basis. The B12 and liver injection can be combined as one injection; the others are taken orally.

Similar accounts of the successful use of Gerson Therapy for the treatment of breast cancer, pancreatic cancer, non-Hodgkins lymphoma and all skin cancers are available.

The abovementioned account highlights the considerable effort and time that the patient personally has to devote to the treatment. This applies in the case of most other alternative treatments.

The updated principles of the Gerson diet or its variations are now widely used in many cancer clinics worldwide. The regimes developed at different clinics often differ little from one another and are broadly based on the Gerson principles.

In these programmes, digestion is improved by means of hydrochloric acid supplements (eg betaine hydrochloride) to start the digestive process, followed by pancreatic enzymes to assist the pancreas. Raw fruits and vegetables and their juices add to the level of enzymes, and improve digestion. Cooked vegetables provide soft bulk and nutrients; cooked grains (mostly oats) add bulk, protein and additional minerals. Injections of B12 and multinutrient supplements are given to eliminate deficiencies. Colon cleansing and coffee enemas are common features. Emphasis is placed on carrot juice and Vitamin A. Also attention is given to infected teeth and the removal of mercury amalgams from teeth, which are regarded as a major stumbling block to recovery.

Possible improvements to the Gerson diet

It is now possible to make certain improvements to the Gerson diet, using up to date research which was not available in Dr. Gerson's day.

High blood sugar levels are very undesirable in the cancer patient because it is generally accepted that "cancers are sugar feeders". High blood sugar levels benefit cancer cells more than normal cells. In selecting vegetables and especially fruits for the cancer patient, it is advisable to select those with a GI below 60 (86). In the case of most of the vegetables used by Gerson, this would not be a problem; among his choice of fruits, though, it would be better to exclude bananas (especially ripe ones), grapes and peaches.

The supplements he suggests are in order (especially with the accent placed on thyroid function) but other vitally important supplements should be included: selenium (400mcg), chromium (400mcg), Coenzyme Q10 (100-200mg), Vitamin C (5000mg), magnesium (300mg), zinc (25mg), and Vitamin E (400mg), in addition to a good multinutrient supplement (38).

The coffee enema: procedure

First go on a 2-day juice fast as described elsewhere in this book. Then do a cleansing enema to clean the colon. For this, use an enema bag or similar equipment available at most pharmacies. To do the colon cleanse, dissolve one teaspoon of salt in 2 liters of luke warm water (35ºC). Allow this solution to flow into the colon and then retain the enema for a few minutes before flushing it out to clean the colon. Repeat if necessary.

Note: Never use an enema if there are signs of bleeding, in which case, immediately consult your doctor.

First, it is strongly advised to use organically grown coffee beans in order to avoid introducing pesticides, fungicides and other toxic agricultural chemicals into the body.

The coffee solution to be used in the enema is prepared by adding 7 heaped tablespoons of freshly ground organic coffee beans (not instant coffee) and the contents of 2 B-complex capsules to 2.5 liters of purified water. Boil for 15 minutes, then cool and strain. Use 600-700ml of the strained solution at a time for the enema and keep the rest in a closed container in a refrigerator. To do the enema, preheat the solution to a comfortable lukewarm temperature and pour into the enema bag. Use Vitamin E oil (obtained by puncturing a capsule) to lubricate the tip of the enema tube before insertion. Allow the solution to flow in gradually while kneeling with your head down and your buttocks raised. After introduction of the liquid, roll on to your right side, and lie in this position for 15-20 minutes before expelling it. If you experience no urge to expel the solution, walk around until an urge to do so arises.

The coffee enema is usually used as a retention enema where the enema fluid is retained in the body for about 15-20 minutes. Under these circumstances the coffee does not go through the digestive tract, and substances in the coffee such as caffeine are not absorbed into the bloodstream. Administered as an enema, the caffeine stimulates the liver and gall-bladder so that toxins are released and flushed out of the body. In the case of the cancer patient, this is a valuable method to stimulate and assist the body to dispose of toxins in the liver and those that may be liberated systemically.

- Do not use coffee enemas for more than 4-6 weeks at a time, since they may cause anaemia.
- The coffee enema may be used safely every third day while following a purifying diet.
- In the case of cancer patients, coffee enemas should preferably be carried out under medical supervision, since up to 3 enemas per day may be required.

For further detailed advice on colon cleansing and coffee enemas, consult a health professional.

Further remarks on the coffee enema: if you experience symptoms of toxicity (nausea, headache, fever, intestinal spasms, drowsiness, etc.) you may increase the frequency of the enemas. Eat a piece of fruit before the first coffee enema of the day to activate the upper digestive tract.

Much stored waste will be excreted after a few days on coffee enemas. To assist in the process of eliminating these, you may take several steps:

- Drink at least 4 glasses of chlorine free (purified) water per day.
- Mix one tablespoon of psyllium husks (available from a pharmacy or health shop) with 250ml of pure water in a jar, mix thoroughly then drink immediately before the mix solidifies. Then follow up with a glass of water and 200ml of clay solution previously prepared.
- To prepare the detoxifying clay solution, mix 60g of white clay (available from a pharmacy or health shop) with 300ml of water and let the mixture stand for 12 hours.
- Take the doses of psyllium and clay between meals 3 times a day for 5 days while continuing with daily coffee enemas.

- When you have finished the 5-day period as above, eat yoghurt 2-3 times daily to replenish your gut microflora.

Note that a lot of toxic material will be excreted in the process of cleansing. You may feel discomfort (nausea, headache) and bloating due to the expansion of the psyllium in the gut. You may also pass (as part of the cleansing process) dried mucus and dead cells from the surface of the gut wall. These are wastes that have possibly accumulated over many years of a destructive lifestyle and may seriously interfere with your gut function.

More on coffee enemas

Since coffee enemas play an important role in this protocol, the interested reader may want to consult two sources especially devoted to coffee enemas:

- Wilson, SA: *"A coffee blended specifically for use in coffee enemas"* (*Amazon.com*).
- *"Healing Arts: History of coffee enemas"* by Ralph Moss (*Amazon.com*).
- Further information on coffee enemas is available in the section on the "Kelley Metabolic" protocol elsewhere in this book.

11. The Budwig Diet: flaxseed oil plus cottage cheese

Dr. J. Budwig was born in Germany in 1908 and passed away in 2003 at the age of 95. She was considered one of the world's foremost authorities on fats, the influence of fatty acids on biological membranes, the resulting lowering of the voltage in the cells of our bodies by certain fatty acids and the implications this has on disease processes. The cell nuclei are positively charged, while the outer cell membranes are negatively charged. When unsaturated fats have been chemically treated, such as in margarine, their unsaturated qualities are changed and their electronic fields altered. The ability to absorb protein, and thereby to achieve water solubility in the fluids of the body, is destroyed. As Budwig put it:

" . . . the battery is dead because the electrons in these fats and oils recharge it and when the source of electrons is destroyed the fats are no longer active and cannot flow into the capillaries and fine networks."

This is when circulation problems arise.

For these reasons, hydrogenated fats and margarine should never be used by the cancer patient or by any person interested in health.

Cottage cheese is a critical ingredient of the Budwig diet. The two key ingredients of the protocol are flaxseed oil and cottage cheese. The latter is required because of sulphur-containing proteins which it contains and which form water-soluble complexes with the water-insoluble fatty acids in the flaxseed oil. These then bind oxygen to promote aerobic metabolism. The flaxseed-cottage cheese complex attaches to the cell wall (membrane) of the cancer cell, surrounding it with little magnets which suck oxygen into the cell. The red blood cells carrying carbon dioxide (CO_2) from the tissues give up the carbon dioxide in the lungs and take on oxygen, which is transported via the circulation to the cells, where the oxygen is released into the plasma. The released oxygen is attracted to the cell membranes by the resonance of the pi-electrons in the double bonds of the unsaturated fatty acids, which therefore enhance oxidation. In the absence of these fatty acids, oxygen cannot pass through the cell membranes to the interior of the cells where it is required for energy production.

- We have previously referred to the fact that cancer cells hate oxygen, and it has been known since the 1930s that feeding oxygen into cells is the primary way to protect healthy cells against cancer and to kill cancer cells.
- For those who for some reason cannot use cottage cheese: skim milk powder or whey powder are possible second-best substitutes for the cottage cheese.
- The usual ratios are cottage cheese: flaxseed oil: 2:1, and when skim milk is used the ratio is 4:1. To achieve this, mix one cup of organic cottage cheese with 2-4 tablespoons of flaxseed oil and 1-3 tablespoons of freshly ground flaxseed. Mix well manually and let it settle for a few minutes before use.
- You may add some water or apple juice to make it soft, but do not heat. Store this mix in the fridge in a tightly closed container and consume during the day. Do not let it stand over until the next day.
- The flaxseed oil should be virgin, cold-pressed, organic, liquid, refrigerated, unrefined and contained in dark colored amber bottles. It should be exposed to air as little as possible by closing firmly after opening and returning it to the refrigerator immediately.

Without the proper metabolism of fats in our bodies, every vital function of every organ is affected.

This includes the generation of new life and new cells. Our bodies produce millions of new cells daily, and in growing cells there is a critical relationship between the positively charged nucleus and the negatively charged cell membrane, which is high in unsaturated fatty acids. During cell division, the cell and the new daughter cell must contain electron-rich fatty acids in the cell's surface area to divide off completely from the old cell. If this process is interrupted, the body begins to die. In essence then, these commercially produced fats and oils are shutting down the electrical field of the cells, allowing chronic and terminal conditions to take hold of our bodies.

Dr. Budwig points out in her book that she often took very sick cancer patients from the hospital with only hours or a few days left to live. She had very good results with her protocol in these terminally ill patients, unless they were too badly damaged by chemotherapy and/or radiotherapy. In some of these patients she would start therapy with an enema using an oil mixture that resulted in "their subjective awareness of well-being increased immediately." She found that many of these patients could not urinate, produce bowel movements, or when coughing, bring up mucus. Once the protocol was initiated, this started reactivation of these vital functions, and the patient immediately began to feel better. The Budwig protocol then appears to allow cancer cells to start breathing again, according to Dr. Budwig.

Dr. Budwig personally sums up the position rather well in her book *Flax Oil as a true aid against arthritis, cancer and other diseases*:

> *What we need today in Europe . . . what we need are electron rich highly unsaturated fatty fats. The moment two unsaturated double links occur together in a fatty acid chain, the effects are multiplied and in the unsaturated fats, the so called "linoleic acids" generate a field of electrons and electric charge which can be quickly conducted off into the body thus causing a revival of the living substance—especially of the brain and nerves. It is precisely exactly those highly unsaturated fatty acids which play a decisive role in the respiratory function of the body. Without these fatty acids, the enzymes in the breath cannot function and we asphyxiate even given oxygen . . . The lack of these highly unsaturated fatty acids affects many vital functions. Primarily it cuts off the air we breathe . . . we cannot survive without these fatty acids . . ."* Thus Dr. Budwig's words.

With today's knowledge and insight, we would perhaps word it slightly differently, but the message remains clear.

Much more information is available in Dr. Budwig's book referred to above, including an interesting discussion of the link between the sun's energy and the pi-electron systems in our bodies.

Many authorities scoff at the idea that a serious medical condition such as cancer, which has defied the best efforts of the medical profession, can be treated with a simple mixture of flaxseed oil and cottage cheese. Behind this simple mixture lies a much more complex scientific scenario than meets the eye. This includes the complex interaction of the pi-electron systems in the polyunsaturated oil and cellular energy levels and the interaction between the sulphur proteins in the cottage cheese and the oil which increases its absorption into the cells.

It is remarkable that Dr. Budwig recognized all of this many years ago, before much was known about pi-electron systems in polyunsaturated fatty acids, and how these help in promoting access of oxygen to the interior domain of cells. In a later section I will return to the theoretical aspects of the polyunsaturated fats and the vital role they play in cellular oxygenation.

The Budwig protocol

The flaxseed oil must be of the very best quality with no flavoring added and kept in dark containers which are only opened for a moment when daily portions are taken. It must be refrigerated and the expiry date must be checked. Flaxseed oil is very unstable when exposed to light, heat and air. Therefore, store in a dark place (refrigerator) and keep firmly closed when not in use. Flaxseed oil goes rancid rapidly when exposed to air.

Mix two tablespoonfuls of low fat cottage cheese with one tablespoon of flaxseed oil in a cup and stir well. Mix only one dose at a time. The oil and the cottage cheese must be thoroughly mixed in a low-speed blender until no standing oil is visible in the mixture. The mixture should then be immediately consumed. Do not use commercially flavored, lignum or high lignum flaxseed oil.

The mixture can be flavored differently every day to avoid monotony by adding nuts to the mix before mixing in the blender. Preferably use organic nuts (almonds, walnuts, but not peanuts). You may also use pineapples, bananas (not overripe), organic cocoa, blueberries, raspberries or freshly squeezed fruit juice (only pineapples and apples) to improve the flavor.

For terminally ill patients, Dr. Budwig used up to 4-8 tablespoons of oil daily (with an upper limit of 6-8 tablespoons) mixed with an equal amount of cottage cheese. Once the cancer is under control and the patient is in remission, a maintenance dose of 1 tablespoon of oil plus 1 tablespoon of cottage cheese should be taken for at least 1 year or longer.

The Budwig diet takes time to work: it may take months before the cancer starts to disappear. It is therefore not suitable as a principal and first treatment protocol for very advanced cases (eg pancreatic cancer).

Other conditions may respond sooner. Cancer patients should consider taking 1 tablespoon of flaxseed oil daily as in the abovementioned formula as a life-time commitment.

The dairy component in the Budwig Protocol is important because of the presence of sulphur-containing proteins in dairy products. Patients who are lactose sensitive must experiment to find other sources of dairy products that they can tolerate and although they are less desirable than cottage cheese, they are essential. Some possible alternatives are:

- Use goat's milk products instead of cow's milk: cottage cheese made with goat's milk may be the preferred product.
- Raw milk or raw milk products.
- Use yoghurt instead of cottage cheese, but in this case you have to use 3 times more yoghurt than cottage cheese to ensure an adequate intake of sulphur proteins. This is not ideal but if nothing else is available then use it.
- Take the enzyme lactase (commercially available) with cottage cheese or quark if you are lactose sensitive.
- Use yoghurt quark or cottage cheese if normal cottage cheese is not available.
- Prepare your own kefir quark (strain kefir to get a cream cheese consistency). Explore the Internet to learn more about kefir. Kefir cottage cheese (or quark) is apparently the preferred solution for lactose intolerant patients.
- For those that have to be fed by feeding tube, ¼ cup of kefir and 1 tablespoon of flaxseed oil are mixed to a uniform consistency and poured down the feeding tube several times a day.
- After the flaxseed oil has been thoroughly blended with the cottage cheese, you may add organic fruit such as bananas (not overripe), strawberries, pineapple, etc. to improve the flavor and to avoid monotony. These should be ground into the mix or even blended in.
- You may also use whole flaxseeds available in health food stores. Dr. Budwig used 2-3 tablespoonfuls of whole flaxseeds daily, which are

ground up and mixed with cottage cheese as above. The mix obtained in this manner must be consumed within 15 minutes. Taste may be improved by the addition of fruits as mentioned previously.
- More details are available in Dr. Budwig's diet cookbook *The Oil Protein Diet Cook Book*, which is available from Amazon.com or possibly from large book shops in South Africa. Ref 22 is also a good source of information on the Budwig method.

Forbidden items

The following items are absolutely forbidden in the Budwig Diet (as in most other anti-cancer diets). These items lower the cellular voltage, thereby destroying the anti-cancer effects of the polyunsaturated oils as explained above.

- Sugar and any food with added sugar
- All animal fats
- All meats
- Margarine (even the newer varieties which are claimed to contain no trans-fatty acids)
- Butter
- Salad-dressing oils—with the exception of virgin olive oil
- All chemical additives and preservatives
- All products made of white flour

Additional health-promoting steps to consider

Dr. Budwig strongly promoted the following for her patients (which are similar to those in other health regimens):

- Sunshine for relaxation and mineral absorption. If regular exposure to the sun is impossible, then a daily dose of 1 tablespoon of codliver oil should be taken.
- Exercise—individualized according to the patient's condition. Don't overdo it—a brisk daily walk may be sufficient.
- Strictly avoid all unhealthy foods (18).
- Avoid leftover foods. Food should be prepared fresh and eaten soon after preparation.
- Drink 3-4 glasses of clean purified water daily, as well as herbal teas.
- Avoid all stress and anxiety and enjoy each day. Listen to your favorite music, laugh and spend time with people who are pleasant to be with.

- Do regular meditation exercises. This is not part of Dr. Budwig's protocol, but I consider it of vital importance, since so many highly stressed people find it extremely difficult to relax in such a manner that they derive therapeutic benefit. There are good books available to guide you and teach you how to meditate and to derive maximum benefit from your meditation sessions (88). Remember, you do not have to become a Buddhist in order to benefit from Buddhist meditation techniques.

You should also attend to your spiritual needs according to your own preferences.

Testimonials

Although, for reasons given before, there remains a dearth of strictly scientific clinical studies which support the Budwig Protocol, there are nonetheless numerous case reports and personal accounts of the effectiveness of the method in the treatment of various cancers, much of it collected by Cliff Beckwith (89). The following are some examples.

The first concerns a woman diagnosed with breast cancer on October 8, 2003. At that stage the cancer was painful. She then started on the Budwig Protocol; by mid-November the pain was gone and she has remained pain free ever since. Subsequent CAT and PET scans confirmed that the cancer had shrunk dramatically. After a while, she had only scar tissue left and she has remained cancer free.

This woman decided to go onto the Budwig regimen because of the success her husband had with the protocol in 1994 with a very large, metastasized pancreatic cancer. After surgery, his surgeon said that he would die and probably had less than 3 months to live. After several other treatments had failed, he went onto the Budwig Protocol as well as vegetable juices according to the Gerson protocol. To his surgeon's astonishment, he was well in 5 months.

Here is another remarkable case study in Dr. Budwig's book *Der Tod des Tumors* (*The death of the tumor*, available from Amazon.com.) A Mrs. Harriet had a malignant melanoma cut out of her thigh. After a while, the cancer returned in the form of lymph node metastases on her left temple, which was treated with radiotherapy. Four months later, lymph node metastases reappeared on the left side of her neck, which was again brought under control by means of radiotherapy. Thereafter skin metastases reappeared at other sites on her body. At this stage she came to see Dr. Budwig on her own. What follows are excerpts of a letter from the woman's doctor to Dr. Budwig.

The doctor wrote: "A patient of mine, Mrs. Harriet, has recently been treated by you.

> *"After your treatment, all lymph nodes and skin metastases went into remission. Also all blood indicators were normalized. I have never seen this happen with metastasized malignant melanoma. I would be extremely grateful if you could tell me which treatment you used. Since I have another patient with the same illness, I would be glad to send her to you to extend her life . . ."*

Dr. D.C. Roehm is an oncologist with experience of the Budwig method. He comments as follows (from *Townsend Letter for Doctors and Patients*, 1990):

> *This diet is far and way the most successful anticancer diet in the world. What she (Dr. Johanna Budwig) has demonstrated to my initial disbelief but lately to my complete satisfaction in my practice is: cancer is easily curable.*

Dr. Budwig specifically also commented on preterminal patients who had been unsuccessfully treated with conventional methods. She said that: ". . . even in these cases it is possible to restore health in a few months at most, I would truly say 90% of the time."

Dr. Roehm's comments are based on his own clinical experience with patients in his practice.

There are numerous reports of this nature available, but in medical terminology they have become known as "anecdotal evidence" which is not acceptable as evidence of clinical efficacy. Admittedly, a few such reports would not mean much. But when literally hundreds are available, they do become significant.

My advice is to include the Budwig protocol as part of the treatment of many cancers, but specifically for the treatment of malignant melanoma. Note, however, that it cannot be combined with some treatments (eg the CsCl/DMSO protocol) while it combines well with those treatments which depend on stimulation of the immune system (eg Glyconutrients and Dr. Kelley's protocol.)

The importance of diet in the Budwig protocol

This is a subject that we have previously referred to more than once. Therefore what follows are my summarized recommendations, specifically for those who have chosen the Budwig Protocol to treat cancer.

Before doing so, I would like to point out once again that there are some absolutely forbidden items for the cancer patient (and anybody interested in good health): no smoking, no recreational drugs, no alcohol, no sodas and other cold drinks, no margarine, no fast foods, no sugar or sugar-containing foods.

In addition to these, there are certain other things that the cancer patient should not do and there are others that the cancer patient should do.

What the cancer patient should not do

- Absolutely no sugar or sugary foods (use Stevia or xylitol as sweetener if absolutely necessary).
- No processed food or fast food of any kind.
- Limit animal protein strictly: limit red meat. Also limit fish, chicken, shell fish, eggs. These should be limited until your cancer is under control.
- Dairy products: absolutely no milk or ice cream. Cottage cheese in the Budwig Protocol is permitted since it loses all its dairy properties once it is combined with flaxseed oil, according to Dr. Budwig. This even applies to lactose sensitivity. Again, these can be relaxed somewhat once your cancer is under control.
- Gluten containing foods: bread, cereal, pasta. Apart from the gluten problem which may cause allergic reactions (often hidden); many of these products are high GI foods which result in high blood sugar values. They therefore feed cancer cells. Some gluten-free products are now available and could be considered if they also have low GI values (86).
- No undiluted fruit juices: these are high in sugar and do not provide fiber.

What the cancer patient should do

- Eat as much as possible of raw, green vegetables and low GI fruits such as pineapple, as specified in the cancer diet.
- Cereals made from quinoa or millet are allowed. Use almond milk, not soya milk.

- Fruit: berries, pineapple and apples (one per day) are permitted. Select low GI fruits and when in doubt limit your intake of other fruits to one portion per day.

The Budwig protocol can be used as a primary treatment of cancer (Stage IV). It is more frequently used as treatment during remission to prevent the return of cancer because it has no side-effects and is well suited to long-term treatment (1-2 years).

12. Glyconutrients treatment

Immunity does not only depend on the number of immune cells, but also critically on how well these cells communicate with one another. There are 8 essential sugar derivatives that have become known as "Glyconutrients" which occur *inter alia* in the aloe plant species. Analogous to the essential amino acids, 8 essential sugar derivatitives have been recognized. These are glucose, galactose, mannose, fucose, xylose, N-acetylglucosamine, N-acetylgalactoseamine and N-acetylneuraminic acid. These 8 essential sugars combine with proteins and fats at the cell surfaces to form a code that resides on the membrane of every cell. The term "essential" indicates that they cannot be synthesised in the body and that they therefore have to be obtained from food.

This code identifies the cell and helps the body recognize "self" and "non-self". It therefore plays a vital role in connection with immunity and auto-immune diseases. Differences in this code also help the body identify different blood types. It is an important part of the body's internal communication system.

Sugars combined with proteins and fats are called glycoproteins and glycolipids respectively, and collectively these are known as Glyconutrients.

Glycoproteins play an important part in the body for many essential purposes, eg for synthesizing enzymes when required, and also hormones, immunoglobulins and antibodies. For example, glycolipids play a role in building the brain and nervous system, while fucose and mannose can provide significant suppression of growing tumors.

Transformation of these sugars from one form to the other in the body requires both enzymes and energy.

Such transformations generally involve many intermediate steps, each step requiring specific enzymes and energy in the form of deficiency of energy (ATP). A diet of cooked and "prepared" foods from fastfood outlets is deficient in enzymes since food manipulation and heat destroy the enzymes present in natural foods. Only fresh food contains enzymes. A ATP and enzymes will ultimately lead to a deficiency of Glyconutrients and a consequent breakdown in the body's communication systems, which is an important factor in many diseases including cancer. For example, it has been shown that adding Glyconutrients to the human diet increases the production of stem cell production in the bone marrow. (90). Stem cells have the ability to be transformed into any other cell in the body.

Another sugar derivative, Acemannan, appears to be of particular significance in the treatment of cancer. While most Aloe Vera products contain the 8 Glyconutrients referred to above, not all of them contain Acemannan. The product recommended by the *Cancer Tutor* is called Ambrotose. More information is available from Mannotech, a company which is also represented in South Africa.

13. The Robert Barefoot Ca/CsCl protocol

Warnings and notes

- Much of the information on this protocol which follows was obtained from the book by Barefoot and Reich (75), which I consider highly recommended reading.
- This treatment should be clearly distinguished from the CsCl/DMSO protocol previously discussed. It is not nearly as strong a treatment as the former, and it can at best be considered a strong Stage III treatment. It is definitely not a Stage IV treatment. This protocol runs for 33 days only, and at the end of this period, treatment should be continued using another strong Stage III treatment.
- A terminally ill cancer patient may have only a few weeks to live. Therefore, in such a situation, a much stronger protocol such as the IPT or CsCl/DMSO protocol previously discussed should be used. The Barefoot protocol does, however, have value in situations where a Stage IV treatment has been used but a less drastic follow-up treatment is required to prevent the cancer from returning.
- In any protocol involving CsCl, you should take the same precautions as before: do regular (every 10—20 days) blood determinations of potassium, magnesium, electrolytes, uric acid and calcium. This you should do even if you take potassium and other supplements such as coral calcium.

- We have previously pointed out that uric acid, if its concentration in the blood becomes too high, may damage the kidneys. Uric acid is formed by the decomposition of the nucleic acids in the dead cancer cells. At a dosage level of 3g of CsCl a day, it is unlikely that the uric acid levels will rise too high, but if they do, there are drugs to correct the situation (Xyloprim; ask your doctor). As pointed out before, potassium levels may either rise too high or fall too low, and in both cases a dangerous irregular heartbeat may ensue. The symptoms to look out for are irregular heartbeat, fatigue or significant changes in blood pressure.
- Because cesium accumulates in the cancer cells and cesium levels may remain elevated for periods of up to 3 months, the abovementioned precautionary measurements should be continued for at least 3 months.
- The treatment consists of the combined use of coral calcium (for systemic alkalinization), CsCl to alkalinize the inside of the cancer cells and a few other supplements.

The protocol (35)

- *Coral Calcium.* Take 9 coral calcium tablets (4.5g) in 3 divided doses: 3 tabs in the morning, 3 with the midday meal and 3 tabs in the evening. Make sure that you use the best coral calcium that comes from the coral reefs in Okinawa, containing approximately 20 % Calsium and 10 % magnesium (32).
- *CsCl.* Take 3g of CsCl (6 caps) a day with meals in divided doses of 1g (2 caps) in the morning, 1g (2 caps) with the midday meal and 1g (2 caps) with the evening meal. Take these caps at the same time that you take the coral calcium capsules.
- *DMSO.* Take one tablespoonful of 70 % DMSO every time you take the CsCl. Consult the section on DMSO for safety precautions when using DMSO.
- *Vitamin D.* Take 6 Vitamin D tablets (5000IU) daily in divided doses: 2 in the morning, 2 at midday and 2 in the evening (32). This is *essential* to ensure absorption of the minerals in coral calcium.
- Do not take CsCl orally for more than 33 days.
- Also take 200mg of Coenzyme Q10 daily.
- Also take CellFood daily as prescribed (32).
- Increase your intake of potassium-rich foods (bananas, prunes, potatoes, tomatoes, spinach) but take extra potassium in the form of

supplements if your blood potassium decreases too much. Regularly (weekly in the beginning) check your blood potassium levels.
- In order to further assist in the absorption of minerals, expose your skin and face to at least 2 hours of direct sunshine (without sun block) every day. This is critical for the absorption of minerals.
- The treatment will alkalinize the body's fluids. This causes the toxins bound to the outer cell surfaces to be detached and to enter the blood, causing flu-like symptoms (headaches, stomach aches and possibly diarrhea in the beginning). This is no reason to be alarmed.

14. The Bob Beck Electro-Treatment: removal of toxic micro-organisms

- Cancer-causing micro-organisms are difficult to remove. They may hide in the teeth (root canals), lymph system, stomach lining and possibly elsewhere. There are drugs that can be used to kill them, but this may not be fully effective because these organisms may hide in places not readily accessible to the drugs. However, the Bob Beck Magnetic Pulser is a machine that will kill them no matter where they are hiding (32). In order to remove the organisms hiding in the root canals of the teeth, the Magnetic Pulser must be used on all the teeth, not just the front ones. If you have root canal silver (mercury) fillings (have a dentist check to make sure) you should have them removed by a competent dentist who knows how to do this safely.
- Every cancer patient, regardless of other treatments that he/she may be receiving, should consider two or more treatments (28 days each) with this machine (except for a few kinds of cancer).
- The equipment (with magnetic pulser) is expensive but only needs to be purchased once and can be shared with others. You need to be fully informed on the use of the machine and to attend meticulously to detail if you are to achieve the best results.
- The Bob Beck Protocol was originally used to treat AIDS, but is has turned out to be an effective killer of most micro-organisms (including the pleomorphic ones inside cancer cells) that invade the human body. It has turned out to be a superb cancer treatment.
- According to the *Cancer Tutor* (32), the Bob Beck machine is superior to other similar machines on the market, including the Rife machine, due to the work of two medical doctors, Drs. Kaali and Lyman, in

1990. They discovered that a small electric current destroys a key enzyme on the surface of the micro-organisms, which prevents them from multiplying thus rendering them harmless.
- Unfortunately, even though several patents exist and the technology is well documented, orthodox medicine is not interested in using it, although there are few infectious diseases where it could not be usefully applied. If the machine were to become well-known and generally used by doctors, many drugs would become obsolete, with enormous financial losses to the pharmaceutical companies. The problem also seems to be that it does not treat symptoms but addresses causes, meaning that patients are cured. Of course, every patient cured in this inexpensive manner is a customer lost to Big Pharma; worldwide this may amount to billions of dollars.
- The machine creates a very small alternating current (polarity changes 4 times every second) which destroys a key enzyme on the surface of the cancer microbe, thus preventing the microbe from multiplying.
- The body then safely excretes the inactivated microbes because they are no longer able to attach to cells.
- In order to reach the microbes hiding in inaccessible sites, Dr. Beck (a physicist) then developed a Magnetic Pulser which effectively destroys microbes that are not circulating in the blood.
- The entire treatment consists of four parts. Two of these (the electro-medicine component) disable the microbes from multiplying before being excreted. The third component consists of colloidal silver, which is known to kill microbes. The fourth component (Ozonated water) does the same.
- At least in the USA, it is dangerous for doctors to use this equipment—some have already landed in jail.
- One of the final steps in the process of carcinogenesis is that a microbe enters the cell, thereby breaking the energy-producing Krebs cycle and electron transport chain which occur in all normal cells. Both of these processes require oxygen and produce large amounts of energy, so that if they are interfered with, the cell proceeds to produce energy via a less efficient energy-producing mechanism, but one that does not require oxygen (fermentation). The once normal cell has now become anaerobic (does not require oxygen) and cancerous. The presence of the microbe inside the cancer cell maintains the cell's inability to restore the Krebs cycle and the electron transport chain.

- The next step is that the Bob Beck Protocol removes all critical cellular microbes in the body with the exception of the intracellular ones. Because of this, the body's immune system now has a chance to recover, and it is this that finally kills the last of the cancerous cells (32). Bob Beck personally postulated this scenario and stressed that his treatment supercharges the immune system in this way. It is therefore a powerful mechanism of restoring the patient's immunocompetence.
- Much depends on how fast the microbes multiply, which can be very fast or very slow depending on the biochemical milieu in which they find themselves. An acidic environment in the body (the "inner terrain") creates an ideal medium for the microbes to multiply; this critically depends on the diet.
- Typical acidifying foods are animal products (meat), sugar, white flour and the many other foods which we have previously referred to. All of this boils down to the simple fact that the cancer patient should have a strongly alkalinizing diet and treatment should also be aimed at restoring the pH inside the cells as, for example, in the case of the CsCl/DMSO protocol.
- It is therefore recommended that, while on the Bob Beck protocol, you should eat as much raw (live) foods as possible, which provide electrons that are important for the functioning of the magnetic pulser. Do not, however, overdo this, because of the danger of excessively elevated Vitamin K levels previously referred to.
- The question then, is which foods and when to take them while on the Bob Beck protocol. The consensus of opinion seems to be that many foods, herbs and even supplements can be taken, provided they are taken after the series of Bob Beck treatments are finished for the day. If this is done, there will be many hours for the body to use them normally before the next series of electro-medicine treatments begins on the following day. All of this is because of electroporation (to be discussed later) which occurs during electro-medicine treatment and which allows many substances to enter healthy cells unrestrictedly which otherwise would not happen, at least not to the same extent. Electroporation, however, is quickly reversed (15 minutes) after the electro-medicine treatment is stopped.
- In this manner, there will be at least 20 hours before the next treatment (and therefore electroporation) begins, and by that time the drugs, food and herbs which could cause problems have already

left the bloodstream. You should make sure that all these potentially harmful substances have left the body before starting the next Bob Beck treatment.
- If you feel that there are things that you take but feel unsure of how they can best be combined with the Bob Beck treatment, it is best to experiment. For example, 15 minutes after the last Bob Beck treatment of the day, take a small dose of the substance in question (10 % of the normal dose) and see how you feel on the next day. Then gradually continue with daily increasing doses until you reach the full dose. This will provide an early warning system of whether the substance in question can be incorporated into the Bob Beck protocol.
- Only fairly mild drugs, supplements and herbs should be experimented with in this way.
- Highly potent drugs such as the chemotherapy drugs, certain heart drugs, etc. should never be experimented with in this manner. You must get off any strong prescription drugs (with your doctor's permission) before going on the Bob Beck protocol.
- The Budwig Protocol is considered food and can be used with the Bob Beck protocol.
- The Bob Beck treatment creates a lot of debris by killing the parasites but it does not cure cancer quickly; that is something the immune system must do after the parasites have been removed, but this takes time.

Guidelines for using the Bob Beck protocol

The following rules should be strictly adhered to, as electroporation may cause excessive and rapid absorption of many substances in the blood, which may be lethal (91).

- Use the Bob Beck protocol alone: no other medical drugs, herbs, etc. should be used concurrently. This does not apply in the case of food-based treatments such as the Gerson diet, Budwig diet, etc.
- No other alternative cancer treatment should be used with the Bob Beck protocol. Stop these at least 3-5 days before you start with the Bob Beck treatment. CsCl treatment should be stopped 14 days earlier.
- The main reason is not only electroporation, but especially the excessive toxin load created in this manner, which may overtax the liver and kidneys.

- No other drugs (orthodox or otherwise).
- No painkillers.
- No anti-coagulant drugs.
- No pacemakers.
- No orthodox treatments (radiation, chemo, surgery).
- Do not use on pregnant women.
- No alcohol, tea, coffee, recreational drugs.
- No supplements (vitamins, etc.).
- No garlic, spices, onions.
- Use only healthy foods, but with the above exceptions.
- No acidifying foods.
- Drink a lot of purified water (to eliminate all the toxins).

Note that both the blood electrifier and the magnetic pulser can cause electroporation.

Electroporation will allow substances to enter cells at a rate 20-30 times higher than normal. Thus the effects of taking a normal dose of paracetamol of 300mg will be magnified to that of a 6000mg dose during electroporation.

These rules do not apply to colloidal silver, provided that it is taken after the two electro medicine treatments of the day.

Summarizing the four phases of the Bob Beck treatment
The Bob Beck protocol consists of 4 independent treatments, all of which have been designed to kill cancer-causing microbes in the body. These are:

1. *Blood Electrification.* This disables cancer-causing microbes in the bloodstream which are present in cancer cells.
2. *Magnetic Pulsation.* Most of the cancer cells which contain the cancer microbes are, however, not in the blood. Magnetic pulsation is necessary to kill these organisms which hide elsewhere in the body (lymph system including lymph nodes, root canals, and cells lining the stomach area). This is therefore a very important part of the treatment.
3. *Colloidal silver.* This is a much used antimicrobial (especially antiviral) product which has been shown to be perfectly safe for

human use. Its main purpose is to kill the microbes in the blood and most of those hiding in the tissues. It is not known whether it also penetrates cancer cells.
4. *Ozonated water.* Ozone is a well-known and widely-used antimicrobial agent. It is even used for that purpose to sterilize swimming pools. Like colloidal silver, it is used in cancer patients to kill the circulating microbes and those in hiding. It is not yet known whether or not it will kill microbes inside cancer cells.
5. As in the case of 3 % hydrogen peroxide, Ozonated water can be used to kill microbes hiding in root canals by letting it sit in the mouth for a few minutes, taking care to immerse the affected teeth.
6. Killing cancer cells can cause swelling and inflammation. If the patient becomes aware of this, the abovementioned treatments should be temporarily stopped and medical advice sought. This is of special significance in the case of cancers in anatomically limited areas (eg the brain, gastrointestinal system).

Warning

- It is important not to use the magnetic pulser at the same time as the blood electrification treatment, because the former may damage the latter. The blood electrifier should be switched on 20-30 minutes after completing the treatment with the pulser.
- We suggest that you use the pulser before the electrifier because the pulser may break loose colonies of microbes hiding in the root canals and elsewhere, releasing them into the bloodstream where they can be disabled by the electrifier.
- Take the colloidal silver about 15 minutes after finishing the two electro medicine treatments. These treatments (through electroporation) will create holes in the cell membranes, thus promoting entry of the colloidal silver in both normal as well as cancerous cells. The normal cells will not be affected, but under these conditions the maximum amount of colloidal silver will be absorbed by the cancer cells, thus promoting the therapeutic effect. There is a VHS tape available which has a demonstration on how to use the Bob Beck equipment. Information on how to make your own ozonator and colloidal silver is also available in the *Cancer Tutor* (32).

Example of a daily treatment schedule

- Note: the distilled or purified water used should contain 1-2 teaspoons of sea salt to supply the electrolytes which are required by the magnetic pulser.
- If you decide to make your own colloidal silver, however, use only distilled or purified water.
- 17h00 (5.00 pm): Take ozonated water (1 liter or more) with added sea salt.
- 17h30 (5.30 pm): Take more ozonated water with sea salt (make a new batch).
- 18h00 (6.00 pm): Start magnetic pulser.
- 20h00 (8.00 pm): Finish magnetic pulser.
- 20h00 (8.00 pm): Start blood electrifier.
- 22h00 (10.00 pm): Finish blood electrifier.
- 22h15 (10.15 pm): Drink colloidal silver.
- 22h30 (10.30 pm): Start taking supplements, juices, etc.

Side-effects

The instructions and safety precautions regarding the use of the Bob Beck equipment should be adhered to meticulously. If you do this, the only side-effects of the treatment that you may expect are those related to detoxification. Many microbes and cancer cells are killed during the treatment, and these appear as debris in the circulation that must somehow be eliminated, mainly through the liver and kidneys. In extreme cases in some patients, the situation may be so bad that pus oozes out of the body by way of lesions that resemble sores. This is a good sign and you should not be upset by it. If toxin production and elimination becomes excessive, it may be necessary to stop the treatment and start all over again using less severe conditions. You may also have to protect the friendly bacteria in your gut by taking probiotic supplements.

Detailed articles on the four legs of the Bob Beck treatment are available in the *Cancer Tutor* (32). The same source also provides much general information on the Bob Beck protocol, as well as directions on how to make your own Electrifier and Pulser. Information on where the apparatus can be purchased is also available.

15. The Kelley metabolic protocol (enzyme therapy)

In this protocol the focus is on enzymes secreted by the pancreas: chemotrypsin and trypsin. These enzymes are normally required for the digestion of proteins in the small intestine. The method focuses especially on improving the immune system, but also makes provision for supporting liver function. This is achieved by means of coffee enemas, similar to the one described in the Gerson therapy, but there are also other methods to cleanse the liver which depend on herbs (silimarin).

Cancer cells are in many ways similar to placental cells that occur in pregnancy (trophoblast theory). There are many similarities between early placental trophoblast and cancer cells. Both grow in a protected environment and have provision for a specialized source of nutrition. In the case of the trophoblast these are the placenta (protected environment) and the umbilical cord (specialized source of nutrition), and in the case of cancer cells the tumor structure which provides protection and angiogenesis (development of new blood supply network) provides extra nutrition. It is also not by mere coincidence that the placental trophoblast starts to grow slower in the 8th week of pregnancy and later. This coincides with the functional completion of the fetal digestive system and the activation of the fetal pancreas to produce digestive enzymes. The trophoblast cells also secrete the hormone HCG. The quantity of this hormone starts to decline at the same time that the fetal pancreatic enzymes are produced.

> *This hormone (as well as a glycoprotein layer) coats the trophoblast cells and also the cancer cells to protect them against attack by the immune system. HCG is present in all cancer cells but not in other cells.*

This is the principle upon which the Navarro test for cancer (discussed elsewhere) is based.

The decline in the production of HCG exactly coincides with the production of the pancreatic enzymes trypsin, chymotrypsin and amylase which have been shown to break down the negatively charged coating on the trophoblast cells. In view of all this, we can understand why cancers of the duodenum are so rare (presence of pancreatic enzymes). In those cases where pancreatic cancers do develop, the pancreatic enzymes have not been activated in the small intestine, which also explains why pancreatic cancer has such a high mortality rate (the pancreas has lost its ability to produce these enzymes).

Dr. Kelley's theory is supported by the fact that the pancreas secretes these enzymes not only into the pancreas but also into the small intestine and into the circulation, from where they can reach all cells in the body including cancer cells, which they can subdue and digest.

At one stage in his life, Dr. Kelley personally developed pancreatic cancer and was given 4-8 weeks to live.

However, after switching to the cancer diet given above, he began to improve, but again stopped improving after a further 6 months, at which stage he also started to develop serious digestive problems. He then began taking a high dose (50 tablets per day) of digestive enzymes to improve his digestive problems and in due course he fully recovered from his cancer.

> *His experience suggested to him that cancers progress as a result of the lack of pancreatic enzymes which would normally digest the cancer cells as explained above.*

He lived for many more years, in the course of which he successfully treated 33 000 cancer patients with pancreatic enzymes.

Dr. Kelley claims a 97 % cure rate of the 33 000 patients he treated.

The core of his protocol consisted of high-dose pancreatic enzymes, but in addition he advised patients to follow the cancer diet as detailed above and prescribed individualized treatment for each patient.

Typical enzyme doses may for example be 4-5 Wobe-Mugos tablets with water 4 times a day, starting with a low dose of 1 tablet 4 times daily and gradually increasing the dose to 4 tablets 4 times daily.

By taking mannitol (2-3g) with each dose, the absorption of the enzymes is improved.

Alternatively, the patient may use 10-30 tablets of Intenzyme 3 times a day, starting with the low dose and gradually increasing the dose.

Dr. Kelley restricted protein intake and included coffee enemas as in the Gerson diet.

Dr. N. Gonsalez was sent by the medical establishment to investigate Dr. Kelley's patients and records, with the intention of discrediting him. Instead, Gonsalez became so impressed that he not only refused to discredit Kelley, but instead continued to do a study of his own on patients with pancreatic cancer for which standard medical treatments were totally ineffective, with a 5-year survival rate of 0 %. In this study, the median survival rate in pancreatic cancer patients treated according to the Kelley protocol was found to be 9 years as opposed to the 6 months usually given these patients to live after conventional treatment. In the end, he was harassed and ultimately thrown in jail and legally prevented from publishing his results. He eventually moved to Mexico where he died in 2005. Before he died, he wrote his last book entitled *Cancer: Curing the Incurable without Surgery, Chemotherapy and Radiation*, which is available from *Amazon.com*.

Detailed information is available in Dr. Kelley's book and on the website (available from the book).

An important aspect of enzyme therapy is that it effectively reduces the invasive and metastatic potential of cancer cells. By removing the sticky, outer coating of cancer cells, enzymes reduce the risk of such cells adhering to other tissues in the body to initiate new cancer growths. Many doctors in Europe know that enzymes play an invaluable role in keeping cancers from spreading and developing into terminal tumors—those capable of spreading and killing their host.

> *Thus the reduction of the adhesiveness of blood is seen to be an over-all important step in the cancer patient, no matter what other treatments may be used, since it also improves immune function.*

Interestingly, adhesiveness depends on the stickiness of blood or its ability to coagulate. The greater the adhesive quality of the blood, the greater is the tendency of the tumor to develop metastases.

Thus it is not surprising to find that anti-coagulants, in addition to enzymes, both reduce the invasive and metastatic potential of cancer cells (92).

In the light of this, it is now thought that the cancer cell uses a fibrin or fat coat to mask its identity, to hide it from detection by the immune system.

In addition to these effects of enzymes, they remain what they were originally considered for: agents to digest food. This is no mean property. In the absence of adequate levels of enzymes in the digestive tract, dietary proteins are only partly digested and these partly digested protein molecules are nonetheless absorbed into the bloodstream. The immune system "sees" these partly digested protein molecules as invaders (foreign to the body) causing antibodies to be formed against them and to couple them with the antibodies produced to form immune complexes that circulate in the bloodstream. In a healthy person such antigen-antibody complexes are neutralized and removed in the lymphatic system. In the cancer patient, however, these complexes tend to accumulate in the blood where they may precipitate in certain areas (eg the joints), and where they may also burden the immune system thus decreasing its ability to fight the cancer and possibly causing allergic reactions. If the load of these complexes becomes too great, the kidneys may become overburdened, with the result that the complexes may be precipitated in certain soft tissues, causing inflammation and bringing unnecessary stress to the immune system. In this process, adequate amounts of proteolytic enzymes will not only prevent the whole process from taking place, but will also break down the immune complexes if they do form. In the cancer patient, the situation may become serious. In most cancer patients, the circulating immune complexes become more numerous as the cancer advances, because tumors (and the dying tumor cells) release large amounts of antigens contributing to the load of immune complexes. As this process progresses, the circulating immune complexes impose a serious burden on the immune system and it has been shown clinically that cancer patients with high concentrations of circulating immune complexes have a particularly poor prognosis (93).

It has also been shown that supplementation with proteolytic enzymes is an effective and practical way of reducing the level of these complexes in the blood, and that the rate of reduction of the complexes in the blood parallels the increases in enzyme dosage levels (94). It has also been reported that as the level of the immune complexes in the blood declines, the patients experience marked improvements in their well-being (improved appetite, increased vitality, weight gain, increased mobility, and even improvement in the level of depression and anxiety).

When the diet is of such a nature that too much of the proteolytic enzymes are required for digestion, less are available for protection against cancer and for reduction of the circulating immune complexes. Dr. J. Taylor points out that if you assist the process of digestion by providing enzyme-rich foods (pineapple, paw-paw) you can assist the body's ability to fight cancer.

On the other hand, in a diet rich in over-cooked (which destroys the natural enzymes) animal products, such as meat and dairy products, most of the pancreatic enzymes that are naturally produced will be used up in digesting food. The active enzymes present in many raw foods can similarly assist the body to fight cancer.

Several proteolytic enzyme preparations are available in Europe and Germany, where they were originally developed. These include preparations such as Wobenzyme, Wobe-Mugos and others (Vitalzyme). These preparations generally contain pancreatin, bromelain, trypsin, chymotrypsin, lipase, amylase and ruin. Different galenic formulations are available for injections, suppositories and oral administration. The oral forms generally are enteric-coated to allow liberation of the enzymes in the small intestine. Pancreatic enzymes can attack cancer cells during their reproductive phase, when they are still developing and therefore more susceptible to destruction.

Dr. M. Wolf first started to use Wobe-Mugos in cancer patients in 1949 when he treated 1000 patients with Wobe-Mugos and other multi-enzyme formulas. Initially, doses varied from 200-4000mg daily in divided doses. He reported that the enzymes appeared to curtail the spread of the cancer and to moderately prolong survival. For example, in one study on 108 women who had undergone mastectomy, the 5-year survival rate was 84 % in the enzyme treated subgroup as against 43-48 % in the other subgroup who had received conventional treatment. In this case it was also shown that enzyme therapy produced the best results in stopping the spread of the cancer.

In another study it was shown that pancreatic cancer responded well to enzyme therapy, confirming the original results of Dr. Kelley. In this study 30 patients were still alive 2 years after enzyme therapy. Some of these patients survived for 5-9 years, whereas the usual survival time for this type of cancer is 7 months.

Since enzyme treatment depends heavily on the immune system, this method is not suitable for terminally ill cancer patients who have little time available. It may be suitable for the treatment of a patient in remission after successful treatment with a more powerful protocol.

More on enzyme therapy and the other provisions of the Kelley protocol

Various digestive enzyme preparations are available that are suitable for cancer treatment, according to Dr. Kelley. These are enteric-coated enzyme formulations generally available in tablet form under various names (eg Wobenzyme, Wobe-Mugos, and Intenzyme). Potencies vary and generally 3-10 tablets are used 3 times a day between meals. The enzymes (trypsin, pancreatin and chymotrypsin) break down the protein coat of cancer cells, thus exposing the cancer cells to the action of the immune system.

Bromelain (500-1500mg) 2-3 times a day between meals can also be used for this purpose.

Enzyme therapy is especially indicated for the treatment of pancreatic, liver and GI tract cancers.

It is contra-indicated with certain other therapies and especially in patients on blood clotting medication.

Other aspects of the Kelley protocol call for a diet of whole grains, fruit, vegetables and raw juices. He also advised patients to strictly avoid pasteurized milk, peanuts, white flour, sugar, chlorinated water and all processed foods. The diet should consist of 70 % raw foods such as fresh raw salads. He also developed 25 nutritional formulations for hard tumors and 29 for soft tumors such as leukemia, melanoma and lymphoma which the patients had to take until they have been cancer free for 2 years.

The capacity to absorb nutrients differs widely from patient to patient, so that the therapy has to be carefully individualized.

Subsequently the success of the Kelley protocol was confirmed by other workers such as Dr. Gonsalez. As an example, the following results were obtained in the case of pancreatic patients. The 5-year survival rate for pancreatic cancer with conventional medical therapies is 0 %, as well as a life expectancy of 2-3 months after diagnosis. Five patients with pancreas cancer, who followed the Kelley programme precisely, survived for 9 years and continued to live normal lives, but in the case of others who followed the programme only partly, the survival times were better than those on conventional therapy but not as good as those who had followed the programme closely. Dr. Gonsalez modified the Kelley programme slightly as follows:

- A diet appropriate to each individual
- Intensive nutritional support including supplements
- Digestive aids such as hydrochloric acid
- Proteolytic enzymes as described above
- Raw beef organs and glands
- Thorough detoxification.

Dr. Gonsalez claims an 80 % success rate of patients previously treated by conventional means and given up as total failures with only weeks to live.

The three main advantages of using enzyme therapy in the treatment of cancer may be summarized as follows:

- To remove the fibrous and/or lipid covering to expose the cancer cells, thus making the cancer cell an easier target for the immune system
- To reduce the adhesiveness of cancer cells, thus reducing their tendency to adhere to different sites in the body to start new cancer growths (metastases)
- To reduce the level of circulating immune complexes which tend to reduce the immune system's ability to deal with the cancer and to reduce the tendency of inflammation.

16. Oxygen and hydrogen peroxide therapy in the treatment of cancer

I have previously referred to the importance of oxygen in the treatment of cancer and the fact that cancer cells do not thrive in an oxygen rich environment. If the oxygen level in the environment is high enough, all cancer cells will eventually die (through the process of apoptosis) because they cannot live in an oxygen rich (aerobic) environment.

Oxygen, either derived from the element oxygen in gaseous form or from hydrogen peroxide, provides a source of free radicals that kill not only cancer cells but also bacteria, viruses, fungi and other micro-organisms.

It is also known that oxygen suppresses the dissemination of cancer cells and stimulates the immune system.

As previously mentioned, Dr. Otto Warburg first discovered the pivotal role of oxygen in relation to the process of carcinogenesis. He summarized his work over many years in this field in his book *The Prime Cause and Prevention of Cancer* in 1967. In summary, Dr. Warburg suggested that, as a first priority of cancer treatment, all growing body cells should be saturated with oxygen. A second priority is to avoid further exposure to toxins and carcinogens as a means of shifting the metabolic pattern and enzyme balance in the cancer cells (predominantly anaerobic) towards normal aerobic pathways, thereby restoring the cancer cells to normality. In relation to oxygen therapy, it is necessary to distinguish clearly which tissues are targeted by the treatment. In the conventional forms of oxygen therapy (hyperbaric oxygen, hydrogen peroxide), oxygen levels in the circulation and extracellular spaces are increased. The resulting reduced growth of cancer cells is explained below. Mainly as a result of the work of the two-time Nobel Prize winner Dr. Otto Warburg, more recent work has concentrated on increasing intracellular oxygen levels. Although the principles of the method were established more than 70 years ago, its practical clinical application has only recently assumed prominence as a result of the work of Peskin and Habib, previously discussed in relation to the various cancer therapies.

One older form of administering oxygen is by means of hyperbaric oxygen therapy, which introduces oxygen into the body by means of a pressurized chamber. Oxygenation applied in this manner should be carefully controlled; it is essential to undergo the treatment with an experienced therapist in a clinic. It is important to prevent over-oxidation when an excess of free radicals is produced.

If used carefully under controlled conditions, it is able *inter alia* to kill off old and devitalized cells to make way for new, healthy cells that are better able to resist the cancer. It does not, however, specifically target the intracellular spaces.

17. Hydrogen peroxide (H_2O_2)

Hydrogen peroxide is a natural substance that occurs in small quantities in the body where it is used *inter alia* by normal cells to regulate metabolism and as a poison to destroy invaders.

It is one compound that will increase the available oxygen content in the body to a level that will kill cancer cells and prevent metastases. It was first used intravenously in India in the 1920s to treat influenza, and since then it has been experimented with to treat a number of conditions including emphysema, angina, lung infections, cancer and other conditions. Apart from its use as a source of oxygen free radicals, it has also been shown to stimulate natural killer cells, the immune cells that will attack cancer cells wherever they may occur in the body. It is produced in normal cells during metabolism by enzymes called oxydases. Dr. Farr, a specialist on the use of hydrogen peroxide, states that it has other wide-spread effects on cellular metabolism, including

- Regulation or tissue repair
- Cellular respiration
- Normalization of energy metabolism
- Production of cytokines, including cytokines which assist the body to combat cancer cells
- Macrophages and other immune cells produce hydrogen peroxide to help kill micro-organisms, parasites, etc.
- It stimulates the detoxifying effect of detoxifying enzymes.

Hydrogen peroxide, given in the correct dosage, can have an oxidizing and cleansing effect. As might be expected, the American Cancer Society and the FDA still dispute claims regarding the benefits of hydrogen peroxide in medicine without any real scientific evidence on which to base their claims. Hydrogen peroxide, like Vitamin C, represents a potentially grave threat to the financial interests of Big Pharma because it is in direct competition with chemotherapy and the drug industry. As a natural substance, it is inexpensive, readily available and effective when used correctly. Hydrogen peroxide in medicine is only used in very dilute solution (eg for intravenous administration) in which form it is harmless (0.3 %). Some practitioners use hydrogen peroxide together with antioxidants, for example by alternatively giving hydrogen peroxide with Vitamin C via the intravenous route.

DILUTED **hydrogen peroxide** *MUST NOT BE USED ORALLY.*

Several authors have warned against the oral use of hydrogen peroxide in the treatment of cancer. It may be wise not to use hydrogen peroxide orally or intravenously as a source of oxygen except in a clinical situation.

However, used in a nebulizer or inhaler the procedure is safe and uncomplicated.

For this purpose, mix 30ml of medical grade 35 % hydrogen peroxide in 4.5l of chlorine-free pure water to prepare a 0.23 % hydrogen peroxide solution and use this solution in a vaporizer. This improves night-time breathing tremendously and improves the quality of life of the patient with a lung condition. But intravenous hydrogen peroxide holds the real key to permanent relief in lung patients, because it has the ability to clear the inner linings of the lungs thus restoring the ability to breathe.

The safety aspects of intravenous hydrogen peroxide in human patients have been studied by several authors including Dr. R. Pelton and the medical staff of the Santa Monica Hospital in Mexico, who reported on their experience gained from the treatment of 30 000 infusions of dilute hydrogen peroxide without a serious reaction (95).

There are many reports of lung patients who had used the nebulizer treatment, who no longer needed a wheelchair and supplemental oxygen. Similar benefits can be expected in cancer patients when oxygen supply to the tissues is improved. Fortifood can help you find a doctor who has experience in this technique.

Dr. Farr in America is one of the main proponents on the use of intravenous hydrogen peroxide in the treatment of lung conditions. He and others report many subjective benefits of hydrogen peroxide. Patients frequently report increased mental clarity and an increased sense of well-being. This may be because of the improved saturation of intracellular spaces with oxygen derived from hydrogen peroxide.

Several studies have demonstrated the benefits of using hydrogen peroxide therapy in combination with conventional cancer treatments. One study showed improved therapeutic outcome if chemotherapy (vinblastin) was combined with hydrogen peroxide (96).

18. Germanium sesquioxide

This compound helps the body activate and use oxygen. It also enhances the natural killer cell activity of the immune system which is an important immune component against cancer cells (97).

19. Sodium chlorite ($NaClO_2$)

This is one safe and effective way of increasing oxygen in the extracellular tissues that can be used at home safely. Although not accepted by the FDA in America and other official bodies (as might be expected), there are many convincing reports on the Internet on the success of this method in treating cancer.

The method consists of the use of a dilute sodium *chlorite* solution in water (0.5 %) in a nebulizer or inhaler.

It is very important to note that we are not talking about sodium *chloride* (NaCl), which is ordinary salt.

Sodium chlorite is a precursor of chlorine dioxide (ClO_2) which is a vehicle by means of which oxygen is delivered to the tissues. Chlorine dioxide is generated from sodium chlorite in acid medium. For this purpose an acid stronger than $HClO_2$ is needed. Citric acid solution is preferred and is used as detailed below. What follows is a summary of information from the literature. More information is available on the Internet (98).

Protocol for Sodium Chlorite

Chlorine dioxide may be generated from an aqueous solution of sodium chlorite by acidifying the solution with a strong organic acid. For this purpose, the procedure is as follows (adapted from the literature (96, 97) and from the Internet):

- The sodium chlorite is provided as a powder (7.5g of sodium chlorite) in a 25ml bottle. By filling this bottle with pure chlorine-free water, a 30 % solution of sodium chlorite is obtained, which is used to generate chlorine dioxide by acidification. This is done by using the other 25ml bottle containing citric acid crystals (2.5g) and filling it up with pure, chlorine-free water to yield a 10 % solution of citric acid.
- To prepare the Chlorine dioxide solution, the sodium chlorite and citric acid solutions should be mixed in a 1:5 ratio. The actual treatment protocol calls for increasing Chlorine dioxide doses depending on the patient's reaction. This is achieved by using increasing quantities of the two reagents, but always in the fixed 1:5 ratio.
- For measuring the two solutions, use a 1ml calibrated syringe with 0.1ml calibrations.
- *Baseline dose:* In a clean glass, put 0.1ml of the sodium chlorite solution, add 0.5ml of the citric acid solution, mix well, leave for 4 minutes then add ½ glass of preservative free fruit juice (preferably pure apple juice) and drink.
- *Procedure:* Always start treatment with the baseline dose in the morning as detailed above. If you do not become uncomfortable after the base-line dose, then take the next dose in the evening before

going to bed, using 0.2ml of the sodium chlorite solution mixed with 1.0ml of the citric acid solution as detailed for the baseline dose. If you become nauseous, then reduce the next dose again to 0.1ml sodium chlorite + 0.5ml citric acid solution the next morning as in the baseline dose. The next dose (the following evening) must again be 0.2ml sodium chlorite + 1.0ml citric acid solution, before going to bed. The idea is to continue at a dosage level that you can tolerate, and then to increase the dose by another 0.1ml sodium chlorite + 0.5ml citric every time to the next higher dose, until you can tolerate that dose and then to continue increasing the doses until you reach a dose level of 1.5ml of sodium chlorite + 7.5ml of the citric acid solution twice a day without nausea or diarrhea (use larger syringes, eg 2.0 or 5.0ml to conveniently measure off the larger doses). This is your maximum dosage level.

- The next step then is to take the maximum dose three times a day instead of twice a day. Thereafter increase dosage interval to 3 times a day and stay at this higher dose for at least 7 days. It may take weeks to achieve this level without nausea. Whenever, during the course of treatment, symptoms of side-effects reappear (eg nausea, diarrhea), reduce the dose temporarily for the next lower dose as above and then continue. You should always look for the nausea-level dose and adjust dosage levels accordingly, constantly increasing dosage levels slowly as determined by patient reaction to the maximum dosage level.
- The maintenance dose consists of 0.6ml of sodium chlorite + 3.0ml of citric acid solution per day for normal patients (if you choose to go on a maintenance dose). Reduce the dose for the weak and the elderly people and children as required.
- Cancer patients may have to take more of the chlorite protocol. Build up to the maximum dosage level in the usual manner as described above. This you may achieve by increasing the dose as described above but also by increasing the dose frequency that will permit maximum dose level just short of nausea. Thus you may increase the dosage level from 0.5ml + 2.5ml every 12 hours to taking this dose every 4 hours and later even every 2 hours. If nausea develops at this level, reduce the frequency to one dose every 6 hours or more.
- Try to maintain the dosage at 0.5 + 2.5ml every 2-4 hours for as long as you can, preferably for 6 months or more.

Notes:

- To speed up absorption and therapeutic effect, some of the sodium chlorite citric acid mixed with every dose may be applied to the gums and palate before the rest is mixed with juice and drunk. This may be of special importance in cancer patients. After preparing the mix (eg 0.5 +2.5ml), and waiting for 3 minutes for the conversion of the chlorite into Chlorine dioxide by the citric acid, dip your finger into the solution and apply part of it to gums and palate. Then add juice and drink the rest.
- Although apple juice is much to be preferred, you may use other low-sugar juices which are also low in antioxidants. Do not use any fruit juice to which anything has been added in the form of preservatives or anything else. Also do not use juices that are high in antioxidants such as orange or naartjie juice. Read the label carefully.
- Side effects to be expected in the beginning when on this treatment: nausea, vomiting, diarrhea, stomach cramps. The diarrhea is not a sign of gastro-intestinal infection. These are signs of detoxification and therefore not bad. You should feel much better after these have passed.
- Normally the best time for this treatment is 1 hour after meals. In this manner nausea may be reduced
- Do not take any antioxidants (multinutrient, Vitamin C, etc.) for at least 3 hours before or after taking the chlorite dose.
- Take at least 5-8 multi-enzyme caps daily during treatment with chlorite.
- You must continue with your existing anti-cancer diet while on the abovementioned treatment, but do not eat any food for 1 hour before your daily doses. Extend this to 3 hours in the case of supplements which contain antioxidants such as Vitamin C.
- Depending on the type and stage of cancer, you may have to continue for 9 months on this protocol.
- During treatment you must take copious quantities of purified water (eg 1-1.5l daily) to assist the body in disposing of the toxins and the debris of dead cancer cells.
- You must expect to develop nausea and some of the other side-effects mentioned at some stage during your treatment. As stated, this is a good sign. It develops as a result of the toxins liberated by the dead cancer cells. If the body cannot clear these toxins fast enough through

the liver and kidneys, the accumulated toxins are responsible for the side-effects. If you find that you can gradually increase your dosage level with time, it is a sign that you are winning the battle, but you may have to persist for a long time before that happens. The rate at which your body generates cancer cells must not be greater than the rate at which successive applications of chlorite destroy the cancer cells.

- If for some reason you do not seem to be able to reach that point, you have to look at some other, additional, treatment, which brings up the matter of how the chlorite treatment can be integrated into the overall programme suggested in this book.
- First of all, consider your diet. No cancer treatment can succeed if the diet is not correct. Follow the cancer diet strictly.
- As in all cancer treatment programmes, it is highly desirable to undergo detoxification of the colon, liver and kidneys before starting the chlorite programme. Details are available elsewhere in this book.
- In general, the chlorite protocol should be considered a strong Stage III; for some patients it may even be regarded as a Stage IV treatment. It should not be combined in general with any of the other Stage IV treatments discussed in this book. Depending on patient reaction, however, it can be combined with the Budwig, Kelley, Gerson, and other similar protocols which strengthen the immune system.
- As complementary treatment to the chlorite protocol, you should always alkalinize your blood by taking coral calcium (4-6 caps = 2.0-3g) daily or more until your salivary pH reaches 7.5 or more.
- You may determine whether you are winning the war against cancer by doing the tests discussed in this book. You may also gain a (less accurate) impression by your reaction to the treatment. You are not winning if you get nauseous every time you take a dose of the chlorite + citric acid no matter what that dose is, and also if the body never seems to adapt to a lower dose before going on to a higher dose. For example, if you can tolerate the 0.3+1.5ml dose, but you get nausea if you go to the next higher dose, you may have to tolerate the 0.3+1.5ml dose for a day or two. But if the nausea persists at this dose, it shows that the cancer is growing faster than you are killing the cancer cells. In this situation, try increasing dose frequency instead of dose level for a day or two. If you can overcome the nausea in this manner, it indicates that you have to proceed very slowly, at each level increasing dose frequency instead of dose level until you can tolerate the dose. In extreme cases, you may have to

consider another protocol such as IPT or the CsCl/DMSO protocol, or one of the other Stage IV protocols previously discussed.

Warning: If you have a stomach or duodenal ulcer, have the ulcer treated by your doctor before going on this treatment.

20. Ozone (O_3) in the treatment of cancer

Oxygen is one of the key elements in the overall functioning of all cells in the body.

It is required to feed the chemical reactions in the cells, including the energy-producing mechanisms in the mitochondria and for the detoxifying pathways in the liver. When oxygen levels in the cells drop by 35 % of normal, many things can go wrong, including a significantly increased cancer risk (refer to Warburg's work on the relationship between oxygen and cancer). Warburg stated that:

> *Cancer has only one prime cause (which is) the replacement of normal oxygen respiration of body cells by anaerobic respiration.*

Oxygen destroys 99 % of toxins, and many pathogens like most bacteria, viruses, moulds, fungi and parasites are destroyed by oxygen, but it is not harmful to normal cells.

Ozone therapy is another valuable cancer treatment that depends on increasing the available oxygen tissue levels. The ozone molecule (O_3) is relatively unstable and readily loses one oxygen atom:

$$O_3 = \ddagger O_2 + O \text{ (oxygen atom)}.$$

It is the reactive oxygen atoms that are so beneficial for the cancer patient, because as a result of its high activity, it alkalinizes cells and kills cancer cells. In this respect, ozone treatment differs from oxygen therapy which does not provide this extra oxygen atom. Included in the beneficial effects of ozone is the fact that it stimulates the production of cytokines, which are the messengers of the immune system. In this manner, the concerted action of the various arms of the immune system is ensured.

- Millions of people in Europe have been successfully treated with ozone in spite of objections by the conventional medical establishment.

- The highly selective effect of ozone in killing cancer cells was highlighted in a study published in the journal *Science* by several medical doctors (99). These doctors found that: " . . . the growth of human cancer cells from lung, breast, and uterine cancers were selectively inhibited in a dose-dependent manner by ozone at 0.3-0.8 ppm of ozone in ambient air." (*Science*, 1987, 236: 280)

The treatment consists of the application of an apparatus that produces medical grade ozone as a gas which is introduced intravenously into the patient. (There are also other ways of introducing ozone into the body). The procedure is not dangerous when used correctly. Minor problems may arise if your lungs contain a lot of microbes. If you wish to use ozone therapy, I advise you to find a clinic in your area where the procedure can be safely and effectively performed.

An objection that is often made is that a gas is being introduced into the bloodstream which may cause embolisms that could lead to a stroke or even heart attack. This happens when large amounts of nitrogen gas are introduced into the bloodstream but not with the small amounts of ozone introduced by this technique because ozone (unlike nitrogen) is quickly absorbed into the bloodstream. It therefore never forms bubbles like nitrogen which could cause embolisms (100). Used correctly, it is a safe and very effective Stage IV cancer treatment. Before using it, I suggest that you buy the authoritative book on this subject by Dr. Ed McCane (101). Note that although there are also other ozone protocols available, the McCane protocol is the safest and most effective. For more information, contact Peter Jovan (102) and consult the various sources and testimonials on the Internet.

Ozone is remarkably non-toxic and safe to use, as was shown by a study by the German Medical Society for Ozone Therapy. In this study, Dr. Pressman reported:

> *644 therapists were polled regarding their 384 775 patients with a total of 5 579 238 ozone treatments administered. There were only 40 cases of side-effects noted out of this number, which represents the incredibly low rate of 0.000007 %.*

Ozone has thus proved to be the safest medical treatment ever devised. And yet in many countries like the USA it is still an illegal treatment.

This figure should be compared to chemotherapy (which is a legal treatment) with a success rate of only 3% and a very high mortality rate.

As with hydrogen peroxide, caution should be observed with ozone therapy. The only danger is the possibility of generating excess free radical activity, which can be prevented by taking antioxidants such as Vitamin C.

Dr. J. Wright, a well-known natural practitioner, states that ozone should not be used alone. It should be combined with a good diet (as all other cancer therapies should be) and possibly other treatments. Vitamin C should be given to all patients who are receiving any form of oxygen therapy, since it prevents uncontrolled oxidation.

Some adverse effects with ozone therapy have been reported. These include phlebitis, circulatory depression, and chest pain, shortness of breath, fainting, coughing and cardiac arrhythmias. These are seldom seen if ozone is used correctly by an experienced therapist and under cover of antioxidants.

21. High dose intravenous Vitamin C

The essential role of Vitamin C in the formation of collagen has been known for a long time. It is also known that in the process of collagen synthesis, Vitamin C is *consumed* and not regenerated (unlike other vitamins and co-factors) which explains why such high doses of Vitamin C are required for normal health. Collagen is the cement that holds cells together, and if this intercellular binding is strong enough, it is not easy for tumor cells to spread and invade neighboring structures. Cancer cells produce an enzyme, hyaluronidase, which helps them destroy this intercellular cement.

In addition to this effect, Vitamin C has been shown to be selectively toxic to cancer cells; it also strengthens the immune system and serves as an oxygen transporter in the blood.

I have already discussed the work by Pauling and Cameron on the use of high doses (10g) of oral Vitamin C in terminally ill cancer patients (7). In those studies, these two authors showed that such high oral doses of Vitamin C extended the life expectancy of terminally ill cancer patients (given up on by the medical profession) six-fold (36 months vs 6 months). This bought valuable extra time for the patients to start other treatment programmes and to change their lifestyles.

Since then, studies have shown that similar high doses given intravenously act as an effective anti-cancer treatment. There are several clinics in the USA that have pursued this line of research further (Drs. Riordan and Wassell).

The mechanism of action of Vitamin C under these conditions (studied by Dr. Wassell) is that Vitamin C acts as a pro-oxidant inside the cell (where there are insufficient other antioxidants) in these high concentrations, which leads to the formation of hydrogen peroxide inside cells. In normal cells, this is readily and rapidly disposed of by the enzyme catalase. Cancer cells have a lack of catalase and therefore the hydrogen peroxide and other peroxides accumulate, killing the cancer cells.

The crucial point here is that high enough concentrations of Vitamin C inside the cells must be achieved. Other workers subsequently showed that the rapid intravenous infusion of Vitamin C in combination with alpha-lipoic acid was effective in achieving Vitamin C levels inside cells that were effective in killing cancer cells (103). One comment made by the researchers was that because this treatment rapidly kills cancer cells, it is not recommended for cancers where even small amounts of swelling and inflammation would be dangerous. There are clinics in this country that use this technique.

22. Carrier Molecule Potentiation Therapies (IPT and DMSO-PT)

Many years ago a book appeared with the title *The Magic Bullet*. From the contents of the book it was clear that therapists, even those many years ago, were striving hard to find some means of targeting cancer cells selectively in the presence of normal cells. One way of achieving this would be to find some metabolic difference between cancer cells and normal cells that can be exploited for this purpose. The fact that cancer cells have such a great affinity for glucose offers such a possibility. Cancer cells consume 15 times more glucose than normal cells, which means that they also have very active insulin receptors on their surface. Therefore, if we could attach some toxin to glucose, perhaps the cancer cells would accept this complex just as readily as the untagged glucose. Alternatively, would it not be possible to use glucose and insulin to open the ports of entry to the cancer cells and then push in some toxins through the "open doors" to the cancer cells? These and other similar ideas have been studied by scientists for many years with some positive results. The following two procedures are examples of this.

1. *Insulin Potentiation Therapy*

The rationale behind these therapies is that certain natural substances such as insulin and DMSO can be used to carry lethal cancer-killing drugs (eg chemotherapy drugs) selectively into cancer cells.

Cancer cells are known to be voracious sugar "eaters" and for this reason they also have large numbers of highly active insulin receptors on their cell surfaces. These receptors are "opened up" by insulin to allow access of glucose to the cells. At the same time, chemotherapy drugs that may also be present are also permitted to enter the cancer cells and kill them. The important point is that, because of the presence of insulin, much larger quantities of the drug enter the cancer cells than normal cells, meaning that much less (eg 10 % of the normal dose) of the drug has to be administered to effectively kill the cancer cells. This also means that the numerous side-effects of the chemotherapy drugs are reduced, and similarly makes the treatment more potent. Hence the name Insulin Potentiation Therapy (IPT). The core principle to understand is that it is the insulin that brings the selectivity to the treatment (105).

In normal (without insulin) chemotherapy, the toxic chemotherapy drugs kill both cancer cells and normal cells (hence the side-effects) at the dosage levels used in conventional chemotherapy.

Dr. Stephen Ayre is a well-known specialist on IPT. He comments as follows in his book: "... because of this favorable side-effect profile, cycles of low dose chemotherapy with IPT may be done more frequently..." (104).

Not only is IPT much more effective than normal chemotherapy, it can also be administered more frequently, with fewer and less severe side-effects, thus improving the effectiveness of the treatment significantly.

The following table lists the conventional doses of some chemotherapy drugs vs the same drugs when used in IPT:

Drug	**Normal dose**	**IPT dose**
Cisplatin	150mg	15mg
Cyclophosphamide	1500mg	200mg
Methotrexate	60mg	10mg
Doxorubicin	100mg	10mg

Some mechanisms of action of insulin in IPT

Dr. Ayre further comments as follows:

> "... in those undergoing treatment with IPT, an overall gentler experience promotes the concurrent use of other important elements in a programme of comprehensive cancer care, which includes nutrition and immune support..." (104).

The first potentiating effects of insulin were observed with the drug Methotrexate (106).

There are many diseases of the central nervous system for which good drugs exist, but which cannot be used effectively because they do not cross the blood-brain barrier into the central nervous system.

The barrier retards the entry of many compounds into the brain, including the chemotherapy drugs.

> *The important point is that insulin also facilitates the entry of these drugs into the brain, presumably because the brain needs glucose.*

This effect can be further increased by including DMSO as part of the treatment.

Previously patients had to be put into an insulin coma for IPT, which afforded conventional doctors some basis to object to IPT.

That is no longer necessary. Newer technology allows insulin to be used in IPT without putting the patient into an insulin coma. This may be achieved by administering insulin until blood glucose levels reach a level of 1.7-2.0 mmole/l before administering the chemotherapy dose.

There is therefore now no valid, scientific reason why conventional medicine should not accept and use IPT.

It is unbelievable but true that the American Medical Association has effectively stopped doctors in the USA from using IPT, thus depriving millions of patients of the very real benefits of IPT. According to the *Cancer Tutor*, there is now only one doctor left in the USA who uses the technique. The others have all fled to Mexico.

IPT is a procedure that should only be carried out in a clinic, under medical supervision. Usually it is administered by a trained nurse under the guidance of a medical doctor.

The following procedure has been adapted from that described by Drs. R. Hauser and M. Hauser in their book *Treating Cancer with Insulin Potentiation Therapy*, 2002, Oak Park Ill, USA: Beulah Landpress.

Before treatment, the patient is instructed on the whole procedure including risks, which are minimal. Typically, during the first treatment, a complete blood analysis including all vital blood components is done and the patient's vital signs are registered. Then insulin is given until the blood sugar level reaches a level of 1.7-2.0mmol/L. In addition, provision is made in the intravenous line for the administration of additional supportive Nutraceutical compounds such as multivitamins, Vitamin C, glutathione and DMSO as may be indicated during treatment. Also an acid neutralising agent (eg. Alkalinizing Formula from *Fortifood*) is given orally to prevent any gastrointestinal upsets that may occur. A careful record is kept of all the medications given, and in each case the precise time is noted. After the intravenous insulin has been given, additional Nutraceutical intramuscular supportive therapy is given in the form of testosterone injections and others as deemed necessary by the therapist in charge. About 20 minutes after the insulin, the patient begins to sweat and to feel drowsy and tired and the heart rate may be accelerated. These are hypoglycemic symptoms. At this time the blood sugar level is checked once again to ensure that it remains in the desired range. Generally after about half an hour, the patient begins to sweat profusely and to feel hot. This is when the patient's blood sugar reaches its lowest point, corresponding to the insulin dose given. After checking the blood sugar level once again, which should be within the abovementioned range, the chemotherapeutic drugs are injected intravenously. Usually 3 or 4 different drugs are given, according to the judgment of the therapist. The chemotherapy cocktail given in this manner is critical in determining the outcome of the treatment. Usually several drugs are given in combination and these are selected in such a manner that the different drugs used affect cancer cells by different biochemical mechanisms so that a complementary effect is achieved.

The patient is then held at the low blood sugar level for another 40 minutes according to the preference of the therapist. The patient may then be given a fruit drink or glucose solution to gradually return the blood sugar to normal with the disappearance of the hypoglycemic symptoms. At this stage, most people feel refreshed and may even be hungry.

Positive results (tumor regression) may be expected after 6-10 bi-weekly treatments. In the case of a large tumor load, 20 or more sessions may be needed. It may be wise to check the blood chemistry after every 2 or 3 treatments to check for liver and kidney function. Also, after every 8-10 treatments, the selected cancer markers are checked and a CT scan is done on the cancer status of the patient. At this stage, any other determinations are done such as radiography or mammography as may be deemed necessary.

More specific information on treatment protocol is available in the book by Hauser and Hauser previously referred to.

Some important other information about IPT

Why, if IPT is as good as claimed by those who use it, doesn't everyone use it? This is the age-old problem of bringing new ideas into medicine and science in general. Many doctors fear what they do not know and have no inclination to study the textbooks and manuals. Frequently they lead busy lives in order to survive financially. Drug companies (who sell more than

$6 billion worth of chemotherapy drugs annually) are reluctant to promote a system that would reduce this figure to $1 billion.

In the collective experience of Dr. Garcia and his family (who discovered IPT) of more than one hundred years of clinical use of IPT, no single patient has died as a result of the procedure, during the procedure or after the procedure (see the reference above to the book by Hauser and Hauser).

The success record of the treatment of various cancers by this means is also available in this book. The estimated chances (by Dr. Garcia) of success for some of the cancers listed there are as follows: Hodgkins lymphoma 100 %; Non-Hodgkins lymphoma 80 %; chronic leukemia 80 %; acute leukemia 80%; pancreas cancer 50 %; stomach cancer 80 %; colon cancer 80 %; kidney cancer 50 %; bladder cancer 60 %; uterine cancer 90 %; cervical cancer 100 %; ovarian cancer 90 %; sarcoma 90 %; Glioblastoma multiform 10 %.

If the cancer has already metastasized, can IPT still help? Dr. Garcia says that in fact it can still help, but if the cancer has metastasized, it means the cancer has overcome the immune system and organs such as the liver may have impaired function.

In such cases, what is the likelihood of success? Mostly just improvement of the quality of life for most cases. A few patients can expect 50 % remission (Dr. G).

If the cancer has spread to the brain, can ITP still help? No, says Dr. G.

The quality of life is improved by ITP, even in those where a cure cannot be achieved (Dr. G).

Frequently asked questions

How do I know that IPT will help in my case?
In order to answer this question the following information is relevant

- Biopsy results
- Ct and mri scans
- Details of previous treatments
- Initial pet scan
- Blood tests to evaluate liver, kidney and immune function
- Surgical report.

This information is best evaluated by a health professional with appropriate experience. The ultimate treatment plan should be developed by the patient (and family) under the guidance of the health professional selected.

Who is the ideal patient for IPT?
The following patient details are important:

- Positive mental attitude with strong family support
- No previous treatment
- Small tumor load
- Cancer, newly diagnosed
- No metastases.

This does not mean that patients in whom one or more of these conditions do not apply will not benefit from IPT; only the prognosis may not be so good.

How many treatments will be necessary?
According to Dr. Hauser, the patient is re-evaluated after 6-12 IPT treatments (3-6 weeks). In general, IPT treatment is continued until the following responses occur:

- The cancer goes into remission (or has been completely removed)
- IPT is clearly not working.

Generally, rapidly growing cancers usually respond within the first month, especially if treatment is instituted during the early stages of the cancer. For someone with a slow growing cancer (eg certain breast cancers), response may be slower and in some cases the cancer may not be responding at all.

If the treatment is not working, it may indicate that the wrong combination of chemotherapeutic agents is being used. How this might be changed is best left in the hands of an oncologist who also has experience with IPT, because the problem may be drug resistance.

Preventative chemotherapy is sometimes recommended by oncologists, eg in women after mastectomy. In such cases Dr. Hauser gives 10 weekly IPT treatments instead of conventional high-dose chemotherapy.

It is very important not to stop IPT therapy if the tumor is obviously shrinking. This can be very dangerous because the cancer will certainly regrow, most likely with increased vigour. It may also develop drug resistance if treatment is interrupted.

What other supplements should I take during IPT treatment?
Dr. Hauser uses high doses of vitamins A and D. The latter is particularly important since it may help to prevent the spreading of the tumor. Other sources suggest that high dose intravenous Vitamin C as well as a good multivitamin/mineral may also be beneficial.

It is also relevant here to consider which of the many other cancer treatments discussed may also be used in conjunction with IPT. Most can be used, but it is best to be guided in this regard by an experienced therapist.

First of all, the cancer diet is of the utmost importance. The methods that depend on the stimulation of the immune system (eg laetrile and the Kelley enzyme treatment) can also be used, as well as all the methods that are based on dietary modifications (eg the Budwig and Gerson protocols). In serious cases, the combined IPT and CsCl/DMSO protocols may be used under the guidance of an experienced therapist.

How much must the blood sugar levels be reduced by insulin?
The following values are given in Dr. Hauser's book. During therapy the blood sugar values are reduced to 1.1—2.2mmol/L (normal values are in the range 4.2—6.2mmol/L). Not all patients react to insulin in the same way, therefore some careful prior experimentation may be necessary to determine the appropriate dose in each case.

How long must the patient fast before IPT?
It is better to fast overnight before IPT. If the IPT is given during the day, a 4 hour fast is necessary before treatment. No other drugs should be taken on the day of treatment. Immediately after treatment, small easily digestible meals are usually taken.

What are the side-effects of IPT?
Unlike conventional high-dose chemotherapy, there are no serious side-effects associated with IPT. Fifteen minutes after insulin is given, the patient begins to feel sleepy and even somewhat fatigued. Somewhat later, sweating, a rapid heartbeat and eventually a very hot feeling may follow. The maximum hypoglycemic response is seen 30 minutes after the insulin is given. The typical very hot feeling is felt when the chemotherapeutic drugs are given (intravenously), because it is at that point that the maximum symptoms of hypoglycemia are manifested, and it is also the point where the drugs have their maximum effect.

After the drugs have been given, the patient is given a fruit drink to reverse the hypoglycemic symptoms.

Forty five minutes later the patient may have a light meal.

Are there any contra-indications to IPT?

None. Previous medical treatment by means of conventional methods may reduce the efficacy of IPT.

What other sources of information on IPT are available?

In addition to the book by R. and M. Hauser referred to in the Introduction, there are other valuable sources of information on the Internet. Dr. Garcia is prepared to answer personal questions *(donatopg3@yahoo.com)*.

Another valuable source is available at *www.IPQT.org* where a list of doctors in the USA trained in the use of IPT is given. In South Africa no such list is available at present, but some information is available from *Fortifood* (see the web-site).

What insulin does

Insulin stimulates all those processes in the body that promote anabolism (tissue growth). Glucose receptors on cell membranes are opened up to increase access of glucose to the cells to increase energy production. At the same time, more amino acids are allowed into the cells (increased protein synthesis) and more fatty acids are absorbed (increased energy production). Insulin achieves this by the alteration of transmembrane movement of nutrients, and also by modifying the level of enzyme activity, mostly those that play a role in energy production. The best-known effect is an increase of glucose transport into cells. As blood glucose levels rise, blood insulin levels increase in normal patients. It is well known and widely accepted that persistent high blood sugar levels promote the growth of a variety of cancers such as breast cancer.

In addition to its role in regulating blood sugar levels, insulin also modifies anabolic enzyme levels, which it does by stimulating RNA synthesis. In a similar manner, it also plays a role in embryonogenesis, cell differentiation, as well as growth and replication of cells, especially in cancer cells. The stimulatory effect of insulin on cancer cells is well known, and this in turn is related to the fact that there are more insulin receptors on cancer cells than on normal cells. This immediately offers a possibility of preferentially and selectively targeting cancer cells in the presence of normal cells.

Given the various actions of insulin, the important question in the case of the cancer patient is: how do insulin levels effect cellular absorption of substances other than glucose, eg drugs such as the chemotherapy drugs? If insulin has a similar effect on the cellular absorption of these drugs by the cancer cells, it would make the cancer cells much more susceptible to the killing effects of chemotherapy, at the same time overcoming the lack of selectivitiy associated with conventional chemotherapy. Typically, breast cancer cells have 7 times more insulin receptors on their cell membranes than normal breast cells (*J Clin Invest* 1990, 86: 1503). Further studies have confirmed the presence of increased numbers of insulin receptors in various types of cancer. In this manner, insulin increases the growth rate of cancers and it was known at the time that fast-growing cancers respond better to chemotherapy drugs than slow-growing cancers. Therefore, at the time when Dr. Donato Perez Garcia started his work on IPT, it was found that the sensitivity of cancer cells to insulin would increase the toxic effects of chemotherapy to cancer cells. Subsequent work by Dr. Garcia proved this to be true beyond expectations. This is partly also related to the alterations in cell cycles that take place in the presence of insulin. Normally, cancer cells go through four different phases during which their susceptibility to chemotherapy drugs is altered. These are two rest phases, a phase with accelerated DNA synthesis and a phase during which mitosis and cell division take place.

With IPT therapy, the two rest periods become shorter, while the two phases during which the cells become increasingly penetrable by chemotherapy drugs (the two phases during which increased DNA synthesis and mitosis take place) are significantly increased (S-phase). This means that the susceptibility to the drugs is also greatly increased, which in turn means that smaller amounts of the drugs (with lesser side-effects) are required for successful therapy as shown above. This represents a great advance in cancer treatment, which was confirmed by many subsequent studies (see Hauser and Hauser, *Ibid.*).

Some mechanisms of action of insulin in IPT

- Enhanced cell permeability, especially in cancer cells with the large lumber of insulin receptors
- Increased cellular oxygenation, which is unfavorable for cancer cells
- Recruitment of cancer cells into the S-phase with increased susceptibility to chemotherapy drugs

- Increased permeability to drugs of the blood-brain barrier
- Increased access of nutrients into the cells
- Increased absorption of drugs into the cell.

IPT and the blood-brain barrier

There are numerous conditions of the central nervous system which could theoretically be treated using existing drugs and natural compounds, but which in practice are refractory to treatment. Brain cancer is a notable example. This is because the blood-brain barrier retards or entirely prevents the entry of many compounds (including the chemotherapy drugs) into the brain. This protective mechanism developed over thousands of years to protect the brain from the harmful effects of foreign environmental compounds. The mechanisms involved include both restrictive anatomical structures and biochemical transport systems. Part of the system includes the tight junctions between the capillary endothelia in the brain. The system as a whole operates in such a manner that access to the brain is only possible for biochemically essential molecules for which special transport systems have been developed. Interestingly, the blood-brain barrier also contains receptors for insulin (which permits entry of glucose into the brain) and other biologically essential molecules. Although the entire process of molecular access is not only restricted to the role that insulin receptors play, it is well documented that insulin promotes the entry of drugs (including the chemotherapy drugs) to the brain, thus promoting the therapeutic effects of these substances in the brain.

Interest in the possible use of insulin to treat brain cancer was stimulated when Dr. Garcia Sr. found, more than 60 years ago, that insulin given prior to the injection of mercury and arsenic salt could greatly enhance their absorption into the central nervous system (*Revista Medical Militar* 1938, 2: 1). This led to the successful treatment of patients with syphilis of the central nervous system by means of anti-syphilitic agents (Hauser). This work was subsequently extended to the treatment of brain tumors by means of IPT and chemotherapy drugs. Successful treatments for highly aggressive brain tumors such as gliomas (Grade IV) were reported.

The standard reference work on the technical details regarding IPT is a book by Drs. R.A. Hauser and M.A. Hauser (Amazon Books). See also Dr. Hauser's website *www.caringmedical.com*. These sources should be consulted by doctors who contemplate the use of the method on their patients.

2. DMSO and DMSO Potentiation Therapy

DMSO is another molecule that can be used to carry toxins into cancer cells because of its high affinity for cancer cells. The following facts regarding DMSO are relevant:

- DMSO, because of its great affinity for cancer cells, targets cancer cells in the presence of normal cells for reasons that are not fully understood.
- DMSO binds chemically to certain kinds of chemotherapy drugs to form complexes.
- The DMSO-drug complexes thus formed will draw the drug into the cancer cells.
- The toxic chemotherapy drug in the complex is still able to kill the cancer cells, and, at much reduced dosage levels, toxicity and side-effects are virtually non-existent.
- On their own, the chemotherapy drugs are so toxic and non-selective that they kill far more normal cells than cancer cells, which is why toxic side-effects are such a problem with chemotherapy.
- DMSO is especially valuable in brain cancer patients, but is also valuable in the treatment of other cancers. DMSO readily crosses the blood-brain barrier.
- DMSO is remarkably non-toxic. It has been used in doses of 2-4g/kg per day without noteworthy side-effects.
- 5-10 % DMSO solutions have been used as a carrier vehicle for a variety of drugs, including the usual chemotherapy drugs.
- The first studies which demonstrated the potentiating effect of DMSO on drug action were done with the aid of a dye haematoxylin (Hauser and Hauser, *Ibid.*). The researchers were able to show that only cancer cells were colored by the dye in the presence of DMSO, indicating that DMSO carried the dye, so to speak, into the cancer cells. This showed that DMSO specifically targeted the cancer cells.
- A further great advantage of DMSO is that it readily crosses the blood-brain barrier, thus making it possible to use drugs (including many chemotherapy drugs) in combination with DMSO to treat brain conditions that would have been impossible otherwise.
- The DMSO effect has been demonstrated with other compounds such as hydrogen peroxide, CsCl, MSM and other products. It

does not combine with all the chemotherapy drugs, but it works in synergy with most other treatments.

The great problem with chemotherapy drugs is that they do not specifically target cancer cells in the presence of normal cells, which explains the serious toxicity problem that goes with chemotherapy for cancer patients. This means that, as in the case of IPT, very much smaller doses of the drugs can be used with DMSO-PT with little or no side effects.

Tragically, these developments have been violently suppressed by the authorities. It is easy to see why. Using these methods, the amount of chemotherapy drugs sold would be reduced by 90 %, a loss of billions of dollars to the industry.

DMSO as such may be of great value in the treatment of different types of cancer. It has been shown to promote differentiation of malignant bone marrow cells, and therefore may be of value in patients who require bone marrow transplants (107).

DMSO has also been shown to retard cancer of the bladder (108), colorectal cancer (109), ovarian cancer (110), breast cancer (111) and skin cancer (112).

DMSO stimulates various parts of the immune system and scavenges hydroxyl radicals, the most dangerous of all free radicals. It also increases the flow of essential minerals across cell membranes and may diminish the effects of carcinogens by cleansing cell membranes.

Increased percentage kill of Adenocarcinoma breast cancer cells by various antineoplastic agents has been demonstrated in tissue culture in the presence of DMSO (5-10 %). This was demonstrated by Dr. Pommier and associates at the University of Portland (USA). (*Am J Surg* 1988, 155: 672). Dramatic results on patients with various cancers by chemotherapy drugs in the presence of 10 % DMSO were subsequently shown by Hauser *et al.* (*Ibid.*, p 154). More than 90 % objective remissions were seen in the case of lymphoma and breast cancer patients using DMSO was found to cause a twofold increase in the concentration of labeled Cyclophosphamide in plasma, brain and liver tissues. The elevation persisted for about 2-3 hours, but subsequently returned to normal levels.

Similar effects are seen in humans. Typically in one experiment, instead of giving 2000mg of Cyclophosphamide, only 150-200mg was given per dose. This is similar to the doses used in IPT.

Remarkable results were obtained with breast cancer patients: 13 of 15 inoperable breast cancer patients with metastases were induced to remission with the DMSO-Cyclophosphamide protocol. Of 65 other patients, 44 achieved remission. No side-effects were seen and pain was relieved to such an extent that no morphine was required (*Annual New York Acad Sc* 1975, 243: 412). Although these promising results were obtained more than 30 years ago, no adequate follow-up studies have been conducted to confirm these very promising results due to medical skepticism and behind the scenes financial interests.

In Dr. Hauser's institute, DMSO low-dose chemotherapy in the presence of 10 % DMSO, demonstrating the effect of DMSO *in vivo*.

According to Dr. Hauser *et al.* (*Ibid.*, p 153), DMSO appears to be particularly useful in the treatment of brain tumors and metastases because of the ease with which it crosses the blood-brain barrier.

Orally ingested DMSO was found to cause a twofold increase in the concentration of labeled Cyclophosphamide in plasma, brain and liver tissues. The elevation persisted for about 2-3 hours, but subsequently returned to normal levels.

Similar effects are seen in humans. Typically in one experiment, instead of giving 2000mg of Cyclophosphamide, only 150-200mg was given per dose. This is similar to the doses used in IPT.

Remarkable results were obtained with breast cancer patients: 13 of 15 inoperable breast cancer patients with metastases were induced to remission with the DMSO-Cyclophosphamide protocol. Of 65 other patients, 44 achieved remission. No side-effects were seen and pain was relieved to such an extent that no morphine was required (*Ann New York Acad Sc* 1975, 243: 412). Although these promising results were obtained more than 30 years ago, no adequate follow-up studies have been conducted to confirm these very promising results due to medical skepticism and behind the scenes financial interests.

In Dr. Hauser's institute, DMSO is often mixed in the syringe with the chemotherapeutic agent used, or in the saline bag in the intravenous line.

Quercetin as a potentiator
Quercetin is a bioflavonoid with antioxidant properties, but it is also a potentiator of chemotherapy drugs. In an *in vitro* study using human ovarian and endometrial cancer cell lines, it was found that the addition of 0.01-10mM

of quercetin caused a 1.5-30 fold potentiation of the cytotoxic effects of cisplatin. It is one of the favorite nutrients used by Dr. Hauser (*Ibid.* p172).

23. Singlet oxygen in the treatment of cancer

In his book *Cancer: Step Outside the Box* (1), Dr. T. Bollinger reproduces a protocol referred to as the "Overnight Cure for Cancer" (OCC). The main ingredients of this treatment are DMSO and MSM, given in frequent small doses over a period of 12 hours. This is done after an induction period of three days, during which toxins are removed from the body, involving *inter alia* a colon cleanse. The entire protocol was developed by W. Kehr of the Independent Cancer Research Foundation in conjunction with Dr. Darrell Wolfe of Canada.

The theoretical background

The procedure is based on the microbe theory of cancer as developed by A. Beauchamp and others presented elsewhere in this book, and postulates that the primary cause of cancer is the metabolic interference by cancerous microbes in the normal cellular metabolism. This results in the suppression of the Krebs cycle and the electron transport chain in the mitochondria of healthy cells, which leads to a switch to fermentation as a means of extracting energy from glucose.

According to this thesis, the key to a solution to the cancer problem lies in *killing the microbes inside the cancer cell without killing the cell itself.* But the question is: how to achieve this without killing the cancer cells *en masse,* which may cause all sorts of problems we have previously referred to. If this could be achieved, the cancer cells would naturally revert to normal cells, which can be considered the prime objective in any cancer treatment programme. Once reverted, the cells are subject to normal regulatory control including apoptosis (programmed killing) as a means of getting rid of unwanted cells. Apoptosis does not cause the massive killing of cells at once, accompanied by the swelling and inflammation previously referred to.

It would seem that the DMSO-MSM therapy proposed by Kehr and Wolfe comes close to achieving this.

Amongst a variety of natural substances that cause cancer cells to revert back to healthy cells, DMSO has been found to be the most effective. MSM is a product closely related to DMSO and which has a similar effect.

Several substances have previously been described as able to reconvert cancer cells into normal cells. To date, DMSO-MSM appears to be the most effective, but the precise mechanism by means of which they work remains unclear. DMSO is known to readily enter cancer cells where, together with MSM, the pair may act as an oxygen delivery system, since both compounds may readily lose their oxygen atoms.

- MSM = methylsulfonylmethane = $CH_3SO_2CH_3$ = $DMSO_2$
- DMSO = dimethylsulfoxide = CH_3SOCH_3 = DMSO

Therefore, inside the cells and acting as an oxygen delivery system, the following happens:

$$DMSO_2 \longrightarrow O + DMSO \longrightarrow DMS \text{ (dimethylsulfide)} + O$$

The oxygen atoms liberated in this manner will then kill the microbes inside the cancer cells without killing the cells themselves. In formulating this process, Kehr as well as others refer to these single atoms as "oxygen singlets" (O_1) as opposed to oxygen molecules as they occur in air and correctly designated by these authors as oxygen pairs (O_2).

To designate O in the abovementioned scheme as an oxygen singlet is not entirely correct, and a fine distinction here is called for between what they call oxygen singlets (O_1) which are in fact oxygen atoms with a particular electronic configuration, and what in physics has been called oxygen singlets based on the electron spins in the oxygen molecule (O_2).

An oxygen bi-radical contains two unpaired electrons on each atom and when these have opposite spins, the bi-radical is called "singlet oxygen" ($1O_2$), whereas when they have opposing spins, the biradical is called an oxygen triplet ($3O_2$).

> *Thus a clear distinction should be made between O_1 (oxygen atoms referred to by Kehr as singlet oxygen (O_1) and true singlet oxygen ($1O_2$).*

In order to avoid confusion, I will only use the terms $1O_2$ for singlet oxygen and O_1 for oxygen atoms.

Kehr correctly points out that oxygen atoms (O_1) kill microbes and neutralize other toxins; their presence is therefore much desired. However, from what we know of the manner in which certain micro-organisms fight one another, it is also true that certain micro-organisms kill others by means of singlet oxygen $1O_2$.

It has been suggested that by increasing the singlet oxygen ($1O_2$) level in the medium in which DMSO and MSM are used to kill microbes, the antimicrobial effects would be substantially increased.

There is evidence that suppressing the metabolic activities of the cancer microbes inside the cells allows the cells to normalize. Cells not normalized in this manner will eventually be disposed of through the normal process of apoptosis. At the same time, the immune system is gradually restored to normality. As pointed out by Kehr and others, this can be achieved by means of treatment with DMSO and MSM. From what has been said above, much of this effect is achieved by means of oxygen singlets ($1O_2$) and this can be enhanced as shown below.

The treatment protocol

As in the Kehr protocol, the proposed new treatment consists of relatively small doses of MSM (taken orally) and DMSO (applied topically) every 30 minutes over a period of 12 hours based on the age and weight of the patient (see later). In the proposed method, transition metal complexes (to enhance formation of singlet oxygen) are dissolved in the DMSO solution. No food is allowed during the 12 hour period preceding the treatment period of 12 hours and following it. No food is therefore allowed for a total period of 36 hours.

This treatment should not be combined with any other cancer protocol.

The main principles on which the treatment is based

The inclusion of substrates to reactivate the Krebs cycle and the electron transport chain and transition metal complexes with chlorophyll to enhance formation of singlet oxygen ($1O_2$). Singlet oxygen selectively increases the microbe-killing capacity of the treatment.

DMSO and MSM are used as basic treatment to convert cancer cells back into normal cells by selectively killing the cancer microbes. The DMSO is applied externally (dosage given below) as in the CsCl/DMSO protocol and the MSM, as well as the singlet oxygen-stimulating supplements, are taken orally. In this manner the cancer cells and intracellular micro-organisms are starved, which induces them to readily take up the high doses of DMSO and MSM. The microbes and cancer cells are also starved of glucose, which suppresses the microbial production of lactic acid. Under these circumstances, the lactic acid in the cells is bound by MSM and eliminated, thus preventing its reconversion in the liver into glucose.

Pretreatment preparation includes a fast as well as a colon cleanse, and optionally, a liver cleanse.

For a period of 12 hours before treatment, absolutely no food or drink (other than purified water) is allowed

The colon cleanse ensures that putrefying waste in the colon is eliminated to prevent it from supplying nutrients (eg glucose) that could interfere with the abovementioned treatment. Suitable methods for cleasing the colon are discussed in a later section under the heading "Colon Cleanse". These include Royal Tea, as recommended by Kehr and Bollinger.

- The reactivation of the Krebs cycle and the electron transport chain is achieved by the inclusion of Krebs cycle intermediaries (such as oxaloacetic acid) in the MSM solution.
- The restoration of mitochondrial energy production also forms part of the singlet oxygen enhancement programme.
- Consuming repeated small quantities of the principal treatment ingredients (MSM, DMSO), as proposed by Kehr and Bollinger, forms part of the strategy of treatment.
- DMSO: use a 70 % DMSO: 30 % purified water mix
- MSM solution: Use a solution containing 0.25g MSM per ml by dissolving 250g of MSM in purfied water and making up to a volume of 1000ml.

Additional supplements which are required

The principal treatment compounds are MSM, DMSO, Krebs cycle activator (oxaloacetic acid) and oxygen singlet booster (transition metal chelates and chlorophyll).

1. Colloidal silver.

This is a known anti-microbial agent. Different brands are available, usually obtainable from large pharmacies or health shops. In this protocol, the DMSO binds to the microscopic silver particles and transports it to the cancer cells. Dose: 30ml orally as a daily dose.

2. Pancreatic enzymes

Several products are available, but Vitalzym and Wobenzyme are the most popular products; also available from pharmacies and health shops. Use as directed, eg 1-2 caps every hour for 12 hours. These enzymes cleanse the tissues, increase circulation by removing toxins and support the immune system.

3. Green tea
Drink 5—10 cups per day. I prefer the product made in Japan.

4. Royal tea
For a colon cleansing prior to beginning the full treatment: 1 glass in the evening and morning followed by 2 half glasses during the day This product is used to cleanse the gastro-intestinal system. The internet gives sources.

5. Barley Powder.
Twenty tablets per day divided into 3 doses, each taken 15 minutes before every meal.

Build-up period

This is also according to Kehr as reproduced in the book by Bollinger.

The full treatment consists of 25 one-dose treatments (of MSM and DMSO) given every 30 minutes—the full treatment is given over a 12-hour period during the day.

In order to familiarize the patient with the procedure and to detect and eliminate other problems that may arise, an introductory period of three days is provided, during which gradually increased doses are given and during which also the colon cleanse is done using Royal Tea and/or any other procedure that your health professional may suggest. During the entire treatment you may drink as much water as you can, but make sure that you use only the best quality purified water. Under no circumstances should you use tap water or water that contains chlorine or fluoride. They are known carcinogens.

- *Day 1 of the 3-day build-up period*: treatment consists of a 3-hour period, during which a total of 7 doses of the various treatment ingredients are given. During this period colloidal silver, pancreatic enzymes, DMSO, MSM and Barley are all administered for a 3-hour period only.
- *Day 2 of the 3-day build-up period*: As for day 1, but use a total of 13 doses over a 6 hour period.
- *Day 3 of the 3-day build-up period:* As for day 2, but use a total of 19 doses over a 9 hour period.

Dosage levels (for an 80kg patient). One full dose for the introductory period consists of:

- DMSO: 8ml 70 % solution (= 1 tablespoonful). Apply topically over a different area for each application. Include 50 % colloidal silver with the DMSO. Take the rest of the colloidal silver dose orally. Do not take any DMSO orally.
- MSM: 8ml 25 % solution (=1 tablespoonful). Take orally.
- *Krebs cycle activator*: oxaloacetic acid (as indicated below).
- *Singlet oxygen stimulator*: chlorophyll (as indicated below).

Do not touch gloves or anything else made of rubber or plastic when handling DMSO. Everything DMSO comes in touch with will be absorbed through the skin. You may apply it with your finger, but immediately afterwards wash your hands thoroughly.

NOTE: The build-up period with reduced doses is designed to detect complications that may arise at an early stage and to take preventive measures if necessary. For example, a certain amount of dangerous swelling and congestion may arise in the case of some patients (eg brain, colon and lung patients). In such cases, medical advice should immediately be sought and the programme terminated until symptoms subside. The programme can then be restarted at a later date at reduced dosage levels and a more gradual increase in dosage levels. Alternatively, another protocol which is perhaps better suited for the situation could be considered.

The full treatment

- This consists of 25 doses administered over a 12 hour period.
- Treatment schedule for an 80kg patient:

DMSO 70 %: 15ml every 30 minutes for a period of 9 hours, apply locally.
MSM (25 % solution): 15ml taken orally every 30 minutes for a period of 9 hours.
Oxaloacetic acid: 0.5g every 30 minutes for a period of 9 hours.
Chlorophyll: 200mg (half a tablet) every 30 minutes.

- Include the other components of the protocol on the same basis: $1/25^{th}$ of the full daily dose every 30 minutes for a period of 12 hours.

How to apply the DMSO
Do not take orally. Identify six areas of the body, approximately the size of half an A4 page each, to apply the DMSO by means of an eye dropper.

Convenient sites are left and right forearm, left and right thigh and the left and right calf. Do each application on a different site. Repeated applications of DMSO may cause a rash due to dehydration. To alleviate, spray copious amounts of purified water over the area. If desired, you may also cover it with MSM cream. Mix a portion of your daily colloidal silver dose with the DMSO before application.

24. Barley green

This is another product about which many favorable reports are available. It is the type of product that can be taken alone or in combination with other protocols. It is available commercially as Barley Green tablets, at a very reasonable price. The dose is 15-20 tabs daily.

Another important reason why I include it here is that it alkalinizes the body in a gentle way and is therefore suitable for long-term therapy. It is also a rich source of minerals and vitamins.

I would recommend Barley Green as an immune stimulant that is particularly suitable to prevent recurrence of cancer after successful initial treatment.

25. Exercise with oxygen therapy (EWOT)

This is described in more detail by Bill Henderson in his book (p 97). I have considered the procedure and find it suitable for virtually all cancer patients, with the possible exception of the very weak.

The patient simply spends 15 minutes a day on a treadmill while breathing pure oxygen through a mask. The pure oxygen increases the partial oxygen pressure in the lungs, while the exercise promotes tissue distribution. A certain oxygen pressure is required (6 liter/minute) and certain vitamins (niacin, 500-1000mg daily) need to be taken 30 minutes before treatment starts.

Details of treatment may be varied according to the patient's condition. Exercise can be in the form of a treadmill or stationary bicycle while breathing oxygen at a rate of 6 liter/hour by placing the oxygen mask over your nose. The treatment can be done daily or less frequently depending on the patient's condition.

Having read what was said previously about oxygen toxicity for cancer cells, you will realize that this procedure should be part of the treatment of every cancer patient. Exercise with oxygen therapy is similar to Hydrogen peroxide therapy in providing oxygen to the tissues, but it has the great advantage that you can do it at home.

It is not the type of therapy that could be recommended as sole therapy for seriously ill Type IV patients, but it should be part of every other cancer protocol as supporting adjunct therapy. However, and like hydrogen peroxide and ozone therapy, intracellular oxygen levels are not markedly increased by this treatment unless adequate quantities of the correct mix of w-3 and w-6 fatty acids are available.

More information is available on the Internet (113).

It is recommended that the patient should achieve what is called niacin saturation 30 minutes before starting the procedure. Niacin increases peripheral circulation, so that after taking, say, 200mg of niacin initially, a mild, warm pink-eared vasodilatation (known as a flush) results, indicating increased blood circulation. Many people who start taking niacin are disturbed by this, but it is perfectly harmless and decreases in intensity with time, allowing the patient to increase dose levels to 500mg of niacin or more.

26. Essential fatty acid therapy

The patient should understand that raising blood oxygen levels is not enough unless the mechanisms that ensure cellular absorption of oxygen are in place. The role that certain fatty acids (including the w-6 polyunsaturated fatty acids) play in transporting oxygen molecules across cell membranes has received much attention in the recent medical literature (see for example the book by B.S. Peskin. 2008. *The Hidden Story of Cancer*. Houston, USA: Pinnacle Press). This explains the fact that prominent sportsmen also develop cancer. Warburg was the first to show that reduced oxygen levels in cells are the prime cause of cancer. He stated:

We find by experiment that about 35% inhibition of oxygen respiration already suffices to bring about such a transformation during cell growth.

As a result of the work of Peskin (p 40-42) and others, it is now recognized that a deficiency of unadulterated dietary w-6 fatty acids is mainly responsible for suppressed intracellular oxygen levels.

The Peskin protocol is based on the use of a mix of unadulterated w-3 and w-6 fatty acids as discussed elsewhere in this book. The protocol calls for the daily administration of 3-5g of a mix of w-3:w-6 fatty acids in a ratio of 1—2.5 w-6 unadulterated linoleic acid (sunflower oil) to 1 part of w-3, eg as fish oil.

27. Stem Cells

A stem cell is a cell that has the ability to duplicate itself endlessly and to become cells of virtually any organ and tissue of the body. Embryonic stem cells are cells extracted from the blastula, the very early embryo, that have an exceptional ability to duplicate in vitro, that is in a test tube, and to become cells of almost any tissue. Adult stem cells are cells found in an organism after birth. Until very recently, it was believed that adult stem cells could only become blood cells, bone and connective tissue. But recent development over the past 5 years has revealed that adult stem cells have capabilities similar to embryonic stem cells.

The Stem Cell Theory of Renewal proposes that stem cells are naturally released by the bone marrow and travel via the bloodstream toward tissues to promote the body's natural process of renewal. When an organ is subjected to a process that requires renewal, such as the natural aging process, this organ releases compounds that trigger the release of stem cells from the bone marrow. The organ also releases compounds that attract stem cells to this organ. The released stem cells then follow the concentration gradient of these compounds and leave the blood circulation to migrate to the organ where they proliferate and differentiate into cells of this organ, supporting the natural process of renewal.

In the contexts of cancer, stem cells may play an important role in restoring tissues damaged which may lead to cancer.

StemEnhance is a blend of two compounds extracted from the widely consumed aquatic botanical Aphanizomenon flos-aquae (AFA). One extract, which contains an L-selectin ligand, supports the natural release of stem cells (CD34+ cells) from the bone marrow. The other extract, a polysaccharide-rich fraction named Migratose™, may support the migration of stem cells out of the blood into tissues.

Circulating stem cells can reach various organs and become cells of that organ, helping such organ regain and maintain optimal health. Recent studies have suggested that the number of circulating stem cells is a key factor; the higher the number of circulating stem cells the greater is the ability of the body at healing itself.

Cleaning the inner terrain

Detoxifying the body

We are slowly and systematically being poisoned by the thousands of artificially created chemicals that have become a permanent feature of modern living. The extent, to which we nevertheless cope and survive, reflects the remarkable efficiency of human detoxification mechanisms. But toxification is intimately related to the ever-increasing death rate due to chronic metabolic diseases and cancer.

Chemical pollution is a silent killer, the extent and importance of which is appreciated by only a few.

In the Western World, the average person consumes 5kg of food additives each year, as well as 4.5kg of pesticides sprayed on crops. This amounts to nearly 14g (about 3 teaspoonfuls or 15ml) of food additives, 12g of pesticides and 25g of foreign chemicals a day. This needs to be added to all the other toxins such as antibiotics, organic pollutants, nitrates, heavy metals (lead, mercury, aluminum, cadmium, etc.) as well as the numerous other chemicals that are present in food and unpurified water.

At least 6 000 new chemicals have been introduced into our environment during the past 20 years, and we remain largely unaware of them although they are capable of inflicting significant metabolic damage. In addition, we increase our burden of foreign chemicals voluntarily through tobacco products, fried foods, alcoholic drinks, cosmetics, deodorants, sweeteners and numerous other sources. The total burden of foreign chemicals in our environment has been estimated to be in excess of 30 000.

The human detoxification system is remarkably efficient, but we have reached the stage where it has become overburdened.

In order to deal with the problem, the body deposits the excess in various tissues such as the bones, brain and other fatty tissues for "temporary storage" in order to prevent immediate damage to sensitive structures.

All the tissues in the body are constantly being renewed by replacement with new structures as the old ones are "dissolved" to make way for new ones. The toxins lodged there are similarly freed and taken up in the circulation for final detoxification and excretion. In most cases, the toxins undergo chemical modifications (known as Phase I and Phase II detoxification) in order to facilitate excretion. Minerals such as lead lodged in bones are liberated when bone is broken down, while fat-soluble organic chemicals (eg pesticides and insecticides), which are mostly stored in fatty tissues, are mobilized when fats are used for energy production.

After mobilization, these in transit toxins may now reach sensitive tissues such as the nervous system (including the brain), liver, kidneys and other vital organs. Many of the carcinogenic chemicals in our environment belong to this group of fat-soluble organic compounds.

The cumulative effect of toxins

Different chemical carcinogens may enhance one another's action, meaning that the combined effect of two chemicals may be more than an additive. The effects of any one chemical or any combination of chemicals may be cumulative in the sense that these effects are only seen long (even years) after exposure.

This makes it difficult to establish cause/effect relationships that are of particular significance to the cancer patient. The cancer that is currently seen may be the result of low-level exposure over many years, or it may be due to the cumulative effect of different carcinogens acting in an additive manner.

The consequences of exposure to carcinogenic chemicals are greatly aggravated in the presence of critically low levels of vital nutrients that are required for their detoxification and low levels of intracellular oxygen.

There are two ways of dealing with environmental toxins: one is to avoid exposure (which is by far the best) and the other is to remove accumulated carcinogenic chemicals from the body.

Avoiding exposure to environmental toxins

- Wash all commercial vegetables in a bowl of water to which half a cup (125ml) of glycerol and half a cup of vinegar have been added. The glycerol increases the solubility of fat soluble organic compounds (eg pesticides) and the vinegar mobilizes heavy metals such as lead.
- Use only purified water (preferably by reverse osmosis) in food and for drinking. Bottled or fountain water is not acceptable.
- Do not use aluminum foil in the preparation of food.
- Do not use aluminum pots and pans—rather use stainless steel or glass. Many non-stick pans are also made of aluminum and once the covering layer (which is in itself toxic) is removed, the aluminum is exposed.
- Avoid aluminum-containing medicines such as antacids.
- Do not smoke and avoid passive smoking, in other words do not live or work with someone who smokes.
- Discard the outer leaves of commercial vegetables and select a green-grocer or farm stall whose premises are not near a busy highway.
- Eat only organically grown vegetables and fruit; where possible, these should be homegrown on richly manured soil.
- Strictly avoid nitrate and nitrite-containing foods such as preserved meats and sausages.

- Choose fruits and vegetables that can be peeled (eg bananas, apples) and that are fresh and in season.
- Regularly take a reliable multinutrient formulation with optimum quantities of minerals (calcium, magnesium, zinc and selenium) which are heavy metal antagonists. These minerals also help to dislodge heavy metals such as lead trapped in bone.
- Do not supplement with less than 2000mg of Vitamin C per day, regardless of what your doctor or anyone else might say.
- Strictly avoid all foods and drinks that contain synthetic colorants and other additives.
- Develop the habit of carefully reading labels. Approach the manufacturers if you are not sure about any particular ingredient. Be aware that manufacturers often hide dangerous chemicals behind such innocent-sounding names as "emulsifiers", "stabilizers", etc.

Removing accumulated carcinogenic chemicals from tissue depots

Removal of these chemicals may be achieved by increasing the circulation to reach the deeper layers of the tissues where carcinogens may have been deposited over a long period. This is best achieved through the judicious combination of sauna, massage and exercise with the simultaneous use of natural vasodilatory substances such as nicotinic acid (see later). These procedures must be carried out under medical supervision, as some cancer patients may be too weak to undergo rigorous exercise and prolonged exposure to sauna.

For the patient who is judged fit enough to undergo such treatment, the ideal programme would be a 20-minute session of whole-body massage, 10 minutes of running followed by a 1 to 2 hour period in the sauna. Depending on the condition of the patient, the procedure should be repeated twice a day for 20 days or more.

The sequence of the procedures is important, as the idea is to increase the circulation as much as possible before the sauna. The duration of each procedure should be adapted according to the condition of the patient.

The whole procedure should be started on the same day as the intensified supplement programme described later, which also runs for 3 weeks.

If your attending physician judges the exercise and sauna parts of the procedure inappropriate for you, then skip these but follow the intensified supplement programme under medical guidance as described later, in order to promote mobilization of toxic deposits and to stimulate the detoxification pathways in the liver.

Start the sauna immediately after running. In this way carcinogens partly mobilized by running can be physically eliminated from the body through sweating. In addition, since the intensified supplement programme is simultaneously introduced, carcinogens not eliminated through sweating can be detoxified in the liver.

The temperature in the sauna should be high enough to induce sweating (50-60ºC), but you must be able to tolerate it comfortably. It may be advisable to start at a lower temperature and then to gradually increase the temperature until copious sweating is induced

During both the exercise and sauna parts of the programme, it is necessary to ensure adequate intake of fluids to compensate for losses during the treatment and to promote elimination of toxins.

How the detoxification system works

The detoxification process takes place mainly in the liver, in two phases. During Phase 1, toxic compounds are chemically altered through oxidation, reduction and hydrolysis reactions to make the toxin molecules more polar and thus to increase water solubility. Because this phase generates free radicals, adequate antioxidants must be present to detoxify the free radicals. Zinc, magnesium and molybdenum are important co-factors to support the chemical reactions in this phase.

Also, the products produced in Phase 1 may still be toxic and also not suitable for rapid elimination: for this, yet more chemical modifications are required (Phase 2). These occur by means of enzymatic conjugation (joining together) reactions with conjugating agents such as glutathione, glucuronic acid, cysteine, phosphate and glycine. These conjugated molecules are now much less toxic, more water soluble and more readily excreted by the kidneys. Magnesium, riboflavin and nicotinic acid are co-factors required in the Phase 2 conversions.

Glutathione is a key substance in the detoxifying pathways and it plays an important role in other metabolic reactions. It is present in all cells, including the liver, where it acts as a universal scavenger of a wide variety of toxins and as an antioxidant that reacts with numerous free radicals, including those generated in Phase 1.

This multifunctional control of many cellular processes with which it is involved elevates glutathione to the status of one of the controllers of all living systems, especially with respect to their ability to adapt to changing circumstances and threats to cellular survival. It is therefore the cell's first line of defense against many invaders, including foreign chemicals, viruses, cancer cells, etc. In experimental animals, the age-related decline in glutathione levels parallels survival curves. Clearly, glutathione is of the utmost importance to the cancer patient.

Supplementing with glutathione is to some extent problematic, though. Glutathione is a tripeptide (consists of 3 amino acids) of which the sulphur-containing cysteine is the most important. As a peptide (small protein), it is hydrolyzed (broken down) to a large extent in the stomach. Even if some is absorbed into the circulation, it is doubtful whether significant quantities will cross cellular membranes to the intracellular compartment where it exerts its effects. Intracellular glutathione is therefore mainly generated inside cells from its precursor amino acids, of which cysteine is the limiting factor. N-acetyl cysteine is the best available form of cysteine precursor for this purpose.

Nicotinic acid (Vitamin B3)

Nicotinic acid should be clearly distinguished from nicotine, a toxic alkaloid that occurs in tobacco and which has many harmful effects.

In many ways, nicotinic acid, or niacin, has properties that are directly the opposite of those of nicotine.

Nicotine causes vasoconstriction (narrowing of the arteries) while niacin is a vasodilator (increases the diameter of arteries), which therefore increases blood flow in tissues, which is so important in the cancer patient in the light of what was previously said about oxygen supply and the growth of cancer cells.

Niacin also improves peripheral circulation. In the presence of niacin, fewer red blood cells stick together, thus also improving tissue oxygenation. Niacin therefore allows the general circulation to penetrate more freely into the capillary network, thereby facilitating the removal of toxins. This effect of niacin may be increased by taking niacin in conjunction with massage, exercise (running) and sweating (sauna).

When starting niacin supplementation (eg with a dose of 100-200mg), most people will experience red flushes on the skin (especially in the neck area) due to the histamine-induced vasodilatory effect of niacin. This is harmless and will usually disappear after a few days. The flushes will reappear if the niacin dose is increased by 100-200mg increments, only to disappear once more at this higher dose level. By gradually increasing dosage levels in this manner, patients may be able to tolerate doses as high as 1000mg of niacin after a while.

Other nutrients

Niacin, like all other B-vitamins, can create induced deficiencies of other vitamins if large doses are taken in isolation. It is therefore important to take a good multinutrient supplement when high doses of niacin are used to increase oxygen delivery in cancer patients as discussed below.

In the context of detoxification of the cancer patient, mineral supplementation is also very important for several reasons. Minerals like magnesium, calcium and zinc replace toxic minerals such as lead and mercury lodged in the bones, thus promoting their elimination. During prolonged sweating in the sauna, heavy losses of minerals (especially magnesium) may occur, which need to be replaced urgently.

In general, mineral intake needs to be adequate but not excessive. With calcium and magnesium, the relative proportions are also important.

Numerous other nutrients are required for the process of detoxification. For Phase 1 detoxification, the following are of special importance: molybdenum, zinc, copper, iron, ascorbate, Vitamin E and beta-carotene.

For Phase 2 detoxification, the following are important: manganese, magnesium, N-acetyl cysteine, selenium, glucoronolactone, and glutamine.

A good diet and a good multinutrient supplement will supply these.

Putting the detoxification programme into action

The programme is based on the principle of niacin-induced vasodilatation of the capillary network in order to facilitate elimination of carcinogens.

Nicotinic acid is used for a variety of reasons. It is a strong vasodilatory substance with no serious side-effects. The success of the programme depends on a gradually intensified vasodilatory effect (achieved by means of incremental increases in dosage levels, and the similarly staged application of exercise and sweating by means of sauna). These effects are coordinated with a similarly intensified liver detoxification programme, based on supplementation with nutrients, milk thistle extracts and coffee enemas. These procedures in isolation are well-known, but their coordinated use in time, coupled with incremental intensification of each, is a new concept.

Nicotinic acid and its property of causing vasodilatory flushes is used as a "pace maker" to guide the programme and to determine the rate at which the other treatments are increased in intensity.

Before starting the programme the patient is given a good, balanced multinutrient supplement for at least 10 days, and this is then continued during the implementation of the programme and beyond. The whole programme consists of 6 stages as shown in the following example:

Stage	Multinutrient (tabs)	Nicotinic (mg)	NAC acid (mg)	Milk thistle extract (mg)*	Skeletone (teaspoons)	Vit C (mg)	Vit E (mg)
1	2	200	500	300	1	3000	100
2	3	300	500	400	2	3000	150
3	4	400	500	500	2	4000	200
4	5	500	500	500	2	4000	200
5	6	600	500	600	3	5000	200
6	7	800	500	600	3	5000	200

Note: *Milk thistle extract: use the standardized extract containing 70-80 % silimarin

During the entire process the patient should be under medical supervision and dosage levels modified to suit the patient.

The time required for each stage differs widely from patient to patient as this is an individual matter. It should be determined in consultation with your doctor. Generally, patients remain for 3-5 days in each stage.

While you are on the programme, temporarily terminate all other supplements and medicines in consultation with your doctor.

Do not terminate supplementation abruptly after reaching Stage 6. Rather, gradually reduce levels of all supplements by working back through Stages 5,4,3,2, and 1, allowing 3 days for each stage.

Fat exchange

Most carcinogens are fat-soluble and tend to be stored in the fatty tissues of the body. These stores are constantly being replaced by new fats from the diet, and in the process the toxins lodged there are liberated so that they can be eliminated. This process offers an excellent opportunity to rid the body of accumulated toxins. However, the fat depots represent the body's vital energy reserves and are not easily given up or mobilized unless something else is offered in exchange. Fats are easily stored but difficult to remove, as those on slimming programmes may have discovered! In order to store 100 kilojoules (kJ) in the form of fat, only 3.1kJ of energy is required, whereas 23kJ of energy is required to store the same amount of energy in the form of protein or carbohydrate.

The human race has developed these evolutionary mechanisms to store vital energy reserves over centuries as a result of severe and recurring famines. One of these mechanisms involves a dramatic increase of the enzyme lipoprotein lipase, the enzyme that stores fat. It is strongly activated as soon as we try to remove fat, for example by fasting. In attempting to remove the accumulated toxins in fatty depots, our aim must therefore be to *replace* the fat depots, rather than burn them away by means of kilojoules restriction or increased energy expenditure.

Experience gained by cattle farmers in fattening up livestock for the market has demonstrated how easy it is to replace fats in the body. By feeding livestock a ration consisting mainly of maize as a source of energy, the carcasses contain mainly relatively hard saturated fat (lard). When the same animals are then fed a ration consisting mainly of sunflower seed (which contains a higher percentage of oily, polyunsaturated fatty acids), the fat on the carcasses rapidly, within 1-2 months, becomes more oily, illustrating the replacement of body fat by the fats in the diet. I have developed a mixture of oils that is suitable for use by the cancer patient for this purpose. The oils have been selected in such a manner that they also have other advantages for the cancer patient, such as improving the prostaglandin balance.

To make one liter of the mixture, mix:

- Flaxseed oil 150ml
- First virgin cold pressed sunflower oil 450ml
- Wheat germ oil 100ml
- Olive oil 200ml
- Soy lecithin 100ml.

Use 10-15ml (2-3 tablespoonfuls) daily with meals.

You will need to buy the oils individually and prepare your own blend at home or you could ask your pharmacist to do so.

- Buy only cold-pressed, first virgin quality oils with no signs of rancidity in airtight, dark, containers.
- Store them at home in the same containers in a refrigerator, and open only briefly to prepare the mixture. Check regularly for rancidity (smell and appearance) and discard if any of these signs are present.
- Your dosage levels should be such that you experience no discomfort (eg diarrhea) and that there is no increase in body weight.
- The oil blend may be taken on or with food or on its own after meals—most people prefer to use it as a salad dressing as part of the cancer diet.

Bowel function

Putrefaction in the colon and elsewhere in the digestive system plays an important but often overlooked role in cancer prevention and treatment. It is responsible for body and breath odors which we often treat with antiperspirants and deodorants, thus aggravating the problem. One of the reasons so many middle-aged men have oversized bellies ("spare tyres") is that the large intestine (a muscle) is filled with a mass of putrefying, stagnant waste material which causes the abdomen to bulge. It then falls down and bulges out of the abdomen. The average person carries with him about 3-4kg of this putrefying fecal mass. There are many reasons why this happens. One of them is obviously diet and lack of exercise. In addition to this a sluggish ("lazy") colon, an over-burdened liver with compromised function, reduced elimination of waste material by the kidneys and lack of oxygen are some of the other reasons why our sewage disposal systems become overloaded.

Lack of oxygen (exercise) creates the perfect anaerobic environment in which many of these putrefactive organisms thrive.

The main organs that keep our internal environment clean are the colon, the liver, the kidneys and the gall-bladder, and when they function less than optimally, toxins and pollutants start to accumulate, consuming much of the body's oxygen supply, which in turn acidifies the inner terrain and also suppresses immune function.

Thus the scenario is created in which diseases flourish and normal cells can become cancerous due to the prevailing acidic conditions and lack of oxygen.

The organs usually affected adversely by our living conditions are the bowel but also the liver, gall-bladder and kidneys.

The colon

The first step in any health programme must be to clean up the waste disposal organs of the body, and the best place to begin is the colon.

The colon is the source of putrefying toxic material, from where toxins reach the blood, causing *inter alia* acidosis, which is a major cause of disease. It has been estimated that more than 80 % of all diseases originate in the colon. When the blood becomes overburdened with these deadly toxins from the colon, the liver, with already more than 500 metabolic functions, picks up the overload. This in turn continues until the liver becomes overburdened, which results in increased toxin accumulation in the blood (toxemia), which is responsible for a variety of toxic systemic effects (eg headaches). Next the kidneys become involved, and if they cannot cope with the extra load, low back pain is one of the first symptoms. Other signs that may show up are frequent urination, bladder infections, sweaty palms and bags under the eyes. The lymph system may also become involved, in an endless chain of events all of which contribute to ill health.

Colorectal cancer is a common result of an impacted and dirty colon. Many other conditions such as constipation, ulcerative colitis, diverticulitis and hemorrhoids are also involved.

The entire toxin disposal system therefore consists of colon, kidneys, liver/gall-bladder and blood, which form a major part of the inner terrain. The problem of chronic systemic toxicity can only be addressed by cleaning up the entire system, but quite obviously this has to take place in a distinctive order to be effective. For example, it serves no purpose to clean the liver before the colon has been cleansed. Therefore the order in which these organs have to be cleansed as practiced by most health professionals is as follows:

Colon > intestinal parasites > kidneys > liver/gall-bladder > blood

Different products are available on the market to clean the colon. I suggest that you consult your health shop or the local representatives of large pharmacy chains such as Dischem in your area.

In addition, you might wish to look at Dr. Young's basic procedure (13). This consists of a week on fresh vegetable juices accompanied by a green formula composed of vegetable and grass fibres. This is then followed by a mild natural laxative such as Irish moss or Spirulina and/or another suitable laxative.

It is important to realize that cleaning the colon is not a once-off event of, say, 2-4 weeks' treatment with a particular product. This will probably make you feel much better but gradually you will return to your previous unwell condition after a month or two if you persist with your previous lifestyle, during which time your colon has again become clogged up. For optimum health, you have to continually think of keeping your colon clean. Therefore you may have to regularly repeat the treatment.

A complicating and rather serious aspect of bowel function is the fact that even serious bowel problems can go unnoticed. This is due to a lack of awareness of the crucial importance of proper bowel function, and secondly, the lack of knowledge including signs and symptoms to look for. For example, most people, including many doctors, believe that a foul odor in the stool is normal. If you eat fried and over-cooked foods, processed foods, devitalized starches, sugar and other unnatural foods, your colon could not possibly be efficient, even with regular bowel movements.

The main reason is mucoid production. The body produces mucus in response to almost anything ingested. When inferior foods are presented to the body, the result is a mucoid coating of slime on the inner walls of the colon, formed as a protective measure. The colon may then become spastic, resulting in constriction in certain parts of the colon with ballooning. These constrictions can be quite small—they may restrict the passage of food to the extent that partially digested food is passed, the nutritional value of which is lost to the body. This condition is extremely widespread. Dr. H.W. Kellogg, a well-known surgeon, reports that in 22 000 operations personally performed by him, not a single colon was normal.

In addition to cleaning out your colon, you have to attend to two other related matters. First of all, you have to ensure that you have a healthy population of intestinal bacteria. This is one of the essentials of a strong immune system. Most people have had the normal friendly bacteria in their intestines destroyed as a result of antibiotic treatment, other harsh chemicals, chlorine-containing tap water, poor diet, drugs, etc. In order to restore the friendly gut bacteria it is advisable to regularly (daily) include yoghurt in your diet and to take a good supplement of probiotic cultures.

Another important step is to never mix high protein foods and high carbohydrate foods in your diet. These two food groups require different enzyme systems and conditions in the gastrointestinal tract for optimum digestion. If this is not done, food is poorly digested and the conditions favorable for putrefaction are created in the colon.

In this regard, Dr. V.E. Irons, a recognized specialist on bowel conditions, states:

> *"In my opinion, there is only one real disease, and that disease is auto-intoxication—the body poisoning itself. It's the filth in our system that kills us. So I am convinced that unless you clean out your bowel you will never reach vibrant health."*

Suggested procedure

Juice your preferred green vegetables (eg celery, broccoli, cabbage, spinach, carrots, beets, lettuce, etc.) in a juicer. Do not include more than half a beet at first—it may cause diarrhea. Then start the colon cleanse by taking 8-10 glasses of juice a day. Do not eat anything else, but you may drink as much purified water as you want. Strictly avoid tap water. In addition, take a mild natural laxative formula (available from large pharmacies): 3-4 capsules every 4 hours while awake. If hunger compels you to eat some solid food, eat fresh whole vegetables. During the cleansing process, toxins are dumped from storage sites into the blood. For a while, therefore, you may feel worse (nausea, headaches, dizziness) before getting better. This is called a "healing crisis" and must be considered a sign that your treatment is working. However, if it becomes too intense, it is best to seek professional advice. The cleanse should last until the "healing crisis" has passed. This usually lasts for 2-3 days, but not longer than 5 days.

Another practical procedure which you can use at home is given by Dr. Young in his book (13).

Parasite cleanse

Internal parasites are one of the most unrecognized of all diseases.

The parasite cleanse is closely related to the broader problem of colon cleanse. There is reason for us to be concerned about internal parasites—it is not a problem limited to Third World countries. It is estimated that 90 % of the population in Western Countries suffer a load of many different parasites without being aware of it. Parasites are scavenger organisms living in the intestines, which may aggravate many other diseases including cancer. They are found in the intestinal tract, liver, pancreas and many other areas where the type of food they thrive on is abundantly available (eg sugars and refined food). The main danger associated with the presence of parasites lies in the toxic waste products produced and excreted by these organisms. They also have other harmful effects in the body, including consumption of red blood cells. In addition, many unsuspected symptoms may occur, including joint and muscle aches, anaemia, allergy, skin conditions, immune dysfunction, chronic fatigue, constipation, bloating, diarrhea, nervousness and many others. If these symptoms persist with no obvious cause, parasites should be suspected.

To deal with the problem in a comprehensive manner, the following steps are suggested:

- Reduce animal products and totally eliminate all junk food from your diet, and replace with a vegetarian type of diet based largely on vegetables and fruit, but ensure adequate protein intake (nuts, pulses, etc.).
- Remove accumulated waste in the colon, in which parasites may be hiding. You can flush the waste out by using some of the following natural products, preferably in combination: pumpkin seeds, citrus

pectin, paw-paw extract, psyllium husks, agar-agar and bentonite clay in combination with psyllium husks.
- Colon irrigation: irrigate the colon with 400-600ml of chlorine-free water (preferably boiled for a few minutes and cooled) to which you may add black walnut extract, garlic juice or vinegar (2 tablespoonfuls per liter).
- To flush the gall-bladder, take lime or lemon juice in warm water or Swedish bitters before each meal.
- To remove the parasites following the abovementioned cleansing procedures, use a blend of 3 herbs as suggested by Dr. R. Clark. These are black walnut hull tincture (or capsules), wormwood capsules and fresh ground cloves to kill the parasite eggs. Take this blend 20 minutes before meals.
- During the parasite flush, it is advisable to take additional Vitamin C (2000-3000mg per day) with copious quantities of purified water. Also sanitize your environment by washing all clothes and bed linen, and also treat your pets for worm infestation. In addition, modify your diet to a largely vegetarian type of diet, including pineapples and paw-paw. You can also include roasted pumpkin seed ($1/_3$ cup) and 2 cloves of raw garlic daily.

For more information consult the book (69) by Diamond, Cowden and Goldberg (p 974).

Drugs to remove the different types of internal parasites (eg Vermox) are available from all leading pharmacies. It is also a problem you should discuss with your doctor.

Kidney cleanse

The kidneys are basically a filtering system designed to remove and clear the circulation of toxins (eg heavy metals, drugs, urea, creatinine and other metabolic products) as well as surplus water. The filtration process takes place through a delicate system of membranes, in the structure of which certain unsaturated fatty acids (eg linoleic and linolenic acid) play an important role. The surplus water is excreted in the form of urine. If there is too little water, the urine becomes more concentrated and less urine is produced, meaning that the various toxins dissolved in the urine are also more concentrated, carrying with it the potential of greater damage to the kidneys. The minimum daily volume of urine beyond which kidney damage is likely to occur is 500ml. The normal daily adult urine volume is approx 1500ml. When the kidneys are overloaded with toxins, diseases of the kidney and bladder may result. Various deposits and crystals may be precipitated on the inner membranes, and eventually some of these present in the form of kidney stones. The main purpose of a kidney cleanse is to remove these potentially harmful deposits in the kidneys.

A variety of methods to remove these deposits in the kidneys are available. Often whole lemons are used as part of the treatment. Others depend on celery tea.

- *The Lemon Kidney Cleanse.* Do the treatment in the morning and do not eat anything beforehand. Reduce two whole lemons to pulp including the skins and seeds. Add the pulp to 300ml of lukewarm water, add a pinch of Cayenne pepper and mix thoroughly. Drink the mixture immediately.

Kidney cleaners are also available from all large pharmacies and some are also described in the literature (114).

The liver/gall-bladder cleanse

The liver is one of the most important organs in the body. It not only detoxifies numerous toxins and drugs, but also synthesizes many important compounds that the body requires. For these reasons a large safety margin is built into the way the liver performs its functions: up to 80 % of the liver can be damaged without producing symptoms or the patient being aware of it. A healthy liver is the best insurance anyone can have against many of the diseases that threaten mankind.

Here is one good liver cleanse described by Dr. Schulze (115) which I have modified slightly.

- To start the cleanse take 2 liters of organic, unprocessed apple juice each day for 3 days. During this period, only eat raw, organic vegetables and low GI fruits or better still, go on a waterfast. On the evening of the third day, drink 200ml of organic, cold pressed virgin olive oil mixed with the juice of one lemon. Mix well and drink down quickly. Then lie curled up on your right side in the fetal position for 30 minutes.

The next morning you may find a few dark-colored objects in your stool: these are gall stones.

Good foods for the liver are beet juice, wheat grass and parsley. Eat some parsley before each meal in order to get the bile flowing.

Another good 5-day liver cleanse is described by Jon Barron, see (1), p 251.

The blood cleanse

An unhealthy diet and exposure to environmental toxins may lead to the accumulation of toxins in the blood, some of which may precipitate in the vascular system, coating the walls of arteries, capillaries and veins, thus impeding its primary function of delivering nutrients to the tissues. This is one of the prime causes of hardening of the arteries, which is so often seen in elderly people. The originally soft and pliable artery walls then become hard and lose their elasticity, preventing them from expanding and contracting in tandem with the heart beat. Eventually they become weak, brittle with a tendency to break as in some diseases. In the process calcium is also leached out of the artery walls, which further contributes to malfunction. The end result is that oxygen delivery to the tissues is curtailed, which significantly promotes the development of cancer as we have seen.

One of the most effective ways of cleaning the arterial system is to take large doses of proteolytic enzymes on an empty stomach. The enzymes hydrolyze the deposits on the walls of the vascular system (see Dr. Kelley's metabolic protocol in this book).

There are also some good blood cleansing herbs available, such as burdock root, red clover, sheep sorrel and others. Consult your pharmacist and/or herbalist.

Treating the healthy cells in the cancer patient

Treating the non-cancerous or healthy cells in the cancer patient may be just as important as killing the cancer cells. If the patient is to survive, his/her future lies with the healthy cells, which may be under severe stress while the cancer cells are being killed. This is one of the reasons why many (up to 40 %) of cancer patients die, not because of the cancer, but because of malnutrition. The "healthy" cells become so toxic (because of the microbial toxins, lack of oxygen and the decomposition products of the dead cancer cells) and so starved of nutrients (because of the voracious appetite of the cancer cells) and suffer severely from a loss of energy for reasons previously discussed that the patient dies just as if he/she had starved to death (without the toxicity).

Quite often the toxicity results mainly from chemotherapy, but even without chemotherapy, cancerous cells "steal" glucose and other nutrients from the normal cells, leaving them starved. The reason for this is that they obtain energy by means of fermentation of glucose, as previously explained. Fermentation requires about 15 times more fuel (glucose) than the aerobic (oxygen burning) energy metabolism of normal cells. The cachexia cycle further contributes to the shortage of energy. In this cycle, cancer cells ferment glucose to produce lactic acid, which is then expelled by the cancer cells into the circulation from where it reaches the liver. The liver then converts lactic acid back into glucose, which is also liberated into the circulation, by means of which it reaches the cancer cells once again, thereby completing the cycle. The problem is that these two processes or parts of the cycle consume enormous amounts of energy, which is effectively stolen as ATP from the healthy cells, leaving them starved.

Such patients are by definition Stage IV. One of the effective ways of breaking this destructive cycle is by the use of cesium, as in the CsCl/DMSO protocol and hydrazine. The cesium stops the cycle in the cancer cells and the hydrazine stops it in the liver, as further explained in the section on hydrazine sulphate.

The healthy cells in the cancer patient therefore lack both energy and nutrients, and suffer from the induced acidity and the presence of microbes and their toxins. Cumulatively, this damage to the healthy cells is responsible for the fact that 40 % of cancer patients die of malnutrition in the first place, before they succumb to the cancer.

Tragically, conventional oncology does not recognize this fact, but by treating the patient with radiotherapy and chemotherapy, they contribute to the problem by killing more normal cells by these treatments than cancer cells. It is quite possible that it is the toxic damage done to the normal cells that survive the treatment that eventually causes many patients to die.

There is no question that the health and energy of the normal cells in key organs such as the liver and kidneys are of the utmost importance in the treatment of cancer. It is therefore necessary, especially in the case of advanced cancer patients (Stage IV) to flood the body with high-density nutrients both in the form of food and supplements. This will not only make the patient feel better, but will also greatly increase his/her chances of ultimate survival. Many alternative treatments make provision for this in the form of concentrated juice extracts.

Products that provide these nutrients are the same ones used to buy time for the critically ill patient: high doses of Vitamin C, concentrated vegetable and fruit juices (as in the Gerson diet) and others. Buying time for the patient in reality amounts to protecting the normal cells and preventing the patient from dying of malnutrition. In the beginning, when the patient receives such a regimen to feed the normal cells, he/she might experience a burst of mood elevation, improved energy and "feeling good". This must not be seen as evidence that the cancer has been cured. Curing the cancer and feeding the patient are two separate issues, albeit related.

Supplements

Some of these are required because of the poor quality of our processed foods. Others are necessary to remove pathogenic micro-organisms from the body (yeasts, fungi and moulds). I have composed the following programme of supplementation for the cancer patient. Most of these are available from *Fortifood*; others are available from large pharmacies such as Dischem or from health shops. You may have to shop around to locate the best sources.

- Multinutrient supplement (*Fortifood*): 4-6 tabs
- Vitamin C effervescent powder (*Fortifood*): 5g (= 1 heaped teaspoonful) (antioxidant)
- Alpha-lipoic acid (*Fortifood*): 300-500mg (antioxidant)
- N-acetyl cysteine (*Fortifood*): 500mg (source of glutathione)
- Coral calcium (*Fortifood*): Four 500mg caps (calcium, magnesium, trace elements)
- Omega-3 fatty acids (*Fortifood* Fish Oil 1g caps): 3 caps
- Omega-6 fatty acids (*Fortifood* flaxseed oil): 2 teaspoons
- Bromelain (*Fortifood*): 500mg three times daily on an empty stomach (proteolytic enzymes)
- Caprylic acid (*Fortifood*): 3g daily (antifungal)
- Undecylenic acid (*Fortifood*): 3g daily (antifungal)
- Olive leaf extract (*Fortifood*): 4-6 caps (antimicrobial and antifungal) (take only intermittently)
- Garlic: 1-2 cloves daily (antimicrobial and antifungal)
- Magnesium: 300-400mg (4-6 capsules of BioMag, *Fortifood*).

This is a short list of vital supplements that every cancer patient should take.

How to detoxify your food

You must assume that all commercial food that you buy contains pesticides and poisons used in its production. This applies not only to fruits and vegetables, but also to meat products.

- Before cooking, soak your food in a dilute solution of hydrochloric acid, prepared by adding 1 teaspoonful of 10 % hydrochloric acid (chemically pure) and 100ml of glycerol to 5 liters of chlorine-free water. Soak your foods in this solution, using the following immersion times: leafy vegetables: 10-15 minutes root vegetables: 10-15 minutes skinned fruits: 15-20 minutes meats: 5-10 minutes per kg

Prepare the dilute hydrochloric acid solution fresh every time you require it.

After soaking as above, immerse all the foods for 5-10 minutes in chlorine-free water (use purified water, not tap water).

Some general remarks on cancer

In evaluating the success of treatment, it is important to note the difference between "survival time" and "five-year survival time" as previously pointed out. Dr. P. Binzel summarizes the situation rather well:

> *In the past fifty years, tremendous progress has been made in the early diagnosis of cancer. In that period of time, tremendous progress has been made in the surgical ability to remove tumors. Tremendous progress has been made in the use of radiation and chemotherapy in their ability to shrink or destroy tumors. But the survival time of the cancer patient today is no greater than it was fifty years ago. What does this mean? It obviously means that we are treating the wrong thing* (71).

What kills the cancer patient is the spreading of the tumor. The tumor itself presents no danger to the patient, certainly not in the case of solid tumors, unless they block vital fluids in vital areas such as the brain or the common bile duct.

It is necessary to understand the precise structure of a solid tumor. The majority of cells in such tumors are healthy cells, and there are therefore not enough cancer cells in such a tumor to kill the patient. Cancer cells on their own cannot form tissue, since they are autonomous and do not respond to the growth regulatory mechanisms in the body. Typically, in prostate cancer, the cancer is contained inside the prostate, and there is no danger to the patient's life. This sometimes happens in elderly patients. Even if the cancer cells in such a tumor were killed or if the tumor was cut out, it would not save the patient's life if the cancer has already spread, as shown by the breast cancer example previously discussed. Quite clearly, then, it is the spreading of the cancer that kills the patient, not the cancer cells inside the tumor.

Ironically, orthodox medicine focuses on the shrinking of tumors (killing of cancer cells inside the tumor) and often uses this as evidence of successful treatment. This creates false expectations in the patient, who inevitably has to face the consequences of metastases later on, which is the real reason why the patient may die.

A further complicating factor arises in the case of conventional chemotherapy because the drug itself is so toxic (due to insufficient selectivity) that if enough of the drug were given to kill the cancer cells, the patient would also be killed. The doctor is therefore forced to limit dosage levels so as not to kill the patient, but at these low doses, the cancer is not prevented from spreading. We have previously shown how this problem may be addressed, at least partially, by means of IPT.

That is why chemotherapy may put a patient in remission, which is then claimed as successful treatment. However, virtually every cancer patient who goes into remission eventually comes out of remission and dies as a result of the now more widely disseminated cancer.

This scenario is replayed every day in many cancer wards the world over. Frequently, solid cancers may either be surgically removed or treated with radiotherapy even after the cancer has already spread, because they are interested in shrinking the tumor as mentioned above. But the tumor is not the problem—it is the spreading of the tumor that kills the patient.

As a method of saving the patient's life by ensuring long-term survival, some conventional medical treatments are practically worthless, as shown by the recorded survival rates of 3 % previously discussed. However, many alternative treatment protocols are no better, because for financial reasons many alternative practitioners do not use the best treatments, or they do not have sufficient knowledge. In addition, different vendors promote their own product lines, which are not necessarily the best, for selfish reasons.

On the other hand, there are some good alternative doctors and there are some good products, but these have to be identified and found.

Clearly, then, the cancer patient and his/her doctor are in a very difficult situation. They have to wade through a maze of uncertainty and deception, which is further complicated by the fact that drug authorities strictly prohibit doctors from using or even investigating alternative treatment methods. This means that there is no, or very little, reliable information available on which to base decisions. So what must the cancer patient do? Although it may not sound like a million dollar solution to the problem, the only way forward for the cancer patient is the old-fashioned way of finding people with integrity to work with who are interested in curing your cancer and not in their own bank account in the first place. In addition, the patient and doctor must be prepared to study and gather the necessary knowledge in order for them to make the right decisions. Much information is available on the Internet, where very good websites are to be found (32). There is also a number of excellent books which the cancer patient should buy, to which I have referred in the introduction. The book by the Hausers on IPT and the one on intracellular oxygen levels by Peskin and Habib are of special importance.

If you have received conventional chemotherapy prior to remission or before your alternative treatment started, you are in an even more difficult position, because a significant percentage of cancer cells, including those that are difficult to access, will be of the multi drug resistant (MDR) type of cancer cell. These are more difficult to kill than others and you have to react accordingly.

Blood coagulation and the cancer clotting coat

In order to avoid excessive loss of blood resulting from injuries, the body has developed a finely-tuned mechanism which causes the blood to coagulate and thus to stop potentially lethal bleeding (by the thickening of blood or blood clotting). There is also an opposing anti-clotting mechanism which ensures that excessive clotting is prevented. A delicate balance between these two opposing mechanisms ensures normal clotting in the healthy person. Excessive blood clotting is also referred to as coagulopathy. There are several laboratory procedures by means of which such a tendency can be detected, and both drugs and natural compounds are available to correct such a tendency.

The fibrin network which forms a blood clot also forms around cancer cells, which serves to protect these cells against the immune system. It is therefore not surprising to find that, in most cancer patients, excessive blood clotting (coagulopathy) can be detected by means of platelet aggregation studies as well as blood fibrinogen assays and other methods.

> *It is of particular importance to note that conventional high-dose chemotherapy also worsens the excessive coagulopathy in cancer patients, thus further aggravating the problem.*

Studies have shown that cancer patients treated with anti-coagulation drugs, such as dipyridamole and Coumadin, have a better prognosis. In addition to these drugs, there are many natural compounds that can be used to decrease blood coagulopathy, such as codliver oil, w-3 fatty acids (eg fish oil), bromelain, garlic and many others. When these compounds are used for this purpose, it is necessary to check blood coagulation parameters before and during treatment to ensure that these are being corrected.

Many solid cancers (eg prostate cancer) wall themselves off with a cancer clotting coat, sometimes to produce a complete fibrin gel and later stroma of connective tissue components such as collagen. This fibrin stroma has two important functions: it protects the cancer cells against immune detection and destruction and, perhaps more importantly, this fibrin stroma has been shown to be a key step in the process of angiogenesis (formation of a new vascular system for the growing cancer. (*Bioch Biophys Acta*, 1989, 948: 305).

An important study also showed that removal of this fibrin coat through fibrinolysis (eg by means of proteolytic enzymes) terminates the process of angiogenesis (*Adv Exp Med Biol* 1990, 281: 19).

Moreover, the literature reveals that cancer patients as a group experience an increased incidence of blood clotting episodes and that this is aggravated by conventional high-dose chemotherapy (*Cancer*, 1984, 54: 1264). Reduced fibrinolysis has also been reported in cancer patients.

Dr. Hauser states that: " . . . nearly all patients with cancer manifest laboratory evidence of hypercoagulability and some even develop clinical thrombo-embolic disease."

This abnormal clotting tendency has been widely reported in the oncology literature. It is so general and significant that it has even been suggested that measurement of clotting tendency may be a more reliable measure than mammography as an indication for biopsy in breast cancer patients.

There are numerous agents (both allopathic and naturopathic) available to reduce the blood clotting tendency in cancer patients, some of which have been mentioned above. These agents work through different mechanisms and, in addition to the widely used Coumadin, include agents that suppress fibrin formation (eg bromelain), agents that reduce platelet aggregation (dipyridamole, ginger) and agents that reduce vascular permeability. In spite of the fact that several studies have shown that cancer patients treated with anti-clotting agents have an increased survival rate, these agents are seldom used by oncologists in their cancer treatment protocols. However, one remarkable study on the significantly increased survival rate of melanoma patients after treatment with the anti-platelet drug dipyridamole has been described (*Townsend Letter*, May 2000, p 114). In this study, Stage III and IV melanoma patients were treated with 300mg of dipyridamole. After 5 years, the relative mortalities in the 2 groups were as follows: Stage III 0 %, Stage IV 77 % (see Hauser and Hauser).

This illustrates the important role that inhibition of platelet aggregation plays in cancer.

In cancer patients, fibrinolytic activity is suppressed, which promotes coagulopathy. The increased fibrin coat formation that occurs under these conditions prevents the recognition of the cancer cells by the immune system, explaining the increased growth of cancer cells. These examples indicate the importance of cancer patients to do everything possible to prevent excessive blood clotting tendencies, preferably by means of natural methods. Increased blood clotting also reduces blood circulation, thereby reducing tissue oxygenation, which is a particularly serious matter in cancer patients.

The most common cause of increased blood clotting is a diet high in saturated fats and sugar. The cancer patient who goes on a high protein (low fat), low carbohydrate diet which is also rich in low sugar vegetables, will therefore enjoy the advantages of reduced blood clotting. Infections also increase blood clotting.

Excessive deposits of heavy metals in the tissues constitute a particularly important cause of procoagulant activity.

One study found that high mercury levels in the body cause a 56-fold increase in the rate of thrombin formation by platelets. This is therefore one more reason to have the mercury in your dental fillings removed and to consider a course of chelation therapy.

Some supplements of special significance to cancer patients

- *Nicotinic acid or Niacin (Vitamin B3).* Niacin is a strong vasodilator which increases arterial diameter and therefore blood flow. This is of particular significance to cancer patients in view of what was previously said about oxygen supply to cells and cancer. Niacin also increases peripheral circulation and further prevents red blood cells from sticking together (rouleau formation), thus also improving tissue oxygenation in this manner. This desirable effect of niacin can be enhanced by taking it with massage, running and sweating (sauna) as previously discussed.
- When starting niacin supplementation, most people will experience red flushes (especially in the neck area) due to its histamine-induced vasodilatory effect with doses higher than 200mg. This is harmless and will usually disappear after a few days. The symptoms are also

less severe if the vitamin is taken with meals. After initial doses of 200mg, the dosage levels may be gradually increased to 1000mg a day if so desired. It is best to take niacin in conjunction with other vitamins, eg as part of a multivitamin.
- *Glutathione.* This is a powerful intracellular antioxidant which plays an important role in the process of carcinogenesis. Raising the levels in cells of this antioxidant is very beneficial for cancer patients.
- N-acetylcysteine supplementation is used in cancer treatment programmes for this purpose.

How do I know that my treatment is working?
The Navarro Test
Every cancer patient is eager to know whether he/she is winning the battle on a particular treatment programme.

There are some rough, non-specific indicators of cancer status such as body weight, lean body mass and albumin blood levels (which reflect protein levels). When these are maintained, and especially when protein stores are on the increase, the body is in healing mode. Rising cholesterol levels indicate improved liver function.

Whatever you do, do not rely on these and especially not on how you feel. Every patient who: heeds our warnings on diet and stops high sugar foods, eats more vegetables and fruit, and perhaps takes vitamins will feel better, but while the patient feels better, the cancer can be growing and may even be infiltrating other organs. Although a healthy diet will make the vital organs function better and while it may even improve immune competency in a general way, it will not cause the immune system to specifically destroy cancer cells that have grown out of control. It is only by appropriate, objective and scientific monitoring that a patient would know whether he is winning the battle. There is no substitute for this.

A very important aspect in any cancer treatment programme therefore involves methods of monitoring therapy progress by means of appropriate tests. Here are some of the available methods used for this purpose:

Test	**To detect**
*Blood cancer markers	Different cancers
Immune system monitoring	Different cancers
CT scans of tumor size	Different cancers
Body weight	Especially gastrointestinal cancers

PET scans	Different cancers
X-rays of tumor location and size	Different cancers
MRI methods	Different cancers
Alfa fetoprotein	Liver and testicular cancer
AMAS test	Non-specific for all carcinomas
CA 125	Ovarian and other epithelial cancers
CA 19-9, 15-3	Breast, ovarian and other carcinomas
CEA (carcinoembryonic antigen)	GI, breast, lung and ovarian cancers
Human chorionic gonadotrophin test (Navarro Test)	Many cancers

These are some of the many tests that can give you an indication of the presence of cancer in your body. Some of these may be useful in some situations, but generally they are ambiguous in the sense that they may give false negative or false positive results and that you can never be sure unless you do a series of tests. On the other hand, these tests are not entirely safe, nor reliable, as indicated. The CT/PET scans are best avoided as they require you to drink a large amount of glucose to "light up" the cancer cells, something which the cancer patient will be wise to avoid for reasons discussed previously. This and the other tests mentioned also require you to have several chest X-rays, which the cancer patient should also avoid. I therefore recommend that you only use the Navarro and/or the AMAS Tests as previously discussed.

The most reliable test is known as the HCG or Navarro Test. HCG is a hormone that is liberated during pregnancy or when a cancerous growth is present in the body. This test gives a definite yes or no answer. The test detects the presence of abnormally dividing cells regardless of their origin. The result of the test is given in a single number which can be either above 50 (a positive result) or a result between 0 and 49 (a negative result). By doing more than one test, say 8 weeks apart, a trend is usually clear, and if this is upward from 50, you can be sure that the cancer is growing, unless you are pregnant.

You prepare the test sample (as indicated below) by precipitating the hormones in a urine sample, collecting the precipitate on filter paper and mailing that to the Navarro Clinic in Manila, Philippines. The result is available by e-mail in 7 days, and the cost is $50. This may be a bit expensive for South African patients, but I am at present investigating the possibility of doing a similar analysis locally.

Research has shown that the test detects various cancers as early as 24-29 months *before symptoms appear*.

How to prepare the sample

- Take a 50ml sample of early morning urine and add 200ml of acetone (available from your pharmacy) followed by 5ml of commercial 96 % alcohol (also from your pharmacy). Mix well but make sure that you don't lose any of the mix.
- Let the mix stand in the fridge for 2 hours until sediment has formed. Let the sediment sink to the bottom and decant about half the clear supernatant fluid (acetone/urine) without losing any of the sediment. Then filter the remainder through a coffee filter or ordinary lab filter paper, collecting all of the sediment on the filter paper. Dry the filter paper with the sediment in air, fold up the filter paper with the sediment on it and forward to the Navarro Clinic at 3553 Sining Street, Morning Side Terrace, Santa Mesa, 1016, Philippines, with a copy of your money order or other proof of payment.
- Send your full personal details with the sample which includes the patient's name, address, sex, age and e-mail address, with a brief summary of the case and diagnosis. Do not forget to include your own e-mail address.
- Female patients must avoid sexual contact for 12 days and males for 18-24 hours prior to collecting the urine sample.
- Note that the test is positive if a person is pregnant, has a severe injury or has cancer. The test is positive if severe injury is present, due to the fact that trophoblast cells are the first stage of healing an injury. This process stops once the wound is healed. This does not happen in the case of cancer, as cancer is the result of fast-growing cells which the body fails to turn off. These trophoblast cells also appear in the uterus wall during pregnancy, in order to prepare a place where the embryo may attach for further growth.

The AMAS Test

This test measures serum levels of antimalignin antibody. Malignin is a polypeptide that is present in most cancer cells, regardless of cell type and location. Antimalignan antibodies rise early in the course of the disease, and in some cases the AMAS test has been found to be positive 1 to 19 months before clinical detection. The test is elevated in almost all types of cancer. For sera analyzed within 24 hours of being drawn, false positives and negatives are less than 1 % (specificity and sensitivity better than 99 %). For stored sera, false positives are 5 % and false negatives are 7 %.

A negative AMAS test in the case of clinically known cancer signifies a poor immune response with a poor prognosis.

During IPT, the selected cancer markers are determined every 3 months during the first year and thereafter twice annually for the next two years, when monitoring may be terminated if everything is normal.

Thirteen vital steps for the cancer patient

It is extremely important to realize that the situation is not hopeless if you have been diagnosed with cancer. There are now many strategies that will not only prolong life, but may even lead to a complete cure. There are numerous healthy people who have been cured of cancer and are now enjoying a normal life. Thousands of patient reports confirm this. Life expectancy is rapidly increasing among cancer patients who apply the latest scientific information, which is expanding all the time. I believe that a large segment of future development will come from a study of natural medicine or what is now known as alternative medicine. Increasing numbers of medical practitioners now accept such a view and have already made great contributions toward its advancement. The evolutionary process is still retarded by many members of the old school who exert enormous peer pressure on their colleagues, but they represent a diminishing segment of the medical fraternity.

However, you need to be careful not to get carried away by success stories of others who have been cured by means of some or other plant extract or magic formula. Zealousness and unfounded optimism are no substitute for a sound scientific approach to cancer. Cancer can definitely be cured, but treatment becomes difficult if the patient has been pretreated by some questionable conventional treatments such as high-dose chemotherapy and other similar procedures, especially if the patient has not changed his destructive lifestyle and diet.

I strongly support the judicious integration of conventional cancer treatments with alternative methods where such a step can be justified on scientific grounds. The IPT protocol discussed previously is one such example.

The following steps are aimed primarily at the cancer patient who has already had conventional treatment such as chemotherapy or radiation therapy and has now been given up on by his conventional doctors. These steps may, however, be followed by all cancer patients, regardless of the type and stage of cancer. These steps form a vital part of your overall cancer plan and should be followed meticulously, preferably in consultation with your doctor. Having selected your treatment programme based on the information supplied in this book and in consultation with your doctor, you need to attend to the following steps:

Step 1: Find the right oncologist

We are clearly losing the war on cancer. If your oncologist belongs to the old school of cancer treatment, your chances of full recovery are much reduced. One of the principal errors committed by conventional doctors and oncologists is their failure to recognize the extremely important role that diet plays both in the development of cancer and especially during treatment of the cancer patient, regardless of the treatment protocol used.

Nevertheless, the conventional methods are not without merit if used judiciously in combination with other methods. They may help you gain time while correcting your faulty lifestyle and diet and starting to apply alternative methods.

The ideal is therefore to find an oncologist who is a specialist in conventional methods but also understands the potential and importance of alternative methods. Alternatively, and preferably, include several specialists on your cancer caring team as discussed below.

Unfortunately, much of what is generally known as alternative or complementary methods still subsists at a level that might be justifiably termed "quackery" or "hearsay medicine". This is one of the reasons so many doctors are against complementary medical treatments. It will be your task to convince your doctor (using the evidence in this book) that there is another side to complementary medicine which is as much based on rigorous scientific principles as he/she is supposed to be using.

Step 2: Change your diet

Review and apply the dietary principles outlined in the "Cancer Diet" in this book. Remember that no cancer treatment, whether conventional or alternative, can succeed if the diet and lifestyle are not first corrected.

Foods associated with cancer risk

- Fat, smoked, and cured meat (harmful nitrites and nitrates).
- Butter, cream and high-fat cheeses (non-essential fats) containing hormones used in agriculture (toxins).
- Margarine and commercial cooking oils (harmful fatty acids).
- Vegetable shortenings (harmful fatty acids).
- Deep fried, fatty foods such as potato chips/crisps (oxidized fatty acids).
- Rich desserts (harmful sugar, fat and white flour).
- White bread, rolls, buns, pasta, cakes, cookies, pies, etc. (contribute to poor blood sugar control).
- Commercial whole milk (excess fat, allergens, oestrogens, homogenization, pasteurization).
- Highly processed foods (harmful chemicals, colorants, sugar, salt, sweeteners).

Optimum health foods

- Vegetables, fruits, low-sugar fruit juices rich in vitamins, minerals, enzymes.
- Whole low-gluten grains (high in complex carbohydrates).
- Legumes (healthy protein sources).
- Nuts, seeds (essential oils).

Foods in moderation

- Fish (protein, essential fatty acids).
- Low fat meat and poultry (proteins, minerals).
- Free range eggs (high quality protein, lecithin).
- Ordinary garden vegetables, especially dark green veggies, broccoli, cabbage, etc.

Step 3: Remove carcinogenic chemicals and toxins

Follow the procedures previously given for the mobilization and removal of carcinogenic chemicals from your body. It is to no avail treating cancer while leaving in place an important part of its cause.

As part of the process, remove mercury-containing amalgam fillings in consultation with your oncologist and dentist who have experience in this regard. This must be done by a competent dentist who understands the problem and knows the dangers associated with such a process. Also reduce your exposure to the large number of foreign chemicals in our environment including the use of anti-perspirants and deodorizers.

Step 4: Prevent exposure to cancer-causing toxins and medical procedures

- Eliminate environmental toxins discussed in this book as much as possible, even if this entails much cost and discomfort on your side.
- Purify your drinking water by purchasing an effective system (reverse osmosis or double distillation).
- Home-produced, pesticide-free, organically grown vegetables and fruit are ideal but difficult to obtain.
- Commercially available fresh produce may look attractive, but invariably carries a heavy load of toxic chemicals. If you have to use them, thoroughly wash such products as discussed elsewhere in this book and discard the outer leaves.
- Also, make every effort to reduce your exposure to foreign chemicals, whether these come from water, food, air, medicines, cosmetics or other sources.

Step 5: Follow your supplement programme

It is impossible to treat cancer successfully in the presence of nutrient deficiencies. A good multinutrient supplement that supplies at least 300 % of conventional RDA values is essential. Vitamin C is essential—take at least 3000mg daily, regardless of what the popular press or some doctors say. Make sure that you take magnesium (300-400mg elemental) and calcium (500mg elemental) as separate supplements, preferably in the form of citratemalate or chelated amino acid complexes. Coral calcium is also an excellent mineral supplement, since it supplies micro minerals in addition to calcium and magnesium.

Take special supplements, in consultation with your doctor, of any one or more of the nutrients that have been shown to be of special value in your type of cancer such as melatonin (breast cancer), Lycopene (prostate cancer), indole-3-carbinol (breast cancer).

Step 6: Monitor your progress by means of analyses as discussed in this book

No anti-cancer programme can succeed if you do not have the means to check from time to time whether or not the cancer is regressing. These checks serve as a vital warning to change your treatment programme if necessary.

Treating cancer cannot be based on guesswork. The following tests should be performed regularly, preferably monthly.

- Complete blood chemistry, including all the standard tests done by your laboratory for kidney, liver, thyroid and heart function. Have these tests done at the same laboratory every time, since absolute values may differ somewhat from laboratory to laboratory.
- Immune cell subset test. This should include the following: CD4, CD8, CD4/CD8 ratio, natural killer cells as well as other determinations deemed necessary by your doctor.
- Tumor marker tests. Note that the markers are not available for all tumors, and in some cases the information available obtained from the measurement of one particular marker may not be reliable.
- The Navarro test appears to be one of the most useful tests to determine the amount of cancer left in your body. It is unfortunately not available at local chemical pathology laboratories and having it done overseas may be expensive.
- You may also consider the AMAS test, which is cheaper and may be available locally.

Step 7: Strengthen your immune system

No patient with a weak immune system can recover from cancer. If thyroid tests reveal even a mild tendency towards hypothyroidism, vigorous corrective action should be taken. Many cancer patients have a mild form of hypothyroidism which may not be revealed by the ordinary thyroid tests but which may nonetheless aggravate the cancerous condition. The condition may be detected by means of blood thyroid stimulating hormone (TSH) determinations, the normal value of which is 0.35-5.0 mu/l. Any value above 2.0 in a cancer patient should, however, be suspect.

It is important to note that over-production of cortisol as well as T-suppressor cells is a common feature in cancer patients. Cortisol can be controlled as indicated below, and the drug may be used to normalize over-production of T-suppressor cells

One of the most important steps you can take to strengthen the immune system is to suppress free radical activity that may inhibit sensitive immune cells. Free radical activity can be controlled through lifestyle factors: avoid over-exercising, fried foods, smoking, and pollution, correct your diet and attend to the other factors previously discussed in this regard. Also ensure adequate intake of anti-oxidants by ensuring optimal intake of critical nutrients such as zinc and Vitamin C. In addition, supplement with Beta-1.3DGlucan, as previously discussed.

The thymus gland is a key player in the immune system. Thymus extracts can be used to directly stimulate the thymus gland to produce disease-fighting cells of the immune system. Thymex is an American product that provides fresh, healthy tissue from the thymus and other glands. If this is not available, consider the use of thyroid hormone supplements in consultation with your doctor.

- Several procaine containing drugs have been developed in Europe as anti-ageing agents. These products contain procaine, a drug known to suppress cortisol levels, which may be why it works as an anti-ageing agent.
- Elevated cortisol levels suppress the immune system, and cancer patients often have elevated cortisol levels which may facilitate the spreading of cancer. These drugs may therefore play a useful role as part of a strategy to restore immune function, especially if cortisol levels indicate that such a step is justified.
- Melatonin is another substance that could be considered in the context of immune function. Apart from being a strong anti-oxidant which may protect delicate immune cells, it induces differentiation of cancer cells back to normal cells. According to the Life Extension Foundation in America, a combination of low doses of Interleukin-2 (3 million units subcutaneously weekly for 6 weeks) and/or alpha interferon (10,000—30,000 units subcutaneously) weekly for 6 weeks and melatonin (10-50mg nightly sublingually) may be effective against advanced, normally untreatable cancer.

Finally, you should not lose sight of the fact that Beta-1.3DGlucan *has been found by researchers at Princeton University to be the strongest stimulator of the immune system by far.*

This is discussed elsewhere in this book.

Step 8: Promote cancer cell differentiation

High levels of Vitamin D3 may be used to use to induce differentiation of cancer cells back to normal cells, which differs from its normal use to promote mineral absorption. This can be achieved at an intake of 2000-4000IU per day, which is around 10 times higher than normal requirements for mineral absorption. At these high levels of intake, however, it is necessary to monitor blood calcium and PTH levels on a monthly basis and to reduce dosage levels if indicated by the analyses. Consult your doctor.

Step 9: Suppress cancer cell growth

In addition to the various natural treatments discussed in this book to control the growth of cancer cells, whey protein concentrate may be used as a dietary component. This product suppresses the glutathione concentration in cancer cells, making them more susceptible to destruction by therapeutic agents and the immune system. The normal dose is 30-50g daily with food.

When used in conjunction with the previously discussed methods to control acidity in cells, glutathione is an effective agent to suppress the growth of cancer cells.

Step 10: Develop a positive attitude

You cannot beat cancer if you are dejected, depressed and convinced that you are going to die. The significance of a positive mental attitude in overcoming disease cannot be overestimated, although the complex neurochemical processes involved are not fully understood at present.

One way of overcoming negative feelings is by realizing that you are not alone. There are numerous patients who have fully recovered from cancer. Try to spend time with others who have been successfully treated.

The spiritual element in fighting disease is also of great importance. You do not have to be a regular churchgoer to appreciate that there is a Power beyond our understanding which guides our affairs in a subtle way, mainly through the means of natural laws. By understanding and applying these laws, we are in a position to influence our future.

Family and friends should under no circumstances even raise the subject of death in the presence of the patient.

Step 11: Your oncologist

Initially consult your oncologist and let him/her make the diagnosis and procure other important information on your particular cancer (type of cancer, immediate danger of occlusion, etc.). If he then advises immediate conventional chemotherapy, don't do it. Instead get alternative opinions, but make sure that you have at least a natural medicine specialist on your cancer care team.

Step 12: Insulin Potentiation Therapy and enzymes

Make sure that this is part of your treatment programme.

Step 13: Do not stop treatment after apparent initial success

It is very likely that you will experience a remission of your cancer after treatment with one of the methods discussed in this book. It is extremely important not to stop treatment if this happens, but to continue treatment for at least another year or two using a different method from the one initially used. For example, you may experience remission of your cancer after IPT treatment. Treatment should then continue using another method (preferably one that will also stimulate the immune system) such as laetrile or the Budwig protocol.

The cancer patient's rights

Dr. R. Moss deals with this matter in his book *Questioning Chemotherapy* (10). The most important advice he gives in this regard is to question your doctor every step of the way. Don't be afraid to be firm if necessary; if you do not have the energy, get a friend to question your doctor. Remember it is your life that is at stake. The more serious your condition, the more stringent the questioning must be. Ask him in particular what evidence he has that the treatment he proposes will work and on what basis this conclusion is reached. Five-year survival rates, perhaps? Note what has been said previously about 5-year survival rates. Ask him what other therapies are available and how they compare. Does he know about the many alternative cancer therapies? What does he think of the CsCl/DMSO protocol previously discussed? What does he think of Insulin Potentiation Therapy? Don't let him get away by claiming that these have not been properly tested in clinical trials. Explain to him that the reason is that the powers that be in his profession forbid doctors to use such protocols or to test them. Let him understand that you are an informed consumer and that you are prepared to co-operate with him as much as possible, but it must be on a reasonable basis. Some doctors get cross at being questioned in this manner. If yours does this, you must know that he is uncertain and that the time has arrived for you to find another doctor.

Remember that you do not have to talk to your doctor in a submissive way. You have every right to know what he is proposing to do with your body and why.

Also remember that a diagnosis of cancer is not a death sentence, if you go about it in the correct way. There are many thousands of patients who have had severe Stage IV metastasized cancers and who are completely well today.

Suggested treatments for different types of cancer
Note: The following is a list of examples of successful cancer treatments for different types of cancer compiled from the literature. It is not in any way implied that these are the only treatments for the different types of cancer. It is merely a list of treatments which some therapists have found to work successfully for a particular cancer. The most powerful alternative treatments, like the CsCl/DMSO and IPT protocols are likely to be successful in all types of cancer listed, subject to all the limitations discussed in this book, whether these treatments are listed or not in the following table. Also note that in all cancers diet is of extreme importance as well as the correct mix of w-3 and w-6 fatty acids as discussed in this book.

You should never lose sight of the fact that all cancer treatments should be individualized and that the real key to successful treatment lies in finding an experienced health professional to guide you both in the selection of a particular treatment protocol and in its execution.

Type of cancer Treatment

Type of cancer	Treatment
All cancers	IPT and/or DMSO Potentiation therapy;
All cancers	Vitamin C, IPT, Budwig, Laetrile, CsCl/DMSO,
Bladder	IPT, CsCl/DMSO
Bone marrow	IPT, CsCl/DMSO
Brain	IPT, Henderson, DMSO Potentiation Therapy
Breast	IPT, Gerson, Budwig (Henderson), and ozone
Cancers that cause swelling	Henderson, Budwig
Colorectal	IPT, CsCl/DMSO
Fast growing cancers	Brandt alkaline diet, R. Young, esp. IPT
Gastro-intestinal	Enzymes, IPT
Leukemias	CsCl/DMSO, Colloidal silver, detoxification
Liver	Enzymes, Budwig, IPT
Lung	Henderson, ozone, hydrogen peroxide
Lymphoma (Hodgkins)	Enzymes, Gerson
Lymphoma (non-Hodgkins)	Gerson
Melanoma	IPT, Gerson, Budwig

	Nizoral, Diet, CsCl/DMSO
Ovarian	IPT, CsCl/DMSO
	Ozone, Glyconutrients, Kelley
Pancreas	Enzymes, Gerson, Budwig
Prostate	Lycopene, flutamide, lupron, bromocriptin,
Skin cancers (various)	Gerson, IPT,
	Unadulterated w-6 fatty acid therapy
Uterine	Ozone

Abbreviations

ACI	American Cancer Institute
ACS	American Cancer Society
ACT	alternative cancer treatment
AFP	alpha-fetoprotein
Alt Med Dig	Alternative Medical Digest
AMA	American Medical Association
AMAS	Test Antimalignin antibody test
ATP	The main energy storage and transfer molecule in the cell
BB	Bob Beck Electro-Treatment
BBB	blood-brain barrier
Big Pharma	major pharmaceutical companies
BMJ	British Medical Journal
CA	carcinoma
CA	125 test for ovarian cancer
Ca	calcium
CANSA	Cancer Society of South Africa
CCT	conventional cancer treatment
CEA	carcinoembryonic antigen
ClO_2	chlorine dioxide
CN	cyanide
CNS	isocyanate
Cs	cesium
CsCl	cesium chloride
DMSO	dimethylsulfoxide
DPT	DMSO Potentiation Therapy
EDTA	Ethylene diamine tetra-aecetic acid
EFA	essential fatty acids

EWOT	Exercise with oxygen therapy
FDA	Food and Drug Administration
GI	Glycemic index
H_2O_2	Hydrogen peroxide
HCG	human chorionic gonadotrophin
HCN	hydrogen cyanide
HRT	Hormone Replacement Therapy
IGF	Insulin-like Growth Factor
Int J Health Services	International Journal for Health Services
IPT	Insulin Potentiaion Therapy
IU	International Units
J Clin Oncol	Journal for Clinical Oncology
J Mol Neurosc	*Journal for Molecular Neuroscience*
JAMA	*Journal of the American Medical Association*
K	potassium kJ kilojoules
MAO	mono amine oxidase
MCC	Medicines Control Council
MDS	Myelodysplastic Syndrome
Medical Aids	South African Medical Insurance Companies
MM	Multiple Myeloma
MSM	methylsulfonylmethane
NAC	N-acetyl cysteine
NaCl	sodium chloride
$NaClO_2$	Sodium chlorite
NCI	National Cancer Institute
New Engl J Med	New England Journal of Medicine
NKC	Natural Killer Cells
O_3	Ozone
OCC	Overnight Cure for Cancer
PSA	Prostate Specific Antigen
PUFA	Polyunsaturated fatty acids
RNA	Ribonycleic acid
SAOC	South African Oncology Consortium
SON	absorbable amino acid mix
TSH	thyroid stimulating hormone

References

1. Bollinger, T. 2007. *Step Outside the Box*. USA: Infinity 510 Partners.
2. Starfield, B. 2000. *JAMA*, July 26.
3. Moss, R. 2002. *The Cancer Industry*. Equinox Press, p 79.
4. *JAMA*, 2007, 297: 842.
5. *JAMA*, 1996, 276: 1957.
6. *J Orthomol Med* 1992, 7: 5
7. Cameron, E. & Pauling, L. *Cancer and Vitamin C*. Camino Books, 1993.
8. Morishiga, F., Murata, A. 1978. *J Int Acad Prev Med*, 5: 47
9. Creagan, E., Moertel, C. *et al.* 1979, *New Engl J Med*, Sept 27
10. Moss, R. 2000. *The Cancer Industry*, Equinox Press
11. *The Cancer Tutor*, http://www.cancertutor.com
12. Beale, Morris. *The Drug Story*. Amazon.com.
13. Young, R., & Young, S.H. *Sick and Tired*. Pleasant Grove, UT: Woodland Publishing.
14. Foster, H.D. 2002. *What really causes AIDS*. Victoria, Canada: Trafford Publishing.
15. Howe, G.M. *Global Geocancerology*. Edinburgh: Churchill Livingstone Press.
16. University of Cambridge: Cancer Intelligence Unit Report, June 1997.
17. Israel, L. 1989. *Conquering Cancer. Amazon.com*
18. *Lancet*, 1991, 337, 901
19. Moss, R. 2002. *Questioning Chemotherapy/*. USA: Equinox Press.
20. *New Engl J Med,* 1956, 334:1150.
21. *JAMA* 1986, 276:1957.
22. Henderson, B. 2007. *Cancer Free*. USA: Booklocker
23. See ref 11, p101
24. See ref 11, p 5

25. *http://jonbarron.org/*, then free download.
26. *http://altmedicine About.com. /cs/ dietarytherapy/a/Liverflush.htm*
27. http://www.AboutBetaGlucan.com/bsspecial, asp.
28. Cameron, E. & Pauling, L. Camino Books, USA, p 30.
29. Bioce, J.B., Travis, L. 1995. *J Natl Cancer Inst*, 87: 732, (R45).
30. Serfontein, W. 2002. *Beating Cancer*. Cape Town: Tafelberg Publishers.
31. *Natl Cancer Inst J*, 1983, 87: 10.
32. See ref 11, p185.
33. Serfontein, W. 2001. *New Nutrition*. Cape Town: Tafelberg Publishers.
34. *Am J Clin Nutr* 1983, 37: 368.
35. Holford, P. *The Optimum Nutrition Bible*. London: Judy Piatkus.
36. Foster, H. 2002. *What really causes AIDS*, Trafford Publishing.
37. Abel, F. *Chemotherapy of Advanced Epithelial Cancer*. Stuttgart: Hippocrates Verlag.
38. Lymes, B. 1989. *Healing of Cancer. Amazon.com*
39. *Cancer Chemother Pharmacol*, 1994, 24: 285.
40. *Europ J Gyn Oncol*, 1998, 1: 85.
41. *Int Radiotherapy Oncol Biol Physiol*, 1995, 3 : 875.
42. *Prog Biol Clin Res*, 1988, 259: 307
43. *Ann New Y Acad Sc*, 1982, 393.
44. *Folia Microbiol*, 1998, 43: 505.
45. *Oncology*, 1996. 53: 43.
46. Ghadrian, P. 1987. *Cancer*, 60: 1909.
47. *http://www. macrobiotic.org/thalass.htm.*
48. Weaver, J.C.1993. *J Cell Biology*, 51 : 426.
49. Holm, J. et al., 1993. *J Natl Cancer Inst*, 85 : 32.
50. *Brit J Cancer*, 1996, 73: 1552.
51. *Bull Env Contam Toxicol*. 1976, 15 : 478.
52. *Proc Natl Acad Sc USA*, 1976, 73: 3685; 75: 4538.
53. *J Natl Cancer Inst*, 1979, 62: 89.
54. *J Int Acad Prev Med*,1979, 5: 47.
55. *Cancer Detect Prev*, 1990, 14: 563.
56. *Am J Clin Nutr*,1995, 62 (Suppl), 1510S.
57. *Johns Hopkins Med Letter*, Feb 1995, Editorial, p 3.
58. *Lancet*, 1990, 335: 701.
59. *New Engl J Med*, 1988, 319: 1047.
60. *Cancer Detect Prev*, 1990, 14: 563.
61. *JAMA*, 1980, 243: 337.
62. *Alt Therap*, 1995, 1: 29.

63. *Cancer Detect Prev.* 1990, 14: 563.
64. *Bioch Biophys Res Comms,* 1985, 127: 871.
65. *Ann Med,* 1994, 26: 443.
66. *Am J Epidemiol,* 1994, 139: 1.
67. *Gastroenterology,* 1993, 104: 1405.
68. *Internatl J Epidemiology,* 1992, 21: 6.
69. Diamond, W.J., Cowden, L. & Goldberg, B. 1997. *Definitive Guide to Cancer.* Future Med Publ.
70. Weaver, J.C., 1993. *Cell Biology,* 51: 427.
71. Binzel, P. *Alive and Well,* Chapter 14.
72. http://www.essence+f.life.com/info/cesium.htm.
73. Gold, J. 1987. *Nutr Cancer,* 9: 59.
74. www.whale.to/vaccine/quotas2.html/.
75. Barefoot, R. & Reich, C. *The Calcium Factor.* Amazon Publishing
76. Relman, A. 1982. Closing the Book on Laetrile, *New Engl J Med,* 306: 236.
77. Culbert, M. *Vitamin B17: the forbidden weapon against Cancer.* Amazon Publishing.
78. *JAMA,* 1949, 139: 93.
79. *Am Inst for Cancer Res,* 1997. *Food, Nutrition and Prevention of Cancer.* Washington: Amazon.
80. Jacobs, M.M. *Vitamins and Minerals in the Prevention of Cancer* Florida: CRC Press.
81. *Cancer Detect and Prev,* 1990. 14: 563
82. *JAMA,* 1980, 243: 337.
83. *Nutr Supplem,* 1996, 12: 530.
84. Hildenbrand, G.L. *et al. Alt Ther Health Med,* 1995, 1:29.
85. *Cancer,*1993, 71: 1239; 2995.
86. Leeds, G. *et al.* 1998. *The GI Factor.* Aust: Hodder Headline.
87. Balch.
88. Mitchie, D. 2007. *Buddhism for busy People.* Allen Unwin, http://whale.to.a/bec.
89. McDaniels, J. 2003. *JAMA,* Feb.
90. Weaver, J.C. 1993. *Cell Biol,* 51: 426.
91. *Townsend Letter for Doctors,* 1995, p 30.
92. *Crit Revs Clin Lab Sc,*1980, 12: 123.
93. *Wiener Klin Wochenschr,* 1987, 99: 525.
94. Altmann, N. 1995. *Hydrogen Peroxide in Medicine.* Rochester: Healing Arts Press, p 42.
95. *Cancer Res,* 1965, 25: 1839.

97. *http://www.essence-of-life.com/info/stabilizedoxygen.htm*
98. Sweet, *et al.* 1980. Ozone Selectively Inhibits Human Cancer Cells. *Science*,
99. *http://www.ozoneuniversity.com/Chris%20Gupta.htm*
100. McCane, E. *Flood your body with Oxygen.* Amazon Publishers.
101. Jovan, P, *http://www.ozoneuniversity.com.*
102. *http://tomleveymd.com/archiveissue6.htm.*
103. *www.contemporarymedicine.net/ipt_ main.htm*
104. *www.caringmedical.com.*
105. *http://weeksmd.com/article/cancer/Insulin_potentiation_therapy.htm*
106. *Med Hyp,* 199, 41: 495.
107. *Urology Times,* April, 1987.
108. *Cryobiology,* 1987, 1986, 23: 14.
109. *Am J Obst Gyn,* 1988, 159: 849.
110. *Arch Surgery,* 1986, 12: 12.
111. *Brit J Derm,* 1983, 109: 225S,133.
112. *http://www. giocities.com/SeHo/Gallery/6412/EWOT.htm.*
113. *http://P/curezone.com/clark/kidney.asp.*
114. *www.herbdoc.com.*
115. *Life Extension Disease Prevention and Treatment,* Third edn, 2000

www.ingramcontent.com/pod-product-compliance
Lightning Source LLC
Chambersburg PA
CBHW031816170526
45157CB00001B/79